A Clinical Study of Multiple Sclerosis

A Clinical Study of Multiple Sclerosis

Editor: Alfred Galswells

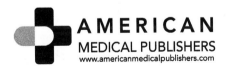

AMERICAN
MEDICAL PUBLISHERS
www.americanmedicalpublishers.com

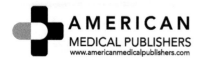
AMERICAN
MEDICAL PUBLISHERS
www.americanmedicalpublishers.com

Cataloging-in-Publication Data

A clinical study of multiple sclerosis / edited by Alfred Galswells.
    p. cm.
Includes bibliographical references and index.
ISBN 978-1-63927-738-4
1. Multiple sclerosis. 2. Multiple sclerosis--Treatment. 3. Multiple sclerosis--Diagnosis.
4. Virus diseases. I. Galswells, Alfred.
RA645.M82 C55 2023
362.196 834--dc23

American Medical Publishers,
41 Flatbush Avenue,
1st Floor, New York,
NY 11217, USA

ISBN 978-1-63927-738-4 (Hardback)

Contents

Preface

I am honored to present to you this unique book which encompasses the most up-to-date data in the field. I was extremely pleased to get this opportunity of editing the work of experts from across the globe. I have also written papers in this field and researched the various aspects revolving around the progress of the discipline. I have tried to unify my knowledge along with that of stalwarts from every corner of the world, to produce a text which not only benefits the readers but also facilitates the growth of the field.

Multiple sclerosis (MS) refers to a neurodegenerative disease. It has been characterized as a chronic immune-mediated disease, with strong neurodegenerative mechanisms in the progressive phase of the disease. Progressive multiple sclerosis is an advanced form of MS, categorized through the slow accumulation of disability over time without relapses. It is often manifested as a neurological development of one or more symptoms. Secondary progressive MS (SPMS) develops after an early relapsing course of the disease, whereas primary progressive MS (PPMS) develops gradually over time. Inflammation can also occur in PMS as aggregates of inflammatory cells in the meninges that includes a follicle-like presence. The diagnosis of PMS might be challenging, as it may remain unnoticed by physicians or patients for a long period. There are presently no recognized therapies for progressive forms of MS. This book aims to understand the clinical perspectives of multiple sclerosis. Some of the diverse topics covered herein address the causes, diagnoses and management of multiple sclerosis. The readers would gain knowledge that would broaden their perspective in this area.

Finally, I would like to thank all the contributing authors for their valuable time and contributions. This book would not have been possible without their efforts. I would also like to thank my friends and family for their constant support.

Editor

Functional Assessment of Outer and Middle Macular Layers in Multiple Sclerosis

Lucia Ziccardi [1], Lucilla Barbano [1,*], Laura Boffa [2], Maria Albanese [2], Carolina Gabri Nicoletti [3], Doriana Landi [3], Andrzej Grzybowski [4,5], Benedetto Falsini [6], Girolama Alessandra Marfia [3,7], Diego Centonze [3,7] and Vincenzo Parisi [1]

1 IRCCS—Fondazione Bietti, Via Livenza 1, 00198 Rome, Italy; lucia.ziccardi@fondazionebietti.it (L.Z.); vincenzo.parisi@fondazionebietti.it (V.P.)
2 Unit of Neurology, Fondazione Policlinico Tor Vergata, Via Oxford 81, 00133 Rome, Italy; dott.boffalaura@gmail.com (L.B.); maria.albanese@hotmail.it (M.A.)
3 Multiple Sclerosis Clinical and Research Unit, Department of Systems Medicine, Tor Vergata University, Via Montpellier 1, 00133 Rome, Italy; carolgabri@gmail.com (C.G.N.); doriana.landi@gmail.com (D.L.); marfia@uniroma2.it (G.A.M.); centonze@uniroma2.it (D.C.)
4 Department of Ophthalmology, University of Warmia and Mazury, Michała Oczapowskiego 2, 10455 Olsztyn, Poland; ae.grzybowski@gmail.com
5 Institute for Research in Ophthalmology, Foundation for Ophthalmology Development, Collegium Maius Fredry 10, 61701 Poznań, Poland
6 Ophthalmology Department, IRCCS—Fondazione Policlinico Universitario A. Gemelli, Catholic University, Largo F. Vito 1, 00168 Rome, Italy; benedetto.falsini@unicatt.it
7 Unit of Neurology and Neurorehabilitation, IRCCS—Neuromed, Via Atinense 18, 86077 Pozzilli (IS), Italy
* Correspondence: lucilla.barbano@fondazionebietti.it;

Abstract: The involvement of macular preganglionic elements' function, during the neurodegenerative process of multiple sclerosis (MS), is controversial. In this case-control observational and retrospective study, we assessed multifocal electroretinogram (mfERG) responses from 41 healthy Controls, 41 relapsing-remitting MS patients without optic neuritis (ON) (MS-noON Group) and 47 MS patients with ON: 27 with full recovery of high-contrast best corrected visual acuity (BCVA) (MS-ON-G Group) and 20 with poor recovery (between 0.2 and 1 LogMAR) of BCVA, (MS-ON-P Group). In the latter Group, Sd-OCT macular volumes and thicknesses of whole and inner and outer retina were measured. MfERG N1 and P1 implicit times (ITs), and N1-P1 response amplitude densities (RADs), were measured from concentric rings (R) with increasing foveal eccentricity: 0–5° (R1), 5–10° (R2), 10–15° (R3), 15–20° (R4), 20–25° (R5), and from retinal sectors (superior, nasal, inferior and temporal) between 0–15° and 0–25°. In the MS-ON-P Group, mean mfERG RADs detected from R1 (0–5°) and from the central nasal sector (0–15°) were significantly reduced ($p < 0.01$) with respect to those of the Control, MS-noON and MS-ON-G Groups. No other significant differences between Groups for any mfERG parameters were found. All Sd-OCT measurements, apart from the inner retina macular volume in the central 1 mm, were significantly reduced in MS-ON-P patients compared to Controls. The functional impairment in the MS-ON-P Group was associated but not correlated with structural changes of the outer and inner retinal layers in corresponding retinal Areas and Sectors. Our results suggest that in MS, exclusively after ON with poor recovery of BCVA, the neurodegenerative process can induce dysfunctional mechanisms involving photoreceptors and bipolar cells of the fovea and of the more central nasal macular area.

Keywords: multiple sclerosis; preganglionic retinal elements; photoreceptors; bipolar cells; multifocal electroretinogram; neurodegeneration

1. Introduction

Multiple sclerosis (MS) is a neurodegenerative disease, characterized by chronic demyelination of the central nervous system, which can result in visual system involvement including retrobulbar optic neuritis (ON) [1].

The ON event is followed by secondary neurodegenerative processes for retrograde trans-synaptic degeneration [2] that involve retinal ganglion cells (RGCs) and their axons [3] forming the innermost retinal layers (IML). In MS patients, an IML dysfunction has been observed by recording abnormal bioelectrical responses with pattern electroretinogram (P-ERG) [4–6] that is a well-known reliable electrophysiological technique for assessing IML function [7].

At the present, it is a debated topic to understand whether the neurodegenerative mechanisms occurring in MS, could involve retinal structures beyond the IML towards the preganglionic elements (i.e., photoceptors, bipolar cells) located in the outer and in middle retinal (O-MR) layers.

The function of preganglionic elements can be assessed by electroretinogram (ERG) recordings [8] that, with its variants, allow us to study the bioelectrical activity of photoreceptor and bipolar cells from the whole retina by Full-field ERG (Ff-ERG) [9], from the central retina by focal ERG (F-ERG) [10] and from multiple localized retinal areas by multifocal ERG (mfERG) [11]. In particular, the mfERG technique provides a topographical map of objective bioelectric responses derived from localized retinal areas, which are driven largely by the cone-related preganglionic components. A "kernel analysis" applied to mfERG responses can be used to assess nonlinear functions of the visual system mainly originating from selected populations of photoreceptors and bipolar cells [12–14].

In MS patients, the Ff-ERG cone a- and b- waves' amplitudes have been found reduced [15–18], thus reflecting post-phototransduction impairment of the photopic system of the whole retina [16], and, by recording F-ERG, impaired photoreceptoral and post-photoreceptoral responses have been found in the macular area [19].

Regarding the mfERG responses in MS, contrasting data have been reported in the recent literature: in fact, mfERG signals have been found either abnormal [18,20,21] or normal [22], due to different types of MS patients (with or without history of ON), acquisition systems and analysis of recordings and limited sample size.

All this contrasting electrophysiological evidence led us to consider that there are no conclusive findings on whether there is or not an O-MR layers dysfunction or functional expression of the extended neurodegenerative process beyond IML in MS.

Therefore, to add information to the debated topic of preganglionic functional involvement or sparing from neurodegeneration, the aim of our work was to assess the function of preganglionic elements in MS patients with the absence or presence of a history of ON, followed by good or poor recovery of the best corrected visual acuity (BCVA).

We attempted to determine whether an O-MR dysfunction could be detected in the central macular area, or whether it might affect more peripheral retinal regions. In addition, we investigated whether the possible O-MR involvement could be observed in specific sectors (Superior (S), Nasal (N), Inferior (I), Temporal (T)) of the central macular region (0 to 15 degrees) and/or in more eccentric retinal areas within the vascular arcades (0 to 25 degrees).

In addition, a morphological involvement of the outer macular layers in MS patients with history of ON was described [20], but with no clear information whether the morphological changes were related or not to the recovery of BCVA after ON. In order to evaluate the macular morphological changes in MS patients with recovery or not of BCVA after an ON, we recently published a work [23] in which a morphological involvement of the outer macular layers was detectable exclusively in those MS patients with poor recovery of BCVA after ON, whereas when a good recovery after ON was reached, the morphology the outer macular layers was not statistically different from those of Controls. Thus, we believed that, in MS patients with poor recovery of BCVA, it could be interesting to evaluate whether a possible preganglionic macular dysfunction could be associated or not to the above-mentioned morphological changes.

2. Materials and Methods

2.1. Study Design and Participants

All research procedures described in this work adhered to the tenets of Declaration of Helsinki. The study protocol (CEC/795/14) was approved by the local Ethical Committee (Comitato Etico Centrale IRCCS Lazio, Sezione IFO/Fondazione Bietti, Rome, Italy) and upon recruitment, informed consent after full explanation of the procedure was obtained from each subject enrolled in the study.

Eighty-eight relapsing remitting (RR) MS patients were enrolled at the Visual Neurophysiology and Neurophthalmology Research Unit, IRCCS- Fondazione Bietti referred by the Multiple Sclerosis center of the Tor Vergata University Hospital in Rome, between September 2016 and 20 October 2020.

In order to obtain homogeneous MS Groups (without ON and with ON followed by good or poor recovery of BCVA, see below) the MS patients were selected form a large cohort (n = 342) based on the following demographic and clinical characteristics:

1.   Age between 28 and 45 years;
2.   Diagnosis of RR MS according to validated 2010 McDonald criteria [24];
3.   MS disease duration (MS-DD), estimated as the number of years from onset to the most recent assessment of disability, ranging from 5 and 15 years;
4.   Expanded Disability Status Scale (EDSS), as ten-point disease severity derived from nine ratings for individual neurological domains [25], ranging from 0 to 3; this score was assessed by two trained [26] neurologists (LaB and MA);
5.   Treatment with disease-modifying therapies (DMT) currently approved for preventing MS relapses. DMT considered in our study were Interferon-β-1a, Interferon-β-1b, Peginterferon beta-1a, Glatiramer acetate, Natalizumab, Dimethyl fumarate and Teriflunomide [27];
6.   Absence of ON, or a single episode of ON without recurrence, that elapsed from the onset of the disease at least 12 months (ranging from 13 to 20 months) before the inclusion in the study. For MS patients with ON, this criterion was chosen, since it is known that the retrograde degeneration following ON occurs over a period of 6 months [28]. When an MS patient was affected by ON in both eyes, we studied the eye affected longer that met the inclusion criteria;
7.   Based on the ophthalmological examination, other inclusion criteria were: mean refractive error (when present) between −3.00 and +3.00 spherical equivalent; intraocular pressure less than 18 mmHg, absence of glaucoma or other diseases involving cornea, lens (lens opacity classification system, LOCS III, stage < 1), uvea, retina; BCVA between 0.0 and 1.0 LogMAR of the Early Treatment of Diabetic Retinopathy (ETDRS) charts; absence of central visual field defects and ability to maintain a stable fixation that allowed performing multifocal ERG (see below); absence of other systemic diseases (i.e., diabetes, systemic hypertension, rheumatologic disorders) that may influence the retinal function.

A Group of selected 41 age-matched healthy subjects (mean age: 40.64 ± 4.83 years, 26 females and 15 males), providing 41 normal eyes, with BCVA of 0.0 LogMAR (mean 0.0 ± 0.0), served as Controls.

The selected MS patients were divided into two Groups for age, MS-DD, EDSS and for previous history of presence or absence of ON.

The 41 MS patients (mean age 41.32 ± 3.72 years, 27 females and 14 males, mean MS-DD 8.53 ± 4.19 years, range 5–20 years; mean EDSS score 1.43 ± 1.06, range 0–3) were without history of unilateral or bilateral clinical signs of ON (i.e., painless reduction of BCVA, contrast sensitivity, color vision and any type of visual field defects) and high-contrast BCVA of 0.0 LogMAR (mean 0.0 ± 0.0). When both eyes met the inclusion criteria, only one eye was randomly chosen for the study. Therefore, we considered 40 eyes from 40 MS patients without ON (MS-noON Group).

The 47 MS patients (mean age 40.64 ± 4.96 years, 29 females and 18 males,) were with previous history of unilateral or bilateral ON (i.e., painless reduction of BCVA -between 0.2 and 1 LogMAR-, contrast sensitivity, color vision and visual field defects). They were further divided in to two Groups on the basis of the recovery of BCVA after ON:

The 27 MS patients (mean age 39.92 ± 4.86 years; 17 females and 10 males; mean MS-DD 9.06 ± 5.58 years, range 5–20 years; mean EDSS score 1.53 ± 1.22, range 0–3) were with previous history of a single unilateral or bilateral ON and with "good" recovery of high-contrast BCVA (0.0 LogMAR; mean 0.0 ± 0.0) after ON. Therefore, we considered 27 eyes from 27 MS patients with ON (MS-ON-G Group);

The 20 MS patients (mean age 41.08 ± 4.66 years; 12 females and 8 males; mean MS-DD 9.96 ± 6.03 years, range 5–20 years; mean EDSS score 1.49 ± 1.18, range 0–3) were with previous history of a single unilateral or bilateral ON with "poor" recovery of high-contrast BCVA (between 0.2 and 1 LogMAR; mean 0.357 ± 0.286) after ON, and reduced P-ERG amplitude with respect to our normative data collected in healthy subjects [29]. Therefore, we considered 20 eyes from 20 MS patients with ON (MS-ON-P Group).

Based on the previous mentioned inclusion criteria, the MS Groups with or without ON were homogeneous for age, MS-DD, EDSS and the MS Groups with ON were homogeneous for number of ON and for the time elapsed from ON. All groups were similar for male/female ratio (see the demographics for each Group in Table 1).

Table 1. Demographic and clinical features in Controls, Multiple Sclerosis patients without Optic Neuritis (MS-noON), with Optic Neuritis and good recovery of best corrected visual acuity (MS-ON-G) and with Optic Neuritis and poor recovery of best corrected visual acuity (MS-ON-P).

	Control (N [a] = 41) (Mean ± 1SD [b])	MS-noON (N [a] = 41) (Mean ± 1SD [b])	MS-ON-G (N [a] = 27) (Mean ± 1SD [b])	MS-ON-P (N [a] = 20) (Mean ± 1SD [b])
Age (years)	40.64 ± 4.83	41.32 ± 3.72	39.92 ± 4.86 [§]	41.08 ± 4.66 [§,#]
Male/Female (Ratio)	15/26 (0.57)	14/27 (0.51)	10/17 (0.58)	8/12 (0.66)
MS-DD [c] (years)	-	8.53 ± 4.19	9.06 ± 5.58 [§]	9.96 ± 6.03 [§,#]
EDSS [d] score	-	1.43 ± 1.06	1.53 ± 1.22 [§]	1.49 ± 1.18 [§,#]
Number of ON [e] episodes	-	-	1.00 ± 0.00	1.00 ± 0.00 [#]
Time elapsed from ON to the mfERG [f] and BCVA [g] assessments (months)	-	-	14.12 ± 2.72	15.87 ± 3.46 [#]

[a] N = Number of eyes of each Group; [b] SD = one Standard Deviation of the mean; [c] MS-DD = Multiple Sclerosis Disease Duration; [d] EDSS = Expanded Disability Status Scale; [e] ON = optic neuritis; [f] mfERG = multifocal electroretinogram; [g] BCVA = best corrected visual acuity; One-way analysis of variance between Groups: [§] $p > 0.01$ vs. Control and MS-noON Groups, [#] $p > 0.01$ vs. MS-ON-G Group.

In all MS patients and Controls, the BCVA and the functional condition of the preganglionic elements, located in the 25 retinal degrees by mfERG recordings, were evaluated in the same session during the same day of the examination. In all MS-ON-P patients, a morphological study of the macular layers by Sd-OCT examination was also performed, in addition to mfERG and BCVA evaluations, in the same session during the same day of the examination.

2.2. Multifocal Electroretinogram Recordings

The mfERG was recorded by using a modified version of Espion system (Diagnosys UK, LTD; Histon, Cambridge, UK) according to our previously published method [14,30,31] following the 2011 International Society for Clinical Electrophysiology of Vision (ISCEV) standards [11]. Briefly, the multifocal stimulus, consisting of 61 scaled hexagons, was displayed on a high-resolution, black-and-white 32″ LCD monitor with a frame rate of 75 Hz. The array of hexagons subtended 50 degrees of visual field (25° radius from the fixation point to edge of display). Each hexagon was independently alternated between black (1 cd/m^2) and white (200 cd/m^2) according to a binary m sequence. This resulted in a contrast of 99%. The luminance of the monitor screen and the central fixation cross (used as target) was 100 cd/m^2. The visual stimulation was performed by correcting BCVA for the distance of the visual stimuli. The m-sequence had 2^{13-1} elements, and total recording time was approximately 8 min. Total recording time was divided into sixteen segments. Between segments, the subject was allowed to rest for a few seconds. Focusing lenses were used when necessary. To maintain a stable fixation, a small red cross target (0.5 degree) was placed in the center of the stimulation field. At every mfERG reported that he/she could clearly perceive the fixation target. The eye's position was continuously monitored by an in-built video system to track fixation losses.

MfERGs were binocularly recorded in the presence of pupils that were maximally pharmacologically dilated with 1% tropicamide to a diameter of 7–8 mm. Pupil diameter was measured by an observer (LuB) by means of a millimeter ruler and a magnifying lens and stored for each tested eye. The cornea was anaesthetized with Benoxinate eye drops 0.4%. MfERGs were recorded between an active Dawson–Trick–Litzkow (DTL) contact electrode and a reference electrode (Ag/AgCl skin electrode placed on the correspondent outer canthi). A small Ag/AgCl skin ground electrode was placed at the centre of the forehead. Interelectrode resistance was <3 KOhms. After automatic rejection of artefacts and post-acquisition processing done by the in-built Espion software, the first-order kernel response was examined. MfERG responses with a signal to noise ≥3 were accepted for the analysis.

In the analysis of mfERG responses, we considered, for each obtained averaged response, the implicit times (ITs) of the first negative peak (N1) and the first positive peak (P1) measured in milliseconds (msec) and the N1-P1 peak-to-peak response amplitude density (RAD) measured in nanoVolt/$degree^2$ ($\eta V/degree^2$).

We considered three possible retinal topographies to explore the bioelectrical responses derived from specific retinal areas. Data were analyzed as follows:

1. Ring analysis: the averaged response obtained from five concentric annular retinal areas (rings) centered on the fovea: from 0 to 5 degrees (ring 1, R1), from 5 to 10 degrees (ring 2, R2), from 10 to 15 degrees (ring 3, R3), from 15 to 20 degrees (ring 4, R4) and from 20 to 25 degrees (ring 5, R5) (Figure 1).

2. Sector analysis 1: the averaged bioelectrical response obtained from the central macular region up to 15 degrees (0–15 degrees) sectioning it in four sectors: superior (S1-S), nasal (S1-N), inferior (S1-I) and temporal (S1-T) with respect to the fovea. In each sector, we included also the responses obtained from the more central macular area (0–5 degrees) (Figure 2).

3. Sector analysis 2: the averaged bioelectrical response obtained from the retinal area from the fovea up to 25 degrees (0–25 degrees) sectioning it in four sectors: S2-S, S2-N, S2-I and S2-T with respect to the fovea. In each sector, we included also the responses obtained from the more central macular area (0–5 degrees) (Figure 3).

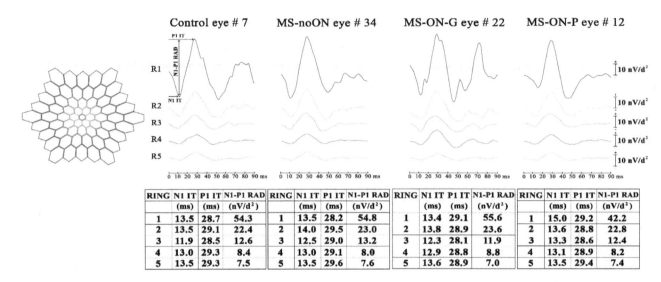

Figure 1. Multifocal electroretinogram averaged recordings obtained in a Control eye (#7), in a patient with multiple sclerosis (MS) without history of optic neuritis (MS-noON#34), and with history of optic neuritis followed by good or poor recovery of visual acuity (MS-ON-G#22 and MS-ON-P#12, respectively) by using ring analysis. For a better comparison, the left eye of representative Control, MS-noON and MS-ON eyes is presented. Ring analysis reports the averaged values of N1 and P1 implicit times (IT, measured in milliseconds -ms-) and of N1-P1 response amplitude density (RAD, measured in nanoVolt/degree^2 -nV/d^2-) obtained from five concentric annular retinal regions (rings) centred on the fovea: from 0 to 5 degrees (ring 1, R1), from 5 to 10 degrees (ring 2, R2), from 10 to 15 degrees (ring 3, R3), from 15 to 20 degrees (ring 4, R4) and from 20 to 25 degrees (ring 5, R5).

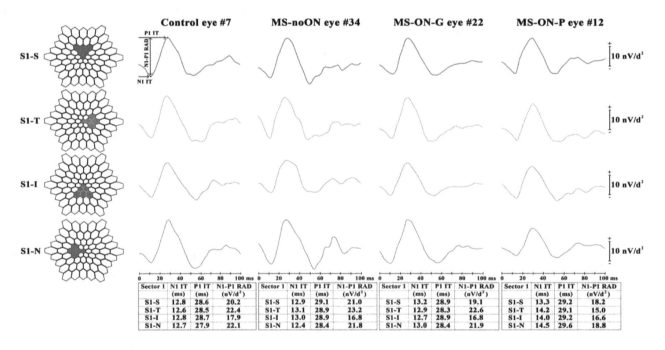

Figure 2. Multifocal electroretinogram averaged recordings obtained in a Control eye (#7), in a patient with multiple sclerosis (MS) without history of optic neuritis (MS-noON#34), and with history of optic neuritis followed by good or poor visual acuity (MS-ON-G#22 and MS-ON-P#12, respectively) by using the sector analysis 1. For a better comparison the left eye of representative Control, MS-noON and MS-ON eyes is presented.

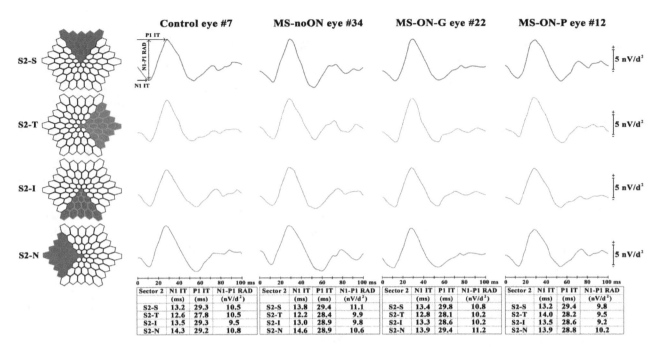

Sector 2	N1 IT (ms)	P1 IT (ms)	N1-P1 RAD (nV/d²)
S2-S	13.2	29.3	10.5
S2-T	12.6	27.8	10.5
S2-I	13.5	29.3	9.5
S2-N	14.3	29.2	10.8

Sector 2	N1 IT (ms)	P1 IT (ms)	N1-P1 RAD (nV/d²)
S2-S	13.8	29.4	11.1
S2-T	12.2	28.4	9.9
S2-I	13.0	28.9	9.8
S2-N	14.6	28.9	10.6

Sector 2	N1 IT (ms)	P1 IT (ms)	N1-P1 RAD (nV/d²)
S2-S	13.4	29.8	10.8
S2-T	12.8	28.1	10.2
S2-I	13.3	28.6	10.2
S2-N	13.9	29.4	11.2

Sector 2	N1 IT (ms)	P1 IT (ms)	N1-P1 RAD (nV/d²)
S2-S	13.2	29.4	9.8
S2-T	14.0	28.2	9.5
S2-I	13.5	28.6	9.2
S2-N	13.9	28.8	10.2

Figure 3. Multifocal electroretinogram averaged recordings obtained in a Control eye (#7), in a patient with multiple sclerosis (MS) without history of optic neuritis (MS-noON#34), and with history of optic neuritis followed by good or poor visual acuity (MS-ON-G#22 and MS-ON-P#12, respectively) by using two different sector analyses 1 and 2. For a better comparison the left eye of representative Control, MS-noON and MS-ON eyes is presented.

2.3. Sd-OCT Assessment

In all MS-ON-P patients, the macular morphology was evaluated by the RTVue-100 Sd-OCT device, following our recently published method [23].

Segmentation analysis was performed in order to measure the macular volume (MV) and macular thickness (MT) of whole, inner and outer retinal layers (WR, IR and OR, respectively) from concentric areas corresponding to the ETDRS topographical map:

(1) the 1 mm central area (named as Area 1, directly provided by the Sd-OCT machine)
(2) the middle 1–3 mm ring (named as Area 2, obtained by subtracting from the displayed volume within 3 mm the ones within the 1 mm),
(3) the external 3–6 mm ring (named as Area 3, obtained by subtracting from the displayed volume within 6 mm the one within 3 mm directly provided by the Sd-OCT machine),
(4) the whole 6 mm area (named as Area 1 + Area 2 + Area 3, directly provided by the Sd-OCT machine).

We also performed a sectorial segmentation analysis of the S, T, I and N sectors within 6 mm (averaging the three values of MV and MT displayed on the machine within the 0.5, 1 and 3 mm of radius from the fovea).

This allowed to compare the electrophysiological data to the morphological ones from corresponding localized retinal areas [32].

Therefore, we considered WR, IR and OR MVs and MTs measured in Area 1 corresponding to mfERG R1, in Area 2 corresponding to mfERG R2, in Area 3 corresponding to mfERG R3 and in Area 1 + Area 2 + Area 3, corresponding to mfERG R1 + R2 + R3. Accordingly, we also compared WR, IR and OR MV and MT values from S, T, I, N sectors to the corresponding mfERG data from Sector analysis 1 (see above).

2.4. Statistical Analysis

We assumed a Gaussian distribution of our data. The normal distribution was assessed by using the Kolmogorov-Smirnov test.

The differences of age, MS-DD, EDSS between MS-noON, MS-ON-G and MS-ON-P Groups were evaluated by the one-way analysis of variance (ANOVA). The differences of the number of ON and the time elapsed from the ON between MS-ON-G and MS-ON-P Groups were evaluated by the ANOVA.

Considering each different mfERG retinal topography (Ring, Sectors 1 and Sectors 2 analyses), the differences of mfERG N1 and P1 IT and N1-P1 RAD mean values between Controls, MS-noON, MS-ON-G and MS-ON-P Groups were evaluated by ANOVA. In addition, mean values of segmented MV and MT from all Areas and Sectors within 6 mm detected in MS-ON-P Group were compared to those of Controls by ANOVA. In MS-ON-P Group, Pearson's test was used to linearly correlate the values of BCVA with those of mfERG parameters and to correlate the individual mfERG values with the segmented MV and MT ones from corresponding retinal Areas and Sectors.

Since for each considered mfERG and OCT parameter, a multiple comparison between Groups (6 comparisons: Control vs. MS-noON Groups, Control vs. MS-ON-G Groups, Control vs. MS-ON-P Groups, MS-noON vs. MS-ON-G Groups, MS-noON vs. MS-ON-P Groups and MS-ON-G vs. MS-ON-P Groups) was performed, the value of statistically significance was calculated by: $p = 0.05$/number of comparison: $0.05/6 = 0.0082$. Therefore, we rounded up to a p-value lower than 0.01 to be considered as statistically significant. Minitab 17 (version 1) software was used for statistical analysis.

3. Results

3.1. Demographic and Clinical Features

In Table 1 are reported the demographic and clinical features observed in Controls, MS-noON, MS-ON-G and MS-ON-P Groups. The descriptive statistics of age, MS-DD and EDSS values were not significantly different between MS-noON, MS-ON-G and MS-ON-P Groups. The descriptive statistics of number of ON and the time elapsed from the ON were not significantly different between MS-ON-G and MS-ON-P Groups.

3.2. Multifocal Electroretinogram Ring Analysis

Examples of averaged mfERG recordings from five rings (R1, R2, R3, R4 and R5), obtained in representative Control (#7), MS-noON (#34), MS-ON-G (#22) and MS-ON-P (#12) eyes, are presented in Figure 1.

In Table 2 are reported the mean values of N1 and P1 IT and of N1-P1 RAD detected in the five rings (R1, R2, R3, R4 and R5) in Control, MS-noON, MS-ON-G and MS-ON-P Groups and the relative statistical analysis between Groups.

On average, when we considered the mean values of N1 and P1 IT obtained in the central retinal areas (R1, R2 and R3, 0 to 15 degrees) and in the more peripheral retinal areas (R4 and R5, 15 to 25 degrees), not statistically significant ($p > 0.01$) differences between all Groups were found.

The mean values of N1-P1 RAD obtained in the most central retinal areas (R1, 0–5 degrees) in MS-noON Group were not statistically ($p > 0.01$) different with respect to those of Controls. In MS-ON-G Group, the mean values of N1-P1 RAD were not significantly ($p > 0.01$) different when compared to those of Control and MS-noON Groups; by contrast, in MS-ON-P Group, the mean values of N1-P1 RAD were significantly ($p < 0.01$) reduced with respect to the ones from Control, MS-noON and MS-ON-G Groups; the reduction of the individual N1-P1 RADs were not significantly correlated ($p > 0.01$) with the corresponding values of BCVA.

In MS-noON, MS-ON-G and MS-ON-P Groups, the mean values of N1-P1 RAD obtained in the other areas (R2, R3, R4 and R5) were not statistically ($p > 0.01$) different with respect to those of Controls, and not statistically significant ($p > 0.01$) differences were found between MS Groups.

Table 2. Multifocal electroretinogram ring analysis in Control (C) eyes and in Multiple Sclerosis patients without Optic Neuritis (MS-noON), with optic neuritis followed by good recovery of best corrected visual acuity (BCVA) (MS-ON-G) or poor recovery of BCVA (MS-ON-P).

		Ring 1: 0–5 Degrees			Ring 2: 5–10 Degrees			Ring 3: 10–15 Degrees			Ring 4: 15–20 Degrees			Ring 5: 20–25 Degrees		
		N1 IT[a]	P1 IT[a]	RAD[b]	N1 IT[a]	P1 IT[a]	RAD[b]	N1 IT[a]	P1 IT[a]	RAD[b]	N1 IT[a]	P1 IT[a]	RAD[b]	N1 IT[a]	P1 IT[a]	RAD[b]
Controls N[d] = 41	Mean	14.693	29.785	56.137	13.863	28.793	22.037	12.890	28.110	12.012	12.815	28.168	8.724	13.459	28.944	7.129
	SD[c]	2.666	2.678	10.771	1.712	1.349	4.816	1.312	1.394	3.090	2.396	1.331	2.090	1.247	1.611	1.778
MS-noON N[d] = 41	Mean	15.078	30.035	54.273	13.743	28.393	21.505	13.193	27.413	12.525	13.115	28.455	9.050	13.198	28.650	7.535
	SD[c]	2.383	1.958	11.665	2.177	1.661	4.556	2.505	3.076	3.409	1.020	1.285	2.573	1.156	1.115	2.321
A[e] vs. C	f(1.81)	0.491	0.234	0.568	0.078	1.432	0.262	0.464	0.913	0.063	0.582	1.002	0.409	0.949	0.902	0.812
	P	0.487	0.638	0.453	0.782	0.235	0.610	0.498	0.343	0.810	0.449	0.319	0.525	0.332	0.345	0.372
MS-ON-G N[d] = 27	Mean	15.748	30.156	53.467	13.741	29.104	21.081	12.800	28.041	12.344	13.089	28.585	8.926	12.963	28.596	7.511
	SD[c]	2.934	2.739	11.053	1.903	1.761	5.121	1.522	1.831	2.755	1.042	1.484	1.906	0.692	1.196	1.622
A[e] vs. C	f(1.67)	2.371	0.029	1.000	0.071	0.672	0.609	0.068	0.032	0.262	0.332	1.423	0.183	3.591	0.879	0.799
	P	0.128	0.563	0.321	0.787	0.415	0.463	0.796	0.859	0.611	0.570	0.238	0.676	0.063	0.352	0.376
A[e] vs. MS-noON	f(1.67)	1.072	0.042	0.079	0.000	2.841	0.164	0.532	0.913	0.063	0.013	0.153	0.042	0.932	0.029	0.009
	P	0.304	0.834	0.776	1.000	0.097	0.693	0.470	0.343	0.810	0.907	0.703	0.836	0.337	0.861	0.954
MS-ON-P N[d] = 20	Mean	15.657	30.012	43.136	13.976	29.464	21.362	12.984	28.524	13.486	13.002	28.648	8.322	13.892	28.027	6.994
	SD[c]	2.572	2.923	10.964	2.023	1.941	6.013	1.937	1.641	3.904	2.474	1.823	3.566	1.721	2.526	2.843
A[e] vs. C	f(1.60)	1.802	0.091	19.36	0.053	2.473	0.221	0.053	1.053	2.570	0.084	1.363	0.311	1.262	2.962	0.051
	P	0.185	0.764	0.000[f]	0.821	0.121	0.638	0.824	0.309	0.115	0.778	0.248	0.581	0.267	0.090	0.821
A[e] vs. MS-noON	f(1.60)	0.753	0.002	12.73	0.162	5.003	0.012	0.111	2.283	0.972	0.064	0.233	0.831	3.482	1.812	0.630
	P	0.389	0.971	0.000[f]	0.690	0.029	0.918	0.744	0.137	0.328	0.801	0.634	0.366	0.067	0.184	0.431
A[e] vs. MS-ON-G	f(1.46)	0.012	0.033	11.41	0.172	0.443	0.033	0.133	0.871	1.383	0.033	0.021	0.562	6.552	1.062	0.626
	P	0.912	0.862	0.002[f]	0.686	0.510	0.864	0.717	0.355	0.245	0.870	0.897	0.458	0.014	0.309	0.434

[a] IT = Implicit Time (measured in msec); [b] RAD = N1-P1 Response Amplitude Density (measured in $\eta V/degree^2$); [c] SD = one Standard Deviation of the mean; [d] N = Number of eyes of each Group; [e] A = one-way analysis of variance. [f] p Values < 0.01 were considered as statistically significant for Group comparisons.

3.3. *Multifocal Electroretinogram Sector Analysis 1 (0–15 Degrees)*

Examples of averaged mfERG recordings from four sectors superior (S1-S), temporal (S1-T), inferior (S1-I) and nasal (S1-N) within 15 degrees of foveal eccentricity, obtained in representative Control (#7), MS-noON (#34), MS-ON-G (#22) and MS-ON-P (#12) eyes, are presented in Figure 2.

Sector analysis 1 reports the averaged values of N1 and P1 IT and of N1-P1 RAD obtained from four macular areas enclosed between 0 and 15 degrees with respect to the fovea on the basis of the retinal topography: superior (S1-S), temporal (S1-T), inferior (S1-I), nasal (S1-N). The bioelectrical responses obtained from the central 0–5 degrees were enclosed in the sector analysis 1.

In Table 3 are reported the mean values of N1 and P1 IT and of N1-P1 RAD detected in the four central sectors (S1-S, S1-T, S1-I, S1-N) in Control, MS-noON, MS-ON-G and MS-ON-P Groups and the relative statistical analysis between Groups.

On average, when we considered the mean values of N1 and P1 IT obtained in the central sectors (S1-S, S1-N, S1-I, S1-T) not statistically significant ($p > 0.01$) differences between all Groups were found.

The mean values of N1-P1 RAD obtained in these sectors in MS-noON Group were not statistically ($p > 0.01$) different with respect to those of Controls.

In MS-ON-G Group, the mean values of N1-P1 RAD from all four sectors were not significant ($p > 0.01$) different when compared to those of Control and MS-noON Groups. By contrast, in MS-ON-P Group, while mean values of N1-P1 RAD detected in S1-I, S1-T and S1-S were not significantly ($p > 0.01$) reduced with respect to Control, MS-noON and MS-ON-G ones, a significant ($p < 0.01$) reduction of N1-P1 RADs in the S1-N sector was observed as compared to Controls, MS-noON and MS-ON-G Groups.

The individual reduced N1-P1 RAD values from S1-N sector in MS-ON-P eyes were not significantly correlated ($p > 0.01$) with the corresponding values of BCVA.

Table 3. Multifocal electroretinogram sector analysis within the 0–15 central degrees in Control (C) eyes and in Multiple Sclerosis patients without Optic Neuritis (MS-noON), with optic neuritis followed by good recovery of best corrected visual acuity (BCVA) (MS-ON-G), or poor recovery of BCVA (MS-ON-P).

		0–15 Central Degrees Superior Sector			0–15 Central Degrees Temporal Sector			0–15 Central Degrees Inferior Sector			0–15 Central Degrees Nasal Sector		
		N1 IT [a]	P1 IT [a]	RAD [b]	N1 IT [a]	P1 IT [a]	RAD [b]	N1 IT [a]	P1 IT [a]	RAD [b]	N1 IT [a]	P1 IT [a]	RAD [b]
Controls N [d] = 41	Mean	13.266	28.800	17.910	13.251	28.917	17.944	13.373	28.327	17.573	13.195	27.698	19.039
	SD [c]	1.712	1.588	4.254	1.659	1.776	4.746	1.747	1.432	4.424	1.742	1.300	4.406
MS-noON N [d] = 41	Mean	13.758	28.319	17.442	13.972	28.508	18.119	13.881	27.997	16.489	13.831	27.506	19.369
	SD [c]	2.058	1.438	3.982	1.996	1.677	4.094	2.167	1.525	4.131	1.679	1.587	4.508
A [e] vs. C	f(1.81)	1.379	2.069	0.262	3.158	1.148	0.029	1.368	1.018	1.308	2.028	0.362	0.108
	P	0.243	0.154	0.608	0.079	0.287	0.859	0.246	0.316	0.255	0.096	0.551	0.738
MS-ON-G N [d] = 27	Mean	13.256	28.459	17.241	13.774	28.356	18.278	13.419	28.648	17.007	13.570	28.037	17.933
	SD [c]	1.430	1.554	3.932	2.042	2.237	4.843	2.027	1.289	4.129	1.610	1.806	4.246
A [e] vs. C	f(1.67)	0.003	0.758	0.432	1.352	1.320	0.079	0.009	0.878	0.282	0.801	0.809	1.002
	P	0.988	0.385	0.516	0.250	0.255	0.779	0.921	0.351	0.598	0.374	0.371	0.321
A [e] vs. MS-noON	f(1.67)	1.222	0.138	0.039	0.162	0.102	0.019	0.779	3.340	0.258	0.408	1.632	1.642
	P	0.274	0.705	0.838	0.693	0.750	0.885	0.381	0.072	0.615	0.526	0.206	0.205
MS-ON-P N [d] = 20	Mean	13.519	29.004	17.828	13.987	28.763	17.874	13.287	28.736	17.232	14.122	28.006	14.892
	SD [c]	2.391	1.738	5.008	2.674	2.222	4.586	2.562	2.876	5.023	1.936	1.964	3.225
A [e] vs. C	f(1.60)	0.222	0.212	0.002	1.75	0.092	0.002	0.022	0.552	0.072	3.542	0.532	14.00
	P	0.637	0.645	0.947	0.191	0.771	0.957	0.878	0.459	0.788	0.065	0.468	0.000 [f]
A [e] vs. MS-noON	f(1.60)	0.161	2.663	0.111	0.002	0.253	0.042	0.901	1.731	0.383	0.372	1.642	15.73
	P	0.688	0.108	0.745	0.980	0.619	0.834	0.348	0.193	0.542	0.548	0.205	0.000 [f]
A [e] vs. MS-ON-G	f(1.46)	0.222	1.284	0.202	0.101	0.386	0.081	0.042	0.022	0.032	1.142	0.002	7.192
	P	0.641	0.264	0.655	0.758	0.539	0.774	0.345	0.888	0.867	0.292	0.956	0.009 [f]

[a] IT = Implicit Time (measured in msec); [b] RAD = N1-P1 Response Amplitude Density (measured in $\eta V/degree^2$); [c] SD = one Standard Deviation of the mean; [d] N = Number of eyes of each Group; [e] A = one-way analysis of variance. [f] p Values < 0.01 were considered as statistically significant for Group comparisons.

3.4. Multifocal Electroretinogram Sector Analysis 2 (0–25 Degrees)

Examples of averaged mfERG recordings from 4 sectors (S2-S, S2-T, S2-I, S2-N) within 25 degrees of foveal eccentricity in representative Control (#7), MS-noON (#34), MS-ON-G (#22) and MS-ON-P (#12) eyes are presented in Figure 3.

Sector analysis 2 reports the averaged values of N1 and P1 IT and of N1-P1 RAD obtained from four retinal areas from 0 to 25 degrees based on the retinal topography: superior (S2-S), temporal (S2-T), inferior (S2-I), nasal (S2-N), with respect to the fovea. The bioelectrical responses obtained from the central 0–5 degrees were enclosed in the sector analysis 2.

The mean values of N1 and P1 IT and of N1-P1 RAD detected in the 4 sectors (S2-S, S2-T, S2-I, S2-N) in Control, MS-ON and MS-noON Groups and the relative statistical analysis between Groups are reported in Table 4.

On average, the mean values of N1 and P1 IT and of N1-P1 RAD detected in all sectors (S2-S, S2-T, S2-I, S2-N) in MS-noON, MS-ON-G and MS-ON-P Groups were not statistically ($p > 0.01$) different when compared with those of Controls. In MS-ON-G and MS-ON-P Groups the mean values of N1-P1 RAD from all four sectors were not significantly ($p > 0.01$) different when compared to those of Control and MS-noON Groups. Furthermore, not statistically significant differences ($p > 0.01$) were found when mean N1-P1 RADs were compared between MS-ON-G and MS-ON-P Groups in all sectors.

Table 4. Multifocal electroretinogram sector analysis within the 0–25 central degrees in Control (C) eyes and in Multiple Sclerosis patients without Optic Neuritis (MS-noON), with optic neuritis followed by good recovery of best corrected visual acuity (BCVA) (MS-ON-G), or poor recovery of BCVA (MS-ON-P).

	0-25 Degrees Superior Sector			0-25 Degrees Temporal Sector			0-25 Degrees Inferior Sector			0-25 Degrees Nasal Sector		
	N1 IT[a]	P1 IT[a]	RAD[b]	N1 IT[a]	P1 IT[a]	RAD[b]	N1 IT[a]	P1 IT[a]	RAD[b]	N1 IT[a]	P1 IT[a]	RAD[b]
Controls (N[d] =41) Mean	13.090	28.783	9.759	13.402	28.027	9.176	13.283	28.680	8.132	13.268	27.985	9.388
SD[c]	1.504	1.357	2.463	1.240	1.405	2.793	1.378	1.613	2.217	1.479	1.227	2.197
MS-noON (N[d] =41) Mean	13.133	28.258	10.192	13.336	28.467	9.181	13.394	28.281	7.994	12.964	27.661	9.994
SD[c]	1.154	1.240	2.789	1.365	1.132	2.606	1.793	1.640	2.558	0.858	1.217	3.022
A[e] vs. C f(1.81)	0.021	3.339	0.561	0.049	2.439	0.001	0.100	1.229	0.069	1.129	1.442	1.082
P	0.896	0.071	0.450	0.819	0.122	0.993	0.754	0.270	0.795	0.258	0.234	0.302
MS-ON-G (N[d] =27) Mean	12.904	28.763	10.022	13.333	28.307	9.437	13.296	28.900	8.322	12.793	27.856	9.552
SD[c]	1.121	1.055	1.857	1.775	1.407	2.224	1.308	1.450	2.246	0.998	1.260	1.963
A[e] vs. C f(1.67)	0.301	0.009	0.219	0.039	0.649	0.168	0.002	0.329	0.118	2.761	0.182	0.104
P	0.585	0.949	0.638	0.851	0.424	0.685	0.969	0.569	0.732	0.101	0.676	0.755
A[e] vs. MS-noON f(1.67)	0.659	3.028	0.079	0.022	0.272	0.178	0.059	2.538	0.092	0.567	0.409	0.448
P	0.421	0.086	0.782	0.994	0.607	0.676	0.808	0.116	0.589	0.454	0.526	0.504
MS-ON-P N[d] = 20 Mean	13.834	28.916	9.786	14.003	28.237	9.924	13.977	28.471	8.976	13.219	28.104	9.812
SD[c]	1.345	1.723	2.923	2.656	1.579	3.512	1.422	1.765	2.784	1.806	3.245	2.782
A[e] vs. C f(1.60)	3.522	0.11	0.00	1.437	0.28	0.812	3.342	0.211	1.644	0.012	0.040	0.422
P	0.066	0.744	0.970	0.231	0.601	0.371	0.073	0.647	0.205	0.911	0.838	0.520
A[e] vs. MS-noON f(1.60)	4.454	2.910	0.281	1.690	0.430	0.871	1.615	0.173	1.874	0.564	0.60	0.051
P	0.039	0.093	0.601	0.198	0.517	0.356	0.209	0.680	0.177	0.456	0.442	0.822
A[e] vs. MS-ON-G f(1.46)	6.673	0.143	0.111	1.073	0.031	0.345	2.892	0.845	0.082	1.076	0.132	0.141
P	0.013	0.708	0.737	0.305	0.874	0.564	0.096	0.365	0.377	0.307	0.718	0.709

[a] IT = Implicit Time (measured in msec); [b] RAD = N1-P1 Response Amplitude Density (measured in $\eta V/degree^2$); [c] SD = one Standard Deviation of the mean; [d] N = Number of eyes of each Group; [e] A = one-way analysis of variance.

3.5. Morphological Data in MS-ON-P Group and Correlations with mfERG Findings

Examples of Sd-OCT map of MV and MT of OR and IR macular layers evaluated in representative Control (#7) and MS-ON-P (#12) eyes are presented in Figure 4.

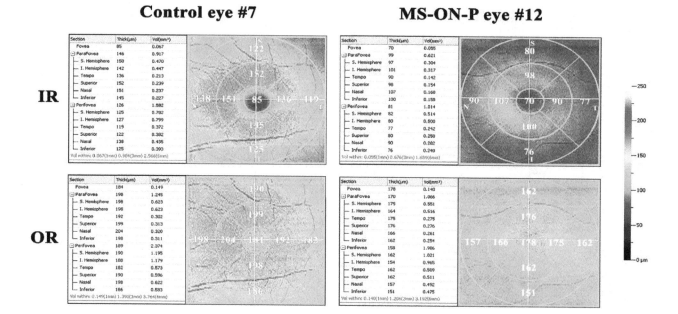

Figure 4. Examples of Early Treatment of Diabetic Retinopathy (ETDRS) topographical map of macular volume and thickness values of inner (top) and outer (bottom) macular layers (IR and OR, respectively) obtained in left eyes of a representative Control (#7) and of a multiple sclerosis patient with history of optic neuritis followed poor recovery of visual acuity (MS-ON-P#12) by using Sd-OCT. On the left side of the ETDRS maps, the volume and thickness numerical values for each sector are reported. On the right side of the Figure, a colorimetric scale is provided to display the macular thickness values. The macular volume and thickness values were measured from concentric circular Areas (Area 1: the 1 mm central area; Area 2: the middle 1–3 mm ring; Area 3: the external 3–6 mm ring; Area 1 + 2 + 3: area within 6 mm) and Sectors (Superior, S; Temporal, T; Inferior, I; Nasal, N) within 6 mm (averaging the three values of macular volume (MV) and macular thickness (MT) displayed on the machine within the 0.5 mm, 1 mm and 3 mm of radius from the fovea). With respect to Control eye, MS-ON-P eye shows reduced MV and MT values in both inner and outer retinal layers (IR and OR) macular layers in each Area or Sector.

In Table 5 are reported the mean values of segmented Sd-OCT MV and MT of WR, IR and OR measured in Area 1, Area 2, Area 3 and Areas 1 + 2 + 3 in Controls and in MS-ON-P patients. We found a statistically significant difference ($p < 0.01$) between these Groups for all structural values but the IR MV from Area 1.

In Table 6 are reported the mean Sd-OCT MVs and MTs of WR, IR and OR measured in the S, T, I and N Sectors within 6 mm from the fovea in Controls and in MS-ON-P patients. We found a statistically significant ($p < 0.01$) reduction of all morphological parameters from each Sector in MS-ON-P with respect to Controls.

In MS-ON-P patients, we found not significant ($p > 0.01$) linear correlations between the reduced mfERG RADs from Ring 1 with the reduction of OR MV and MT from Area 1. No other significant correlations between mfERG parameters from other Rings with Sd-OCT values from corresponding retinal areas were found.

Table 5. Spectral domain-Optical Coherence Tomography macular volume (MV) (A) and macular thickness (MT) (B) segmentation analysis in Control (C) eyes and in Multiple Sclerosis patients with Optic Neuritis and reduced recovery of best corrected visual acuity (MS-ON-P).

A

		WR-MV (mm³)				IR-MV (mm³)				OR-MV (mm³)			
		AREA 1	AREA 2	AREA 3	AREA 1 +2+3	AREA 1	AREA 2	AREA 3	AREA 1 +2+3	AREA 1	AREA 2	AREA 3	AREA 1 +2+3
Controls N[b] = 41	Mean	0.212	2.025	3.656	5.893	0.065	0.824	1.451	2.342	0.146	1.201	2.205	3.552
	SD[a]	0.019	0.135	0.245	0.372	0.018	0.075	0.127	0.199	0.016	0.088	0.233	0.328
MS-ON-P N[b] = 20	Mean	0.189	1.599	2.087	3.875	0.056	0.632	1.217	1.905	0.133	0.967	2.008	3.108
	SD[a]	0.015	0.086	1.412	0.289	0.012	0.038	0.122	0.272	0.008	0.174	0.077	0.131
A[c] vs. C	f(1.60)	22.422	165.532	40.471	453.482	0.112	115.824	46.800	50.661	11.701	49.074	13.482	33.771
	P	0.000 d	0.000 d	0.000 d	0.000 d	0.742	0.000 d	0.000 d	0.000 d	0.001 d	0.000 d	<0.01 d	0.000 d

B

		WR-MT (μ)			IR-MT (μ)			OR-MT (μ)		
		AREA 1	AREA 2	AREA 3	AREA 1	AREA 2	AREA 3	AREA 1	AREA 2	AREA 3
Controls N[b] = 41	Mean	263.866	327.674	299.975	81.134	138.427	114.422	182.732	189.247	185.553
	SD[a]	12.512	12.913	9.572	10.561	8.946	6.566	9.884	9.983	7.002
MS-ON-P N[b] = 20	Mean	243.834	275.179	263.253	69.417	106.667	96.833	174.417	168.512	166.417
	SD[a]	12.999	13.665	10.146	10.227	7.183	9.737	7.225	7.816	5.979
A[c] vs. C	f(1.60)	38.672	213.901	190.280	16.893	191.321	69.202	11.199	86.811	110.000
	P	0.000 d	0.000 d	0.000 d	0.000 d	0.000 d	0.000 d	0.001 d	0.000 d	0.000 d

WR-MV = Whole Retinal Macular Volume; IR-MV = Inner Retinal Macular Volume; OR-MV = Outer Retinal Macular Volume; WR-MT = Whole Retinal Macular Thickness; IR-MT = Inner Retinal Macular Thickness; OR-MT = Outer Retinal Macular Thickness; μ = micron; Area 1 = 1 mm centered to the fovea; Area 2 = annular area 1–3 mm centered to the fovea; Area 3 = annular area 3–6 mm centered to the fovea; Area 1 + 2 + 3 = whole area within 6 mm; [a] SD = one Standard Deviation of the mean; [b] N = Number of eyes of each Group; [c] A = one-way analysis of variance. [d] p Values < 0.01 were considered as statistically significant for Group comparisons.

Table 6. Spectral domain-Optical Coherence Tomography macular volume (MV) (A) and macular thickness (MT) (B) sectorial segmentation analysis in Control (C) eyes and in Multiple Sclerosis patients with Optic Neuritis and reduced recovery of best corrected visual acuity (MS-ON-P).

A		SUPERIOR SECTOR			TEMPORAL SECTOR			INFERIOR SECTOR			NASAL SECTOR		
		WR-MV	IR-MV	OR-MV	WR-MV	IR-MV	OR-MV	WR-MV	IR-MV	OR-MV	WR-MV	IR-MV	OR-MV
		(mm³)	(mm³)	(mm³)	(mm³)	(mm³)	(mm³)	(mm³)	(mm³)	(mm³)	(mm³)	(mm³)	(mm³)
Controls N[b] = 41	Mean	0.551	0.214	0.337	0.537	0.203	0.334	0.551	0.335	0.216	0.579	0.231	0.348
	SD[a]	0.029	0.017	0.019	0.031	0.015	0.02	0.028	0.021	0.012	0.048	0.018	0.024
MS-ON-P N[b] = 20	Mean	0.475	0.168	0.307	0.479	0.172	0.307	0.487	0.310	0.177	0.478	0.175	0.303
	SD[a]	0.029	0.021	0.011	0.028	0.012	0.014	0.021	0.016	0.016	0.028	0.015	0.015
A[c] vs. C	f(1.60)	92.321	84.173	42.642	50.022	64.942	29.312	81.756	22.032	113.55	75.577	144.312	58.801
	P	0.000[d]	0.000[d]	0.000[d]	0.000[d]	0.000[d]	0.000[d]	0.000[d]	0.000[d]	0.000[d]	0.000[d]	0.000[d]	0.000[d]

B		SUPERIOR SECTOR			TEMPORAL SECTOR			INFERIOR SECTOR			NASAL SECTOR		
		WR-MT	IR-MT	OR-MT	WR-MT	IR-MT	OR-MT	WR-MT	IR-MT	OR-MT	WR-MT	IR-MT	OR-MT
		(µ)	(µ)	(µ)	(µ)	(µ)	(µ)	(µ)	(µ)	(µ)	(µ)	(µ)	(µ)
Controls N[b] = 41	Mean	297.124	111.358	185.766	292.804	108.243	184.561	297.078	184.56	112.518	306.789	117.604	189.185
	SD[a]	8.573	7.217	6.755	8.239	7.862	6.561	6.072	6.366	6.756	7.541	8.822	6.341
MS-ON-P N[b] = 20	Mean	271.297	94.442	176.857	271.135	92.052	178.995	268.411	174.221	94.191	274.021	97.834	176.190
	SD[a]	6.580	7.065	5.417	7.742	6.325	5.444	8.341	7.085	9.344	8.033	7.898	5.253
A[c] vs. C	f(1.60)	140.612	68.222	26.427	96.632	64.326	10.755	233.066	32.933	76.457	243.281	72.150	69.390
	P	0.000[d]	0.000[d]	0.000[d]	0.000[d]	0.000[d]	0.002[d]	0.000[d]	0.000[d]	0.000[d]	0.000[d]	0.000[d]	0.000[d]

WR-MV = Whole Retinal Macular Volume; IR-MV = Inner Retinal Macular Volume; OR-MV = Outer Retinal Macular Volume; WR-MT = Whole Retinal Macular Thickness; IR-MT = Inner Retinal Macular Thickness; OR-MT = Outer Retinal Macular Thickness; µ = micron; [a] SD = one Standard Deviation of the mean; [b] N = Number of eyes of each Group; [c] A = one-way analysis of variance; [d] p Values < 0.01 were considered as statistically significant for Group comparisons.

Table 7. Linear correlation (Pearson's Test) between multifocal electroretinogram values from ring analysis (A) and from sector analysis 1 (0–15 central degrees) (B) and the corresponding Spectral domain-Optical Coherence Tomography macular volume (MV) and macular thickness (MT) segmentation analysis individual values in Multiple Sclerosis patients with Optic Neuritis and reduced recovery of best corrected visual acuity (MS-ON-P).

A

	AREA 1 vs. mfERG Ring1			AREA 2 vs. mfERG Ring 2			AREA 3 vs. mfERG Ring 3			AREA 1 + 2 + 3 vs. Rings 1 + 2 + 3		
	N1 IT[a]	P1 IT[a]	RAD[b]	N1 IT[a]	P1 IT[a]	RAD[b]	N1 IT[a]	P1 IT[a]	RAD[b]	N1 IT[a]	P1 IT[a]	RAD[b]
	r; p[c]	r; p[c]	r; p[c]	r; p[c]	r; p[c]	r; p[c]	r; p[c]	r; p[c]	r; p[c]	r; p[c]	r; p[c]	r; p[c]
WR-MV	0.198; 0.535	-0.055; 0.862	0.512; 0.088	0.192; 0.549	-0.103; 0.748	0.245; 0.441	-0.324; 0.303	-0.509; 0.090	-0.163; 0.611	-0.169; 0.599	-0.474; 0.118	0.037; 0.907
IR-MV	0.338; 0.282	0.086; 0.794	0.511; 0.090	0.132; 0.683	-0.160; 0.621	0.283; 0.372	-0.288; 0.365	-0.437; 0.156	-0.061; 0.851	0.185; 0.565	-0.265; 0.405	0.261; 0.413
OR-MV	0.037; 0.910	-0.193; 0.548	0.443; 0.168	0.228; 0.475	-0.348; 0.267	-0.498; 0.099	-0.345; 0.271	-0.567; 0.055	-0.309; 0.328	-0.173; 0.591	-0.308; 0.331	-0.074; 0.819
WR-MT	0.201; 0.532	-0.053; 0.870	0.409; 0.131	0.184; 0.567	-0.100; 0.756	0.254; 0.426	-0.324; 0.304	-0.517; 0.086	-0.167; 0.604	-	-	-
IR-MT	0.331; 0.293	0.073; 0.822	0.507; 0.093	0.134; 0.677	-0.176; 0.585	0.281; 0.376	-0.298; 0.347	-0.435; 0.158	-0.061; 0.851	-	-	-
OR-MT	0.042; 0.896	-0.181; 0.574	0.369; 0.204	0.223; 0.486	-0.021; 0.947	0.169; 0.600	-0.336; 0.285	-0.571; 0.052	-0.309; 0.329	-	-	-

B

	SUPERIOR SECTOR			TEMPORAL SECTOR			INFERIOR SECTOR			NASAL SECTOR		
	N1 IT[a]	P1 IT[a]	RAD[b]	N1 IT[a]	P1 IT[a]	RAD[b]	N1 IT[a]	P1 IT[a]	RAD[b]	N1 IT[a]	P1 IT[a]	RAD[b]
	r; p[c]	r; p[c]	r; p[c]	r; p[c]	r; p[c]	r; p[c]	r; p[c]	r; p[c]	r; p[c]	r; p[c]	r; p[c]	r; p[c]
WR-MV	0.167; 0.602	-0.113; 0.726	0.281; 0.376	-0.331; 0.292	-0.119; 0.711	-0.331; 0.292	-0.045; 0.888	-0.569; 0.053	0.193; 0.547	-0.119; 0.710	-0.036; 0.910	-0.056; 0.861
IR-MV	0.156; 0.627	-0.166; 0.606	0.349; 0.266	-0.363; 0.245	-0.078; 0.809	-0.363; 0.245	0.100; 0.756	-0.341; 0.277	0.171; 0.595	-0.169; 0.598	-0.109; 0.734	0.082; 0.798
OR-MV	0.163; 0.611	0.020; 0.949	0.085; 0.791	-0.125; 0.698	-0.063; 0.845	-0.125; 0.698	-0.168; 0.601	-0.228; 0.407	0.073; 0.819	-0.034; 0.916	-0.060; 0.852	-0.224; 0.483
WR-MT	-0.162; 0.614	0.001; 0.999	0.742; 0.006	-0.159; 0.620	-0.418; 0.175	-0.159; 0.620	0.110; 0.731	-0.549; 0.064	0.131; 0.684	-0.099; 0.759	-0.137; 0.669	-0.074; 0.817
IR-MT	0.145; 0.650	-0.208; 0.516	0.313; 0.321	-0.374; 0.230	-0.082; 0.799	-0.374; 0.230	0.265; 0.404	-0.318; 0.312	0.201; 0.529	-0.117; 0.716	-0.093; 0.771	0.052; 0.870
OR-MT	0.060; 0.852	0.002; 0.994	0.088; 0.785	-0.325; 0.302	-0.164; 0.608	-0.325; 0.302	-0.028; 0.929	-0.391; 0.312	0.055; 0.865	-0.065; 0.840	-0.159; 0.621	-0.186; 0.561

WR-MV = Whole Retinal Macular Volume; IR-MV = Inner Retinal Macular Volume; OR-MV = Outer Retinal Macular Volume; WR-MT = Whole Retinal Macular Thickness; IR-MT = Inner Retinal Macular Thickness; OR-MT = Outer Retinal Macular Thickness; μ = micron; Area 1 = 1 mm centered to the fovea; Area 2 = annular area 1–3 mm centered to the fovea; Area 3 = annular area 3–6 mm centered to the fovea; Area 1 + 2 + 3 = whole area within 6 mm. [a] IT = Implicit Time (measured in msec); [b] RAD = N1-P1 Response Amplitude Density (measured in ηV/degree^2); [c] p values < 0.01 were considered as statistically significant.

When we linearly correlated the mfERG data from Sectors-S1 with the corresponding MV and MT individual values from S, T, I, N Sectors, we found not significant linear correlations between the S1 ITs and RADs and WR, IR and OR MVs and MTs. The results of these statistical linear correlations are reported in Table 7.

4. Discussion

The purpose of this study was to assess the function of preganglionic elements in MS patients, without and with history of ON, adding information on the debated topic of potential O-MR layers dysfunction, expression of the extension or sparing from neurodegenerative process beyond IML in MS.

We studied by mfERG the function of O-MR elements located in different areas of the central macula (0 to 15 degrees) or more peripheral retina within the arcades (0 to 25 degrees), topographically distinguished in rings or sectors. Our results apply to MS Groups with or without ON highly homogeneous for age, MS-DD, EDSS, and when present for number of ON and for the time elapsed from ON to the BCVA and mfERG assessment, differently from all previous reported studies in the literature [18,20–22].

In addition, since a morphological impairment of macular OR has been described in MS-ON patients [20] and in our recent work was confirmed to be detectable exclusively in those MS-ON patients with poor recovery of BCVA [23], we also evaluated in MS-ON-P patients whether a possible preganglionic macular dysfunction could be associated or not to structural OR changes for corresponding retinal areas.

Our mfERG findings showed not statistically significant differences of N1 and P1 IT values in all Groups (MS-noON, MS-ON-G and MS-ON-P) in any considered central circular areas (R1, R2, R3) or sectors (S1-S, S1-T, S1-I, S1-N) and more peripheral circular areas (R4, R5) or sectors (S2-S, S2-T, S2-I, S2-N) either when responses were compared to Controls or with MS Groups. As for N1-P1 RAD values, we found statistically significant ($p < 0.01$) differences in MS-ON-P Group compared to Controls, MS-noON and MS-ON-G only when analyzing responses from Ring 1 (0–5 degrees) and from the S1-N sector, which covers the 0–15 central degrees area. In all other examined central or peripheral rings or sectors, we did not find any significant difference in the values of N1-P1 RAD between Groups. Our results indicate that photoreceptors and bipolar cells of the central fovea, as well as of the more central nasal macular sector within 15 degrees, are functionally impaired in MS only in occurrence of ON and when full recovery of BCVA is not achieved. These results do not apply either to MS-noON nor MS-ON-G Groups, thus confirming that the preganglionic element dysfunction is independent from the event of ON in itself.

As mentioned above, contrasting data are reported in literature about the potential functional involvement of O-MR layers in the MS degenerative process, depending on MS classification, presence or absence of ON and different mfERG signal analyses. As stated by Hanson et al. [33] "similarities or differences between findings in the central and peripheral retina are yet to be definitively elucidated in MS", and therefore we thought reasonable to study O-MR function in our patients by applying not only the standard ring analysis, but also the more innovative sector analyses previously used in other neurodegenerative diseases [30,34].

In MS-noON Group, we found a functional integrity of O-MR elements, in agreement with the results of a previous mfERG study [22] in which, by using the ring analysis, normal function of preganglionic elements in eyes without ON and normal high-contrast visual acuity was found. By contrast, our results differ from those by Saidha et al. [20], who found in five MS-noON patients with an abnormal OCT macular thickness and normal visual acuity, normal mfERG latencies with reduced P1 amplitude. As for the comparison of sector analysis results in MS-noON, Boquete et al. [35] studied, by using a more refined mfERG analysis method, a small cohort of newly diagnosed MS patients with less than 6 months from their first symptoms and no ON. They found an impairment of O-MR function exclusively in the supero-temporal quadrant of the macula. In our study, we analyzed the mfERG responses sectioning the central macular region up to 15 degrees (0–15 degrees, sector analysis 1) and the whole macular area up to 25 degrees (0–25 degrees, sector analysis 2) in four sectors (superior, temporal, inferior and nasal). By adopting this different way to analyze mfERG sector responses [30,34], we did not find statistically significant differences between Controls and MS-noON. Because the exact protocol used by Boquete e al. [35] could not be replicated in our study since, as stated by the Authors [35,36], this method is currently only for research purposes and it is not a commercially available equipment; we could not confirm their data in MS-noON eyes. As for the "primary retinal pathology" process in MS-noON eyes [20], recalled also by Fairless et al. [37], the presence of neuro-retinitis phenomena could interfere with the results. This point therefore needs to be confirmed by a large study cohort.

In a similar cohort of MS-noON patients, we [23] recently observed an absence of WR and IR MVs reduction, and, differently from Saidha et al. [20], we detected that OR MV and MT values were not significantly different from Controls. Taking in account this evidence, our mfERG results may indicate that in MS-noON patients an absence of outer macular layers' morphological involvement together with an absence of O-MR dysfunction can be hypothesized.

In the MS-ON-G Group, when measuring mfERG RADs, we also found absence of O-MR dysfunction either by rings or sectors analyses. Our findings diverge from Hanson et al. [18] who evidenced slight abnormal mfERG responses suggesting inhibitory bipolar cell dysfunction in a mixed cohort of clinically isolated syndrome, primary progressive MS and RR MS eyes, with some cases of ON, and recovery of BCVA. In a very recent study, Filgueiras et al. [21] suggested OR dysfunction based on the exclusive findings of significant shorter mfERG N1 and P1 implicit times in MS with and without ON, and concluding that mfERG may help in differentiating MS-ON from "neuro-myelitis optica" spectrum disorder. In agreement with the commentary by Hanson et al. [33], we also considered as questionable the finding by Filgueiras et al. [21], since "anticipated" N1 and P1 latencies that were on average 1 msec shorter than Controls, cannot be considered as electrophysiological evidence of supernormal bipolar function in MS patients. In addition, in their work, the decision of not including in the mfERG analysis the R5 areas could have affected latency results. Finally, the Authors [21] did not correct their p-values for multiple testing, considering the high number of statistical comparisons, thus overestimating the significance of their results.

As for the MS-noON Group, in a similar cohort of MS-ON-G patients, we recently observed significantly reduced WR and IR MVs and MTs, with OR values similar to Controls; an extensive explanation of these findings was previously discussed [23]. Hence, the presence of mfERG values similar to Controls in this Group, and also considering the previously observed [23] absence of OR morphological impairment, led us to believe that in MS patients with previous history of ON and good recovery of BCVA there are structural changes involving IR but not OR, with also normal O-MR function.

In MS-ON-P Group, together with the above-mentioned mfERG changes (reduced R1 and S1-N RADs), we found, in agreement with our previous work [23], a significant reduction of WR, IR and OR MVs and MTs as compared to Controls. The interpretation of these morphological findings was given elsewhere [23].

These observed reduced R1 RAD values let us consider that when BCVA recovery after ON is poor, the wiring of retinal circuitry in the fovea, where the cones and the RGCs have the highest density [36,38], can be severely impaired. This foveal dysfunction was not significantly correlated with the reduction of OR MV and MT values in the central Area 1 and this might suggest that the O-MR dysfunction is associated but not linearly correlated to the OR morphological involvement. In addition, since not significant correlations between the reduced R1 RADs and the reduction of IR MV and MT values in the central Area 1 were found, it could be hypothesized that the morphological involvement of the inner macular layers does not influence the function of the O-MR layers.

All these findings could have different explanations. First, the absence of a perfect anatomical overlapping between the stratified measurements by mfERG and Sd-OCT assessments. For instance, when segmenting IR and OR layers, our RTVue-100 device software automatically divides the inner and outer neurosensory retinas at the boundary between the inner nuclear layer (INL) and the outer plexiform layer (OPL). The OR encloses the OPL, the outer nuclear layer, and the photoreceptor layer. The IR examines the retinal nerve fiber layer (RNFL), the ganglion cells/inner plexiform layer (GC/IPL), and the INL. On the other hand, the mfERG system allows us to record the bioelectrical activity driven mainly by cones and bipolar cells, specifically mfERG response amplitude values are more correlated with photoreceptors activity whereas peak timing is more associated with the contribution to the signal by bipolar cells [39]. Thus, it could be that as the nuclei of the bipolar cells located into the INL (enclosed in our IR segmentation analysis and resulted reduced) and the relative bioelectrical activity is mainly represented by the mfERG ITs (resulted similar to Controls), there is a not perfect colocalization between the structural and functional tests of the same elements. This could explain the absence of correlation between reduced RADs and reduced OR MV and MT values, as well as the absence of correlation between normal P1 ITs and reduced IR MV and MT values in MS-ON-P patients. A second explanation could be related to the sample of MS-ON-P patients enrolled in the present study. We enrolled a high homogeneous number of 20 patients with MS-ON and poor recovery of visual acuity. Eventually, results from a larger cohort of patients may give different results and different correlations between morpho-functional parameters.

By contrast, since in the more peripheral areas (Area 2 and Area 3) we detected normal mfERG responses (ITs and RADs), but reduced WR, IR and OR MVs and MTs, it should be hypothesized that this morphological involvement is not sufficient to induce functional changes, as suggested by the lack of correlation between mfERG and Sd-OCT data, as reported in Table 7.

In these patients, the observed macular functional changes were not significantly related with the reduced BCVA, as well as we recently reported [23] that the reduced recovery of BCVA is also independent from the morphological condition of the outer macular layers but is correlated with the morphological impairment of the inner macular layers.

Our findings of abnormal mfERG responses specifically in the S1 nasal sector links with Boquete et al. [35] findings (reduced first order kernel RADs in the temporal sectors for their right eyes). The Authors specified that the papillo-macular bundle could be affected earlier in the disease process also in absence of ON, and that this concurs with early Sd-OCT RNFL reduction in the thickest temporal sector in MS [40], as also seen in other neurodegenerative disorders like glaucoma [41], Parkinson's [42] and Alzheimer's [43] diseases.

Moreover, all sectorial WR, IR and OR MVs and MTs in MS-ON-P eyes were significantly reduced as compared to Controls. To our knowledge, no previous reports described similar investigations on Sd-OCT macular sectors. These morphological findings can suggest that in MS-ON-P eyes there is not a prevalent structural involvement of one macular sector with respect to others.

Nevertheless, this morphological impairment cannot influence the functional condition of the S, T and I sectors (that was not significantly different from Controls), as suggested by the lack of correlation between mfERG and Sd-OCT data (see Table 7). In addition, although a morphological impairment of MV and MT and a dysfunction of O-MR layers in the nasal sector were found, the absence of correlation (see Table 7) might suggest that the morphological and functional conditions are independent.

The biological mechanisms underlying the reduction of RADs in our selected group of MS-ON-P, with no previous or present signs of retinal inflammation, can only be hypothesized.

One hypothesis is that in a sub-set of MS-ON patients, a dysfunction of photoreceptors and inhibitory bipolar cells (leading to reduced mfERG RADs) is due to trans-synaptic retrograde degeneration distal to IML. Indeed, the injury that involves the IML (detectable by reduced P-ERG responses [4–6]) could extend more deeply, impairing outer retinal function. This hypothesis, however, on one side is not confirmed by animal studies on the retinal changes after optic nerve transection. In fact, Hollander et al. showed that only the IML are impaired at the light and electron microscopy after optic nerve damage [44]. On the other hand, a full body of evidence in humans supports the fact that trans-synaptic degeneration affects the dorsal lateral geniculate nucleus, but stops at the INL, where the bipolars reside, acting as a potential physiological protective barrier against neurodegeneration [45]. This prominent role of INL is also justified by the occurrence of dynamic and transient phenomena, also in absence of ON, as the microcystic inner retina edema often seen in MS [46,47]. At this level, the homoeostasis of the bipolar system becomes crucial for neurodegeneration processes in MS. Our evidence might suggest that when there is a poor recovery of visual acuity after an ON event, an unbalanced function of the bipolar cells system may occur and this can be detected by recording a reduction in amplitude of mfERG responses.

A second hypothesis that can explain the reduction of mfERG RADs in MS-ON-P patients is a process related to autoimmunity. For instance, in some MS patients with autoantibodies against the retinal protein α-enolase, a reduction of ERG responses has been found [48]. In addition, in validated MS mouse models of ON, it has been reported early altered synaptic vesicle cycling in ribbon synapses, located between outer and inner retinal layers, which are likely targeted by an auto-reactive immune system process [49]. Two adhesion proteins (CASPR1/CNTN1) [50], present at the level of both the paranodal region of myelinated nerves as well as at retinal ribbon synapses [49], could be the specific targets of the auto-immune response in experimental animal models.

Of course, all previous electrophysiological studies done by recording Ff-ERG or flicker ERG in MS eyes, and almost unanimously finding subnormal cone-driven bipolar cell function [16,22,51], are not comparable to our mfERG findings. This is based on the knowledge that mfERG responses are derived from cells localized into the central retina (in our study within the 25 central retinal degrees) [51], whereas Ff-ERG or flicker ERG responses are generated by the preganglionic elements of the whole retina [9].

5. Conclusions

In conclusion, in our study we detected an absence of mfERG abnormalities in MS patients without and with ON followed by full recovery of BCVA. Thus, our results suggest that in MS the function of preganglionic elements located in the O-MR layers is not modified by the occurrence of ON itself. By contrast, the MS neurodegenerative processes could induce a dysfunction of the preganglionic elements of the fovea and the retinal nasal sector after an event of ON followed by permanent impairment of visual acuity (poor recovery of BCVA after ON). This functional impairment was associated, but not correlated, with OR and IR structural changes. In order to better understand the role of middle retinal elements in this process, further studies on both experimental [37,48] and clinical sides [20,44] are needed.

Author Contributions: Conceptualization, L.Z., V.P. and D.C.; methodology, L.B. (Lucilla Barbano), V.P.; software, V.P.; validation, L.Z., V.P., B.F., A.G. and D.C.; formal analysis, G.A.M., D.L., C.G.N., L.B. (Lucilla Barbano) and V.P.; investigation, L.Z., V.P., L.B. (Lucilla Barbano), L.B. (Laura Boffa) and M.A.; resources, V.P., and D.C.; data curation, L.Z.; writing—original draft preparation, L.Z., V.P. and L.B. (Lucilla Barbano); writing—review and editing, L.Z., V.P., B.F. and D.C.; visualization, D.C., and A.G.; supervision, V.P.; project administration, V.P.; funding acquisition, none. All authors have read and agreed to the published version of the manuscript.

Acknowledgments: The contribution of Fondazione Bietti in this paper was supported by the Ministry of Health and Fondazione Roma. Authors acknowledge Maria Luisa Alessi for technical help in electrophysiological recordings and Federica Petrocchi for executing psychophysical measurements.

Abbreviations

MS	multiple sclerosis
ON	optic neuritis
MS-noON	multiple sclerosis patients without optic neuritis
MS-ON-G	multiple sclerosis patients with optic neuritis followed by good recovery of best corrected visual acuity
MS-ON-P	multiple sclerosis patients with optic neuritis followed by poor recovery of best corrected visual acuity

BCVA	best corrected visual acuity
MfERG	multifocal electroretinogram
IT	implicit time
RAD	response amplitude density
P-ERG	pattern electroretinogram
Ff-ERG	Full-field electroretinogram
F-ERG	focal electroretinogram
IML	innermost retinal layers
O-MR	outer and in middle retinal
SD	one standard deviation of the mean
N	number of eyes of each group
A	one-way analysis of variance
MV	macular volume
MT	macular thickness
WR	whole retina
IR	inner retina
OR	outer retina
S-S	sector-superior
S-T	sector-temporal
S-I	sector-inferior
S-N	sector -nasal

References

1. Miller, D.; Barkhof, F.; Montalban, X.; Thompson, A.; Filippi, M. Clinically isolated syndromes suggestive of multiple sclerosis, part 2: Non-conventional MRI, recovery processes, and management. *Lancet Neurol.* **2005**, *4*, 341–348. [CrossRef]
2. Dinkin, M. Trans-synaptic Retrograde Degeneration in the Human Visual System: Slow, Silent, and Real. *Curr. Neurol. Neurosci. Rep.* **2017**, *17*, 16. [CrossRef] [PubMed]
3. Britze, J.; Pihl-Jensen, G.; Frederiksen, J.L. Retinal ganglion cell analysis in multiple sclerosis and optic neuritis: A systematic review and meta-analysis. *J. Neurol.* **2017**, *264*, 1837–1853. [CrossRef] [PubMed]
4. Janáky, M.; Jánossy, Á.; Horváth, G.; Benedek, G.; Braunitzer, G. VEP and PERG in patients with multiple sclerosis, with and without a history of optic neuritis. *Doc. Ophthalmol.* **2017**, *134*, 185–193. [CrossRef]
5. Parisi, V.; Manni, G.; Spadaro, M.; Colacino, G.; Restuccia, R.; Marchi, S.; Bucci, M.G.; Pierelli, F. Correlation between morphological and functional retinal impairment in multiple sclerosis patients. *Investig. Ophthalmol. Vis. Sci.* **1999**, *40*, 2520–2527.
6. Trip, S.A.; Schlottmann, P.G.; Jones, S.J.; Altmann, D.R.; Garway-Heath, D.F.; Thompson, A.J.; Plant, G.T.; Miller, D.H. Retinal nerve fiber layer axonal loss and visual dysfunction in optic neuritis. *Ann. Neurol.* **2005**, *58*, 383–391. [CrossRef]
7. Monsalve, P. Decoding PERG: A neuro-ophthalmic retinal ganglion cell function review. *Curr. Ophthalmol. Rep.* **2019**, *7*, 51–58. [CrossRef]
8. Robson, A.G.; Nilsson, J.; Li, S.; Jalali, S.; Fulton, A.B.; Tormene, A.P.; Holder, G.E.; Brodie, S.E. ISCEV guide to visual electrodiagnostic procedures. *Doc. Ophthalmol.* **2018**, *136*, 1–26. [CrossRef]
9. McCulloch, D.L.; Marmor, M.F.; Brigell, M.G.; Hamilton, R.; Holder, G.E.; Tzekov, R.; Bach, M. ISCEV Standard for full-field clinical electroretinography (2015 update). *Doc. Ophthalmol.* **2015**, *130*, 1–12. [CrossRef]
10. Parisi, V.; Falsini, B. Electrophysiological evaluation of the macular cone system: Focal electroretinography and visual evoked potentials after photostress. *Semin. Ophthalmol.* **1998**, *13*, 178–188. [CrossRef]
11. Hood, D.C.; Bach, M.; Brigell, M.; Keating, D.; Kondo, M.; Lyons, J.S.; Marmor, M.F.; McCulloch, D.F.; Palmowski-Wolfe, A.M. International Society For Clinical Electrophysiology of Vision. ISCEV standard for clinical multifocal electroretinography (mfERG) (2011 edition). *Doc. Ophthalmol.* **2012**, *124*, 1–13. [CrossRef] [PubMed]
12. Bearse, M.A., Jr.; Sutter, E.E. Imaging localized retinal dysfunction with the multifocal electroretinogram. *J. Opt. Soc. Am. A Opt. Image Sci. Vis.* **1996**, *13*, 634–640. [CrossRef] [PubMed]

13. Hood, D.C. Assessing retinal function with the multifocal technique. *Prog. Retin. Eye Res.* **2000**, *19*, 607–646. [CrossRef]

14. Parisi, V.; Ziccardi, L.; Stifano, G.; Montrone, L.; Gallinaro, G.; Falsini, B. Impact of regional retinal responses on cortical visually evoked responses: Multifocal ERGs and VEPs in the retinitis pigmentosa model. *Clin. Neurophysiol.* **2010**, *121*, 380–385. [CrossRef] [PubMed]

15. Papakostopoulos, D.; Fotiou, F.; Hart, J.C.; Banerji, N.K. The electroretinogram in multiple sclerosis and demyelinating optic neuritis. *Electroencephalogr. Clin. Neurophysiol.* **1989**, *74*, 1–10. [CrossRef]

16. Hamurcu, M.; Orhan, G.; Sarıcaoğlu, M.S.; Mungan, S.; Duru, Z. Analysis of multiple sclerosis patients with electrophysiological and structural tests. *Int. Ophthalmol.* **2017**, *37*, 649–653. [CrossRef]

17. Forooghian, F.; Sproule, M.; Westall, C.; Gordon, L.; Jirawuthiworavong, G.; Shimazaki, K.; O'Connor, P. Electroretinographic abnormalities in multiple sclerosis: Possible role for retinal autoantibodies. *Doc. Ophthalmol.* **2006**, *113*, 123–132. [CrossRef]

18. Hanson, J.V.M.; Hediger, M.; Manogaran, P.; Landau, K.; Hagenbuch, N.; Schippling, S.; Gerth-Kahlert, C. Outer Retinal Dysfunction in the Absence of Structural Abnormalities in Multiple Sclerosis. *Investig. Ophthalmol. Vis. Sci.* **2018**, *59*, 549–560. [CrossRef]

19. Falsini, B.; Bardocci, A.; Porciatti, V.; Bolzani, R.; Piccardi, M. Macular dysfunction in multiple sclerosis revealed by steady-state flicker and pattern ERGs. *Electroencephalogr. Clin. Neurophysiol.* **1992**, *82*, 53–59. [CrossRef]

20. Saidha, S.; Syc, S.B.; Ibrahim, M.A.; Eckstein, C.; Warner, C.V.; Farrell, S.K.; Oakley, J.D.; Durbin, M.K.; Meyer, S.A.; Balcer, L.J.; et al. Primary retinal pathology in multiple sclerosis as detected by optical coherence tomography. *Brain* **2011**, *134*, 518–533. [CrossRef]

21. Filgueiras, T.G.; Oyamada, M.K.; Preti, R.C.; Apóstolos-Pereira, S.L.; Callegaro, D.; Monteiro, M.L.R. Outer Retinal Dysfunction on Multifocal Electroretinography May Help Differentiating Multiple Sclerosis From Neuromyelitis Optica Spectrum Disorder. *Front. Neurol.* **2019**, *10*, 928. [CrossRef] [PubMed]

22. Gundogan, F.C.; Demirkaya, S.; Sobaci, G. Is optical coherence tomography really a new biomarker candidate in multiple sclerosis?-A structural and functional evaluation. *Investig. Ophthalmol. Vis. Sci.* **2007**, *48*, 5773–5781. [CrossRef] [PubMed]

23. ZiccardI, L.; Barbano, L.; Boffa, L.; Albanese, M.; Grzybowski, A.; Centonze, D.; Parisi, V. Morphological Outer Retina Findings in Multiple Sclerosis Patients With or Without Optic Neuritis. *Front. Neurol.* **2020**, *11*, 858. [CrossRef] [PubMed]

24. Polman, C.H.; Reingold, S.C.; Banwell, B.; Clanet, M.; Cohen, J.A.; Filippi, M.; Fujihara, K.; Havrdova, E.; Hutchinson, M.; Kappos, L.; et al. Diagnostic criteria for multiple sclerosis: 2010 revisions to the McDonald criteria. *Ann. Neurol.* **2011**, *69*, 292–302. [CrossRef] [PubMed]

25. Kurtzke, J.F. Rating neurologic impairment in multiple sclerosis: An Expanded Disability Status Scale (EDSS). *Neurology* **1983**, *33*, 1444–1452. [CrossRef] [PubMed]

26. Neurostatus.net. Available online: http://www.neurostatus.net/index.php?file=start (accessed on 6 July 2020).

27. Williams, U.E.; Oparah, S.K.; Philip-Ephraim, E.E. Disease Modifying Therapy in Multiple Sclerosis. *Int. Sch. Res. Not.* **2014**, *2014*, 307064. [CrossRef]

28. Huang-Link, Y.M.; Al-Hawasi, A.; Lindehammar, H. Acute optic neuritis: Retinal ganglion cell loss precedes retinal nerve fiber thinning. *Neurol. Sci.* **2015**, *36*, 617–620. [CrossRef]

29. Parisi, V.; Ziccardi, L.; Sadun, F.; De Negri, A.M.; La Morgia, C.; Barbano, L.; Carelli, V.; Barboni, P. Functional Changes of Retinal Ganglion Cells and Visual Pathways in Patients with Chronic Leber's Hereditary Optic Neuropathy during One Year of Follow-up. *Ophthalmology* **2019**, *126*, 1033–1044. [CrossRef]

30. Cascavilla, M.L.; Parisi, V.; Triolo, G.; Ziccardi, L.; Borrelli, E.; Di Renzo, A.; Balducci, N.; Lamperti, C.; Bianchi Marzoli, S.; Darvizeh, F.; et al. Retinal dysfunction characterizes subtypes of dominant optic atrophy. *Acta Ophthalmol.* **2018**, *96*, e156–e163. [CrossRef]

31. Parisi, V.; Ziccardi, L.; Centofanti, M.; Tanga, L.; Gallinaro, G.; Falsini, B.; Bucci, M.G. Macular function in eyes with open-angle glaucoma evaluated by multifocal electroretinogram. *Investig. Ophthalmol. Vis. Sci.* **2012**, *53*, 6973–6980. [CrossRef]

32. Curcio, C.A.; Sloan, K.R.; Kalina, R.E.; Hendrickson, A.E. Human photoreceptor topography. *J. Comp. Neurol.* **1990**, *292*, 497–523. [CrossRef] [PubMed]

33. Hanson, J.V.M.; Schippling, S.; Gerth-Kahlert, C. Commentary: Outer retinal dysfunction on multifocal electroretinography may help differentiating multiple sclerosis from neuromyelitis optica spectrum disorder. *Front. Neurol.* **2020**, *11*, 282. [CrossRef] [PubMed]

34. Ziccardi, L.; Parisi, V.; Picconi, F.; Di Renzo, A.; Lombardo, M.; Frontoni, S.; Parravano, M. Early and localized retinal dysfunction in patients with type 1 diabetes mellitus studied by multifocal electroretinogram. *Acta Diabetol.* **2018**, *55*, 1191–1200. [CrossRef] [PubMed]

35. Boquete, L.; López-Guillén, E.; Vilades, E.; Miguel-Jiménez, J.M.; Pablo, L.E.; De Santiago, L.; Ortiz Del Castillo, M.; Alonso-Rodríguez, M.C.; Sánchez Morla, E.M.; López-Dorado, A.; et al. Diagnostic ability of multifocal electroretinogram in early multiple sclerosis using a new signal analysis method. *PLoS ONE* **2019**, *14*, e0224500. [CrossRef] [PubMed]

36. Verdon, W.A.; Haegerstrom-Portnoy, G. Topography of the multifocal electroretinogram. *Doc. Ophthalmol.* **1998**, *95*, 73–90. [CrossRef] [PubMed]

37. Fairless, R.; Williams, S.K.; Hoffmann, D.B.; Stojic, A.; Hochmeister, S.; Schmitz, F.; Storch, M.K.; Diem, R. Preclinical retinal neurodegeneration in a model of multiple sclerosis. *J. Neurosci.* **2012**, *32*, 5585–5597. [CrossRef]

38. McGregor, J.E.; Yin, L.; Yang, Q.; Godat, T.; Huynh, K.T.; Zhang, G.; Williams, D.G.; Merigan, W.H. Functional architecture of the foveola revealed in the living primate. *PLoS ONE* **2018**, *13*, e0207102. [CrossRef]

39. Hood, D.C.; Frishman, L.J.; Saszik, S.; Viswanathan, S. Retinal origins of the primate multifocal ERG: Implications for the human response. *Investig. Ophthalmol. Vis. Sci.* **2002**, *43*, 1673–1685.

40. Garcia-Martin, E.; Pueyo, V.; Almarcegui, C.; Martin, J.; Ara, J.R.; Sancho, E.; Pablo, L.E.; Dolz, I.; Fernandez, J. Risk factors for progressive axonal degeneration of the retinal nerve fibre layer in multiple sclerosis patients. *Br. J. Ophthalmol.* **2011**, *95*, 1577–1582. [CrossRef]

41. Mousa, M.F.; Cubbidge, R.P.; Al-Mansouri, F.; Bener, A. Evaluation of hemifield sector analysis protocol in multifocal visual evoked potential objective perimetry for the diagnosis and early detection of glaucomatous field defects. *Korean J. Ophthalmol.* **2014**, *28*, 49–65. [CrossRef]

42. Satue, M.; Obis, J.; Alarcia, R.; Orduna, E.; Rodrigo, M.J.; Vilades, E.; Gracia, H.; Otin, S.; Fuertes, M.I.; Polo, V.; et al. Retinal and Choroidal Changes in Patients with Parkinson's Disease Detected by Swept-Source Optical Coherence Tomography. *Curr. Eye Res.* **2018**, *43*, 109–115. [CrossRef] [PubMed]

43. Polo, V.; Garcia-Martin, E.; Bambo, M.P.; Pinilla, J.; Larrosa, J.M.; Satue, M.; Otin, S.; Pablo, L.E. Reliability and validity of Cirrus and Spectralis optical coherence tomography for detecting retinal atrophy in Alzheimer's disease. *Eye (Lond.)* **2014**, *28*, 680–690. [CrossRef] [PubMed]

44. Hollander, H.; Bisti, S.; Maffei, L.; Hebel, R. Electroretinographic responses and retrograde changes of retinal morphology after intracranial optic nerve section. *Exp. Brian Res.* **1984**, *55*, 483–494.

45. Petzold, A.; Balcer, L.J.; Calabresi, P.A.; Costello, F.; Frohman, T.C.; Frohman, E.M.; Martinez-Lapiscina, E.H.; Green, A.J.; Kardon, R.; Outteryck, O.; et al. Retinal layer segmentation in multiple sclerosis: A systematic review and meta-analysis. *Lancet Neurol.* **2017**, *16*, 797–812. [CrossRef]

46. Saidha, S.; Sotirchos, E.S.; Ibrahim, M.A.; Crainiceanu, C.M.; Gelfand, J.M.; Sepah, Y.J.; Ratchford, J.N.; Oh, J.; Seigo, M.A.; Newsome, S.D.; et al. Microcystic macular oedema, thickness of the inner nuclear layer of the retina, and disease characteristics in multiple sclerosis: A retrospective study. *Lancet Neurol.* **2012**, *11*, 963–972. [CrossRef]

47. Gelfand, J.M.; Nolan, R.; Schwartz, D.M.; Graves, J.; Green, A.J. Microcystic macular oedema in multiple sclerosis is associated with disease severity. *Brain* **2012**, *135*, 1786–1793. [CrossRef]

48. Gorczyca, W.A.; Ejma, M.; Witkowska, D.; Misiuk-Hojło, M.; Kuropatwa, M.; Mulak, M.; Szymaniec, S. Retinal antigens are recognized by antibodies present in sera of patients with multiple sclerosis. *Ophthalmic Res.* **2004**, *36*, 120–123. [CrossRef]

49. Dembla, M.; Kesharwani, A.; Natarajan, S.; Fecher-Trost, C.; Fairless, R.; Williams, S.K.; Flockerzi, V.; Diem, R.; Schwarz, K.; Schmitz, F. Early auto-immune targeting of photoreceptor ribbon synapses in mouse models of multiple sclerosis. *EMBO Mol. Med.* **2018**, *10*, e8926. [CrossRef]

50. Stathopoulos, P.; Alexopoulos, H.; Dalakas, M.C. Autoimmune antigenic targets at the node of Ranvier in demyelinating disorders. *Nat. Rev. Neurol.* **2015**, *11*, 143–156. [CrossRef]

51. Hood, D.C.; Seiple, W.; Holopigian, K.; Greenstein, V. A comparison of the components of the multifocal and full-field ERGs. *Vis. Neurosci.* **1997**, *14*, 533–544. [CrossRef]

2

Prevalence of SARS-CoV-2 Antibodies in Multiple Sclerosis: The Hidden Part of the Iceberg

Nicola Capasso [1], Raffaele Palladino [2,3] ⓘ, Emma Montella [4], Francesca Pennino [2],
Roberta Lanzillo [1] ⓘ, Antonio Carotenuto [1] ⓘ, Maria Petracca [1] ⓘ, Rosa Iodice [1], Aniello Iovino [1],
Francesco Aruta [1], Viviana Pastore [2], Antonio Riccardo Buonomo [5], Emanuela Zappulo [5],
Ivan Gentile [5,6] ⓘ, Maria Triassi [2], Vincenzo Brescia Morra [1] and Marcello Moccia [1],* ⓘ

[1] Multiple Sclerosis Clinical Care and Research Centre, Department of Neuroscience,
     Reproductive Sciences and Odontostomatology, University of Naples "Federico II", 80138 Naples, Italy;
     nicolacapasso91@gmail.com (N.C.); robertalanzillo@libero.it (R.L.); carotenuto.antonio87@gmail.com (A.C.);
     maria@petraccas.it (M.P.); rosa.iodice@unina.it (R.I.); anielloiovino@msn.com (A.I.);
     fra.aruta92@gmail.com (F.A.); vincenzo.bresciamorra2@unina.it (V.B.M.)
[2] Department of Public Health, University of Naples "Federico II", 80138 Naples, Italy;
     raffaele.palladino@unina.it (R.P.); francesca.pennino@unina.it (F.P.); vivianapastore10@gmail.com (V.P.);
     triassi@unina.it (M.T.)
[3] Department of Primary Care and Public Health, Imperial College London, London W68RP, UK
[4] Department of Hygiene, Preventive and Industrial Medicine, University Hospital "Federico II",
     80138 Naples, Italy; emma.montella@unina.it
[5] Section of Infectious Diseases, Department of Clinical Medicine and Surgery,
     University of Naples "Federico II", 80138 Naples, Italy; antonioriccardobuonomo@gmail.com (A.R.B.);
     e.zappulo@gmail.com (E.Z.); ivan.gentile@unina.it (I.G.)
[6] Health Education and Sustainable Development, University of Naples "Federico II", 80138 Naples, Italy
*   Correspondence: marcello.moccia@unina.it or moccia.marcello@gmail.com;

Abstract: Background. We compared the prevalence of SARS-CoV-2 IgG/IgM in multiple sclerosis (MS), low-risk, and high-risk populations and explored possible clinical correlates. Methods. In this cross-sectional study, we recruited MS patients, low-risk (university staff from non-clinical departments), and high-risk individuals (healthcare staff from COVID-19 wards) from 11 May to 15 June 2020. We used lateral flow immunoassay to detect SARS-CoV-2 IgG and IgM. We used t-test, Fisher's exact test, chi square test, or McNemar's test, as appropriate, to evaluate between-group differences. Results. We recruited 310 MS patients (42.3 ± 12.4 years; females 67.1%), 862 low-risk individuals (42.9 ± 13.3 years; females 47.8%), and 235 high-risk individuals (39.4 ± 10.9 years; females 54.5%). The prevalence of SARS-CoV-2 IgG/IgM in MS patients ($n = 9$, 2.9%) was significantly lower than in the high-risk population ($n = 25$, 10.6%) ($p < 0.001$), and similar to the low-risk population ($n = 11$, 1.3%) ($p = 0.057$); these results were also confirmed after random matching by age and sex (1:1:1). No significant differences were found in demographic, clinical, treatment, and laboratory features. Among MS patients positive to SARS-CoV-2 IgG/IgM ($n = 9$), only two patients retrospectively reported mild and short-lasting COVID-19 symptoms. Conclusions. MS patients have similar risk of SARS-CoV-2 infection to the general population, and can be asymptomatic from COVID-19, also if using treatments with systemic immunosuppression.

Keywords: multiple sclerosis; COVID-19; infection; antibody; seroprevalence

1. Introduction

On 11 March 2020, the World Health Organization declared coronavirus disease-19 (COVID-19) from severe acute respiratory syndrome coronavirus (SARS-CoV-2) to be a pandemic. In the following months, COVID-19 has caused severe morbidity and mortality worldwide, especially in elderly populations, in males, and in individuals with concomitant diseases (e.g., heart disease, diabetes) [1].

People with multiple sclerosis (MS) might be especially at risk from COVID-19 morbidity and mortality because they are known to suffer and to die more frequently from respiratory and infectious diseases [2]. Additionally, people with MS have higher prevalence of a number of comorbidities (e.g., cardiovascular) when compared with the general population [3,4]. Not least, the use disease-modifying treatments (DMTs), causing different degrees of systemic immunosuppression, might further affect the possibility of preventing and responding to the infection [5]. In line with this, healthcare providers and policy makers have immediately advised people with MS to self-isolate, and the use of immunomodulatory and immunosuppressive DMTs has been postponed [6–8].

Serological tests to detect IgM and IgG immunity, which increase from the second week after COVID-19 onset of symptoms [9], have been used for epidemiological purposes [10] because they can identify all infected individuals, including those with no or mild symptoms [10,11]. In particular, asymptomatic carriers can transmit the virus in the absence of obvious symptoms and could be responsible for keeping SARS-CoV-2 circulating [12]. As such, studying the prevalence of SARS-CoV-2 IgG/IgM in MS can shed light on the risk of COVID-19 infection in relation to MS and/or to the use of some DMTs, on the amount of patients who are still susceptible to infection, and on the possibility of asymptomatic carriers in MS, and can also be used to plan clinical activities accordingly [5,8,13–15]. Thus, in the present study, we aim to: (1) evaluate the prevalence of SARS-CoV-2 IgG/IgM antibodies in asymptomatic MS patients, compared with populations at low-risk and high-risk of COVID-19 infections; and (2) explore possible correlates with demographics, clinical features, treatments, comorbidities, and laboratory findings.

2. Methods

2.1. Study Design

This is a cross-sectional study including all MS patients attending the MS Clinical Care and Research Centre at Federico II University Hospital of Naples (Campania Region, Italy) from 11 May to 15 June 2020. For comparison purposes, we also included a sample of low-risk individuals (university staff from non-clinical departments) and a sample of high-risk individuals (healthcare staff from COVID-19 wards), who underwent the same serological test during the same period.

The study was approved by the Federico II Ethics Committee (355/19 and subsequent amendments). All patients signed informed consent authorizing the use of anonymized data collected routinely as part of clinical practice, in line with data protection regulations (GDPR EU2016/679). The study was performed in accordance with good clinical practice and the Declaration of Helsinki.

2.2. Study Population

During the study period (11 May to 15 June 2020), the COVID-19 Task Force from our University made SARS-CoV-2 IgG/IgM antibody testing compulsory for all patients attending the hospital, for healthcare staff from COVID-19 wards, and for university staff required to come back to office work following lockdown. This policy was driven by the possibility of using serological data to safely deploy healthcare workers, to reduce exposure to the virus in susceptible individuals, and to assess the effect of lockdown at population level [11]. Because this policy was time-limited, we selected the period of time when all individuals were tested; all individuals then consented to study inclusion.

For MS patients, inclusion criteria were: (1) diagnosis of MS [16]; (2) consent to participate; (3) scheduled consultation at the MS Centre from 11 May to 15 June 2020; (4) residence in the Campania Region of Italy.

For low-risk individuals, inclusion criteria were: (1) university staff from non-clinical departments who had been self-isolating at home during lockdown; (2) consent to participate; (3) no history of MS or other central nervous system diseases; (4) no history of chronic diseases and treatments; (5) residence in the Campania Region of Italy.

For high-risk individuals, inclusion criteria were: (1) healthcare staff from COVID-19 wards; (2) consent to participate; (3) no history of MS or other central nervous system diseases; (4) no history of chronic diseases and treatments; (5) residence in the Campania Region of Italy.

For MS patients, low-risk individuals, and high-risk individuals, exclusion criteria were: (1) age < 18 years; (2) incomplete records; (3) previous COVID-19 diagnosis; (4) COVID-19 symptoms (e.g., cough, fever, anosmia, difficulty breathing), either active or in the past 14 days. In particular, as per University policy, all individuals with symptoms of COVID-19 (e.g., cough, fever, anosmia, difficulty breathing), either active or in the past 14 days, were denied access to the University and to the testing.

2.3. Antibody Detection

We used lateral flow immunoassay (LFIA) to detect SARS-CoV-2 IgG and IgM antibodies (Shanghai Kehua Bio-engineering Co., Ltd., Shanghai, China), in accordance with manufacture instructions [17]. LFIA is a rapid method based on immunochromatography that uses colloidal gold conjugated COVID-19 antigens. It comprises a plastic pad where a nitrocellulose membrane is fitted. Three separate lines are created by immobilizing goat anti-human IgM, IgG and goat anti-rabbit-IgG to assess the presence of IgM, IgG, and control (C) lines, respectively. The entire conjugate pad is sprayed with a mixture of AuNP-COVID-19 recombinant antigen-conjugate (colloidal-gold pre-treated with SARS-CoV-2 recombinant protein) and AuNP-rabbit-IgG. A blood sample is applied to the sample pad and, with the aid of a buffer, migrates towards the immobilized lines of antibodies spread with the AuNP-recombinant antigen. When a reaction occurs, a visible line is formed, suggesting the existence of IgM and/or IgG, separately; color in the control line should be formed for a test to be valid [17,18]. The test provides a qualitative result, which was visually examined by a nurse and a physician together (unblinded to group status) 15 min after blood sample application. Though far from perfect (66% pooled sensitivity, 96.6% pooled specificity), LFIA performs the best at our expectedly low prevalence rates (<5%), and is especially indicated for screening purposes [19]. For statistical purposes, we combined IgM and IgG to define SARS-CoV-2 IgG/IgM positive individuals.

2.4. Demographics, Clinical Features, Treatments, and Laboratory Findings

For MS patients, we used clinical records to retrieve age, sex, and expanded disability status scale (EDSS), current disease modifying treatments (DMTs), comorbidities, and most recent laboratory findings (within one month from SARS-CoV-2 IgG/IgM testing) for white blood cell count, total lymphocyte count, and lactic dehydrogenase (these were specifically selected because they have been reported to be commonly changed in COVID-19) [20]. For statistical purposes, we classified DMTs based on the suggested risk of systemic immunosuppression [6,7].

During the same visit, for MS patients who tested positive to SARS-CoV-2 IgG/IgM, we used a standard clinical questionnaire to investigate the occurrence of COVID-19 symptoms (e.g., cough, fever, anosmia, difficulty breathing), and any possible at-risk behavior (e.g., contact with defined COVID-19 cases, travel to high COVID-19 prevalence areas) in the previous three months (corresponding to the beginning of the first wave of COVID-19 infections in the area).

For low-risk and high-risk individuals, we recorded age, sex, and SARS-CoV-2 IgG/IgM status.

2.5. Sample Size Calculation

Based on published data, we estimated that approximately 5500 individuals with MS live in the Campania Region of Italy (among which 30–40% were followed up at our center) [21]. Assuming COVID-19 prevalence ranges from 1% to 10% [22], a sample of 300 MS patients would be enough to estimate COVID-19 prevalence in the MS population with 5% precision and 95% confidence intervals.

2.6. Statistics

To evaluate differences in prevalence of SARS-CoV-2 IgG/IgM between MS, low-risk, and high-risk populations (aim 1), we first calculated raw prevalence. Differences in prevalence rates were further assessed after performing a random matching by age and sex (1:1:1), considering that the three populations (MS, low-risk, and high-risk) had different age and sex distribution. Differences in prevalence were evaluated using chi square test, Fisher's exact test, or McNemar's test, as appropriate.

To evaluate differences in demographics, clinical features and laboratory findings between MS patients with or without SARS-CoV-2 IgG/IgM (aim 2), we used t-test, chi square test, or Fisher's exact test, as appropriate.

Statistical analyses were performed using Stata 15.0. Following Bonferroni correction for multiple comparisons, results were considered statistically significant for $p < 0.005$.

2.7. Data Availability

Data supporting the findings of this study are available if requested to the authors.

3. Results

We recruited 310 MS patients, 862 low-risk individuals, and 235 high-risk individuals. Demographics and SARS-CoV-2 IgG/IgM status are reported in Table 1.

Table 1. Demographics and SARS-CoV-2 IgG/IgM status in multiple sclerosis (MS) patients, low-risk population, and high-risk population.

	MS Patients ($n = 310$)	Low-Risk Population ($n = 862$)	High-Risk Population ($n = 235$)
Age, years	42.3 ± 12.4	42.9 ± 13.3	39.4 ± 10.9
Sex, females (%)	208 (67.1%)	412 (47.8%)	128 (54.5%)
SARS-CoV-2 status, number (prevalence %)			
IgG or IgM positive	9 (2.9%)	11 (1.3%)	25 (10.6%)
Females	6 (2.9%)	7 (1.7%)	14 (10.9%)
Males	3 (2.9%)	4 (0.9%)	11 (10.3%)
IgG positive	9 (2.9%)	5 (0.6%)	9 (3.8%)
IgM positive	0 (0%)	6 (0.7%)	8 (3.4%)
IgM and IgG positive	0 (0%)	0 (0%)	8 (3.4%)

The raw prevalence of SARS-CoV-2 IgG/IgM in MS ($n = 9$, 2.9%) was significantly lower than in the high-risk population ($n = 25$, 10.6%) ($p < 0.001$) and similar to the low-risk population ($n = 11$, 1.3%) ($p = 0.057$). Similarly, after random matching by age and sex, MS, low-risk, and high-risk populations (148 individuals in each group), the prevalence of SARS-CoV-2 IgG/IgM in MS ($n = 6$, 4.0%) was significantly lower than in the high-risk population ($n = 20$, 13.5%) ($p = 0.001$) and similar to the low-risk population ($n = 1$, 0.7%) ($p = 0.130$).

Demographics, clinical features, treatments, and laboratory findings of MS patients are reported in Table 2. MS patients positive to SARS-CoV-2 IgG/IgM were similar to patients negative to SARS-CoV-2 IgG/IgM in age ($p = 0.830$), sex ($p = 0.988$), EDSS ($p = 0.642$), DMTs ($p = 0.486$), comorbidities ($p = 0.605$), white blood cell count ($p = 0.301$), total lymphocyte count ($p = 0.129$), and lactic dehydrogenase ($p = 0.452$).

Table 2. Demographics, clinical features, treatments, and laboratory findings of MS patients.

	MS Negative to SARS-CoV-2 IgG/IgM (*n* = 301)	MS Positive to SARS-CoV-2 IgG/IgM (*n* = 9)
Age, years	42.2 ± 12.4	41.4 ± 12.8
Females, number (%)	202 (67.1%)	6 (66.6%)
Expanded disability status scale (EDSS), median (range)	3.5 (0–8.0)	3.0 (1.0–6.5)
Disease-modifying treatments (DMT), number (%)		
No/Low risk of systemic immunosuppression	187 (62.1%)	5 (55.6%)
Dimethyl Fumarate	8	0
Interferon	3	0
Glatiramer	1	0
Natalizumab	166	3
Teriflunomide	3	1
No DMT	7	1
Moderate/high risk of systemic immunosuppression	114 (37.9%)	4 (44.4%)
Alemtuzumab	16	3
Cladribine	5	1
Fingolimod	12	0
Ocrelizumab	80	0
Rituximab	1	0
Comorbidities, number (%)	32 (10.6%)	0 (0%)
Diabetes	1	0
High blood pressure	19	0
High cholesterol	9	0
Thyroid disease	7	0
White blood cell count, ×10^3/μL	7.43 ± 2.32	6.62 ± 2.07
Total lymphocyte count, ×10^3/μL	2.48 ± 1.35	1.79 ± 1.01
Lactic dehydrogenase, U/L	215.83 ± 49.94	223.44 ± 52.30

Demographics, clinical features, treatments, and laboratory findings of MS patients positive to SARS-CoV-2 IgG/IgM are detailed in Table 3. Only two patients retrospectively reported on possible COVID-19 symptoms, but, at that time, did not undergo SARS-CoV-2 nasopharyngeal-oropharyngeal swab; in particular, one patient reported a cough, which only lasted a few days, and another patient, who had travelled to a high COVID-19 prevalence area (Switzerland through the north of Italy), reported a fever (below 38.5 °C) and anosmia that, again, only lasted a few days. Patients presented with a wide range of clinical disability (EDSS was from 1.0 to 6.5). Eight patients were currently under the clinical effect of DMTs (alemtuzumab, cladribine, natalizumab, and teriflunomide). Looking at laboratory tests, we found values below normal limits for white blood cell count in one patient and for lymphocytes in three patients (one patient had grade 1 lymphopenia (0.8–1 × 10^3/μL) and two patients had grade 2 lymphopenia (0.5–0.7 × 10^3/μL)); lactic dehydrogenase was within normal limits in all patients. Following positive SARS-CoV-2 IgG/IgM testing, all patients underwent SARS-CoV-2 nasopharyngeal-oropharyngeal swab, which resulted negative for SARS-CoV-2 RNA, suggesting previous rather than active infection.

Table 3. Demographics, clinical features, treatments, and laboratory findings of MS patients positive to SARS-CoV-2 IgG/IgM in May–June 2020.

	1	2	3	4	5	6	7	8	9
Age, years	39	54	42	27	35	65	38	57	29
Sex	Male	Female	Female	Female	Female	Female	Female	Male	Male
COVID-19 symptoms	None	Cough	None	None	None	None	None	None	Fever, anosmia
COVID-19 at-risk behaviour	None	None	None	None	None	None	None	None	Travel
EDSS	2.5	3.0	6.5	1.0	4.5	2.5	4.5	4.0	1.5
DMT	Alemtuzumab	Natalizumab	Alemtuzumab	Natalizumab	Natalizumab	Teriflunomide	Alemtuzumab	None	Cladribine
Last DMT administration	January 2019	February 2020	June 2018	March 2020	February 2020	Ongoing	January 2018		July 2019
Comorbidities	None	None	None	None	None	None	None	None	None
White blood cell count *, ×10³/µL	10.27	7.56	7.45	6.93	5.6	7.17	7.29	3.25	4.12
Total lymphocyte count **, ×10³/µL	1.81	2.85	0.90	3.18	3.06	1.97	1.61	0.69	0.71
Lactic dehydrogenase ***, U/L	274	225	215	178	190	332	172	239	186

* Normal range 4–$10 \times 10^3/\mu L$; ** Normal range 1–$4.8 \times 10^3/\mu L$; *** Normal range 140–280 U/L.

4. Discussion

In our population, MS patients, in the absence of overt COVID-19 symptoms, did not present with a significantly higher prevalence of SARS-CoV-2 antibodies when compared with low-risk individuals (2.9% vs. 1.3%). As such, MS patients can develop SARS-CoV-2 immunity, following mild or no COVID-19 symptoms also if using DMTs with high risk of systemic immunosuppression. No significant correlates (e.g., demographics, clinical features, treatments, and laboratory findings) were found for the prevalence of SARS-CoV-2 IgG/IgM in MS.

We specifically set a time frame (11 May to 15 June 2020) and geographical area (Campania Region of Italy) for the three populations in order to study a community undergoing similar infection distribution and lockdown policies; for instance, the conduction of the study within three months from the beginning of the local epidemic reduced the risk of underestimating the prevalence of SARS-CoV-2 IgG/IgM, due to the possibility of antibodies vanishing after this time frame [9]. During the first wave, the Campania Region of Italy was considered a low-prevalence area for COVID-19 [22]. A recent report of the Italian institute of Statistics showed <1% seroprevalence in the Campania region at the time our study was conducted. Accordingly, we found 1.3% seroprevalence in healthy individuals who self-isolated during the lockdown using LFIA, which is at the higher risk of false positive results when compared with CLIA/ELISA, used by the Italian Institute of Statistics [23]. Overall, our estimates are not far from other low-prevalence areas (e.g., 1.79% in Boise, ID, USA) [22,24], and lower than high-prevalence areas (e.g., 4.65% in Los Angeles County, CA, USA) [22,25]. As expected, the prevalence of SARS-CoV-2 IgG/IgM in low-risk individuals (1.3%) and MS (2.9%) was not as high as in high-risk individuals (10.6%). In particular, we selected healthcare staff from COVID-19 wards as a high-risk reference, following previous studies showing high SARS-CoV-2 IgG/IgM in this population [26,27].

The numerically higher prevalence of SARS-CoV-2 IgG/IgM in MS, when compared with low-risk populations, is not surprising. Indeed, MS patients, though possibly worried about risks coming from COVID-19 to individuals with comorbidities, as from national and international recommendations [1,20], have inevitably had hospital access for disease and treatment management during the lockdown, with subsequent risks of COVID-19 infection. Noteworthy, people with MS have been initially classified more at risk of COVID-19 morbidity and mortality [1], and the exposure to DMTs with systemic immunosuppression is thought to further increase the risk of infections [28], though this was not disclosed in our population, possibly due to sample size constraints. Additionally, we did not find any differences in demographics, clinical features, and laboratory findings suggestive of COVID-19 infection in MS patients positive and negative to SARS-CoV-2 IgG/IgM [20].

COVID-19 pandemic has represented a new challenge for neurologists treating patients with MS, as a consequence of possible risks coming from this infection to these patients [5,6,14]. We showed that seven out of nine MS patients using immunomodulatory and immunosuppressive DMTs presented with no symptoms from COVID-19, and two only had mild symptoms. This finding is in line with results on the general population, where up to four fifths of individuals are expected to stay asymptomatic [12], and with previous reports suggesting that MS patients using DMTs have standard COVID-19 morbidity and mortality [29–31]. Unfortunately, the presence of past COVID-19 symptoms was not investigated routinely in our control populations, though they did not have previous COVID-19 diagnosis nor had active/recent respiratory symptoms (as from inclusion criteria). Interestingly, in a UK community-based study including 3907 MS patients and using a questionnaire for self-reported diagnosis, Evangelou and colleagues showed that MS patients (and the use of DMTs) were not at increased risks of COVID-19 [32]. Similarly, French and Dutch studies did not find any association between DMT and COVID-19 severity [33,34]. In another previous study, the Chinese Medical Network for Neuroinflammation conducted a survey on 1804 MS patients and found no cases with formal COVID-19 diagnosis, irrespective of DMTs [35]. However, considering that during the first wave of the pandemic healthcare systems have struggled to guarantee medical care to moderate-severe cases [22], it is possible that MS patients with mild or no COVID-19 symptoms have gone undiagnosed, thus suggesting that future prevalence studies should combine different diagnostic modalities (e.g., clinical history, formal diagnosis of COVID-19, seroprevalence).

Diagnosis of active COVID-19 infection is currently based on nasopharyngeal-oropharyngeal swab and real-time polymerase chain reaction (RT-PCR), which is however unable to detect past infections in prevalence studies [11] and has also a potentially high false negative rate [36]. On the contrary, antibody testing for COVID-19 can support a diagnosis of both active and past infections [13]. A large number of tests have been developed for COVID-19 antibody detection, such as LFIA (used in the present study), chemiluminescent immunoassay (CLIA), enzyme-linked immunosorbent assay (ELISA), and Fluorescence Immunoassays (FIA), all of them targeting IgG and/or IgM antibodies against S and/or N viral proteins of human serum/blood samples [17,18,36,37]. A recent meta-analysis has showed that ELISA and LFIA have the highest specificity, reaching levels >99%, whilst ELISA and CLIA performed better in terms of sensitivity (90–96%), followed by LFIA and FIA with sensitivities ranging from 80% to 89% [10,17]. As such, our test (LFIA) is potentially at risk of false positive results; however, we included MS cases and two control populations, among which the risk of false positive results should have been equally distributed [19]. Overall, we preferred LFIA because it can be quickly used on-site and is particularly attractive for large seroprevalence studies as a consequence of high specificity (e.g., reduced risk of missing positive cases). At the individual level, however, mixed strategies should be adopted (e.g., re-testing a positive case using a different serological test and/or nasopharyngeal-oropharyngeal swab) [10], and, in keeping with this, in MS patients positive to SARS-CoV-2 IgG/IgM, we excluded the presence of active COVID-19 infection with nasopharyngeal-oropharyngeal swab.

The present study raises a number of policy implications for clinical practice. First, there are risks coming from asymptomatic MS patients that could be responsible for COVID-19 spreading to healthcare staff and other patients at MS Centers [12]. Not least, whilst the use of DMTs is generally contraindicated in patients with symptoms of active infection, the use of DMTs causing acute systemic immunosuppression in COVID-19 asymptomatic patients could possibly increase morbidity and mortality, as for the reactivation of chronic asymptomatic infections (e.g., hepatitis, tuberculosis, herpes viruses) [38]. Additionally, the prevalence of SARS-CoV-2 IgG/IgM antibodies in MS is low, and, thus, this population is especially vulnerable to future COVID-19 infections in the case of additional epidemic waves and/or local outbreaks. Safety protocols for accessing the MS centre and for DMT dosing/redosing should then account for additional risks coming from COVID-19. A combination of clinical history (e.g., at-risk contacts, presence of active symptoms), testing (e.g., serology, swab), and non-pharmacological measures (e.g., face masks, self-isolation before/after some DMTs) should be carefully considered within national and international recommendations for MS healthcare organization and clinical practice [5]. Finally, we have also shown the possibility of developing COVID-19 antibodies in MS patients, also if lymphocyte levels were below normal values following DMTs with systemic immunosuppression, suggesting this population would be suitable for vaccination, when available.

Among the study limitations, there is the low sensitivity of SARS-CoV-2 IgG/IgM LFIA testing, with risk of false-positive results in low-incidence settings [10]. False negatives could also have occurred in previously-infected patients who failed to produce antibodies specific to COVID-19 antigens, in patients where antibodies quickly waned, or in patients who have not mounted a specific antibody response yet. However, we performed the same test to both MS patients and controls from the same geographical area and within the same time period and, thus, the risk of false negatives applies equally to different subgroups. Of note, the subpopulation treated with anti-CD20 medications could not have developed antibodies and, therefore, tested negative in our study; this subpopulation could also be more at risk of worse SARS-CoV-2 outcomes and, thus, could have been excluded from the present study that specifically focused on patients with no symptoms/undetected infection. LFIA has already been used for SARS-CoV-2 IgG/IgM prevalence studies worldwide [25] and, considering that IgM and IgG tests have different sensitivity in relation to the phases of the infection (e.g., IgM antibodies increase earlier than IgG) [9], we have combined IgG and IgM testing to improve sensitivity [10].

Our study was cross-sectional and was run within clinical practice, in the absence of actual follow-up to study seroconversion prospectively. We were not able to perform exact matching for the whole populations due to sample size constraints; still, our results were consistent both on raw prevalence estimates and after age- and sex-matching. Our single-center recruitment holds a potential selection bias and, for instance, we cannot exclude the possibility that some older and more disabled patients might have missed the appointment while sheltering at home. Additionally, due to local regulations, hospital access was limited to patients with more complex healthcare needs (e.g., infusion therapy). However, our population is numerically representative of MS patients living in the Campania Region of Italy, and also has a similar age (42 vs. 44 years) [21]. Finally, we were not fully aware of the working conditions and compliance with lockdown/self-isolation policies of our population.

In conclusion, MS patients are not at high risk of SARS-CoV-2 infection, though the prevalence of SARS-CoV-2 IgG/IgM is numerically higher than age- and sex-matched low risk individuals. As in the general population, most MS patients positive to SARS-CoV-2 IgG/IgM did not report on any COVID-19 symptom, also if using treatments with high risk of systemic immunosuppression. In clinical practice, healthcare staff should account for the additional risks coming from COVID-19, while delivering regular care.

Author Contributions: Conceptualization, N.C., R.L., A.C., M.P., R.I., A.I., F.A., V.P., A.R.B., E.Z., I.G., M.T., V.B.M. and M.M.; Data curation, N.C., R.P., E.M., F.P., R.L., A.C., M.P., A.I., F.A., V.P., A.R.B., E.Z., I.G., M.T., V.B.M. and M.M.; Formal analysis, N.C., R.P., E.M., F.P., R.L., A.C., M.P., R.I., A.I., F.A., V.P., A.R.B., E.Z., I.G., M.T., V.B.M. and M.M.; Funding acquisition, N.C., E.M., F.P., R.I., M.T., V.B.M. and M.M.; Investigation, N.C., R.P., M.T., V.B.M. and M.M.; Methodology, M.M.; Supervision, M.M.; Writing—original draft, N.C., E.M. and M.M.; Writing—review & editing, R.P., F.P., R.L., A.C., M.P., R.I., A.I., F.A., V.P., A.R.B., E.Z., I.G., M.T. and V.B.M. All authors have read and agreed to the published version of the manuscript.

Acknowledgments: Authors thank Barbara Satelliti, Maria Sovilla, Donatella Buzzerio, Noemi Strino, and Roberto Buonocore (Multiple Sclerosis Clinical Care and Research Centre, Department of Neuroscience, Reproductive Sciences and Odontostomatology, University of Naples Federico II, Naples, Italy) for performing SARS-CoV-2 IgG/IgM tests in clinical practice.

References

1. Clark, A.; Jit, M.; Warren-Gash, C.; Guthrie, B.; Wang, H.H.X.; Mercer, S.W.; Sanderson, C.; McKee, M.; Troeger, C.; Ong, K.L.; et al. Global, regional, and national estimates of the population at increased risk of severe COVID-19 due to underlying health conditions in 2020: A modelling study. *Lancet Glob. Health* **2020**, *8*, e1003–e1017. [CrossRef]

2. Burkill, S.; Montgomery, S.; Hajiebrahimi, M.H.; Hillert, J.; Olsson, T.; Bahmanyar, S. Mortality trends for multiple sclerosis patients in Sweden from 1968 to 2012. *Neurology* **2017**, *89*, 555–562. [CrossRef] [PubMed]

3. Palladino, R.; Marrie, R.; Majeed, A.; Chataway, J. Evaluating the Risk of Macrovascular Events and Mortality Among People With Multiple Sclerosis in England. *JAMA Neurol.* **2020**, *77*, 820–828. [CrossRef] [PubMed]

4. Marrie, R.A.; Elliott, L.; Marriott, J.; Cossoy, M.; Blanchard, J.; Leung, S.; Yu, N. Effect of comorbidity on mortality in multiple sclerosis. *Neurology* **2015**, *85*, 240–247. [CrossRef]

5. Buonomo, A.; Brescia Morra, V.; Zappulo, E.; Lanzillo, R.; Gentile, I.; Montella, S.; Triassi, M.; Palladino, R.; Moccia, M. COVID-19 prevention and multiple sclerosis management: The SAFE pathway for the post-peak. *Mult. Scler. Relat. Disord.* **2020**, *44*, 102282. [CrossRef]

6. Brownlee, W.; Bourdette, D.; Broadley, S.; Killestein, J.; Ciccarelli, O. Treating multiple sclerosis and neuromyelitis optica spectrum disorder during the COVID-19 pandemic. *Neurology* **2020**, *94*, 949–952. [CrossRef]

7. Amor, S.; Baker, D.; Khoury, S.J.; Schmierer, K.; Giovanonni, G. SARS-CoV-2 and Multiple Sclerosis: Not all immune depleting DMTs are equal or bad. *Ann. Neurol.* **2020**, *87*, 794–797. [CrossRef]

8. Moss, B.P.; Mahajan, K.R.; Bermel, R.A.; Hellisz, K.; Hua, L.H.; Hudec, T.; Husak, S.; McGinley, M.P.; Ontaneda, D.; Wang, Z.; et al. Multiple sclerosis management during the COVID-19 pandemic. *Mult. Scler.* **2020**, *26*, 1163–1171. [CrossRef]

9. Sethuraman, N.; Jeremiah, S.S.; Ryo, A. Interpreting Diagnostic Tests for SARS-CoV-2. *JAMA* **2020**, *323*, 2249–2251. [CrossRef]

10. Kontou, P.I.; Braliou, G.G.; Dimou, N.L.; Nikolopoulos, G.; Bagos, P.G. Antibody tests in detecting SARS-CoV-2 infection: A meta-analysis. *Diagnostics* **2020**, *10*, 319. [CrossRef]

11. Marie, T.-H.; Laurent, B.; Alain, W.; Ingrid, B.; Hugues, M.; Jean-Michel, D.; Jonathan, D. The role of serology for COVID-19 control: Population, kinetics and test performance do matter. *J. Infect.* **2020**, *81*, e91–e92. [CrossRef]

12. Gao, Z.; Xu, Y.; Sun, C.; Wang, X.; Guo, Y.; Qiu, S.; Ma, K. A systematic review of asymptomatic infections with COVID-10. *J. Microbiol. Immunol. Infect.* **2020**. [CrossRef] [PubMed]

13. Goudsmit, J. The paramount importance of serological surveys of SARS-CoV-2 infection and immunity. *Eur. J. Epidemiol.* **2020**, *35*, 331–333. [CrossRef] [PubMed]

14. Ciccarelli, O.; Cohen, J.; Thompson, A. Response of the multiple sclerosis community to COVID-19. *Mult. Scler.* **2020**, *26*, 1134–1136. [CrossRef] [PubMed]

15. Leocani, L.; Diserens, K.; Moccia, M.; Caltagirone, C. Disability through COVID-19 pandemic: Neurorehabilitation cannot wait. *Eur. J. Neurol.* **2020**, *27*, e50–e51. [CrossRef] [PubMed]

16. Thompson, A.J.; Banwell, B.L.; Barkhof, F.; Carroll, W.M.; Coetzee, T.; Comi, G.; Correale, J.; Fazekas, F.; Filippi, M.; Freedman, M.S.; et al. Diagnosis of multiple sclerosis: 2017 revisions of the McDonald criteria. *Lancet Neurol.* **2018**, *17*, 162–173. [CrossRef]

17. Li, Z.; Yi, Y.; Luo, X.; Xiong, N.; Liu, Y.; Li, S.; Sun, R.; Wang, Y.; Hu, B.; Chen, W.; et al. Development and clinical application of a rapid IgM-IgG combined antibody test for SARS-CoV-2 infection diagnosis. *J. Med. Virol.* **2020**, *92*, 1518–1524. [CrossRef]

18. Lou, B.; Li, T.-D.; Zheng, S.-F.; Su, Y.-Y.; Li, Z.-Y.; Liu, W.; Yu, F.; Ge, S.-X.; Zou, Q.-D.; Yuan, Q.; et al. Serology characteristics of SARS-CoV-2 infection since exposure and post symptom onset. *Eur. Respir. J.* **2020**, *56*. [CrossRef]

19. Lisboa Bastos, M.; Tavaziva, G.; Abidi, S.K.; Campbell, J.R.; Haraoui, L.P.; Johnston, J.C.; Lan, Z.; Law, S.; MacLean, E.; Trajman, A.; et al. Diagnostic accuracy of serological tests for covid-19: Systematic review and meta-analysis. *BMJ* **2020**, *370*. [CrossRef]

20. Li, L.; Huang, T.; Wang, Y.-Q.; Wang, Z.-P.; Liang, Y.; Huang, T.-B.; Zhang, H.-Y.; Sun, W.; Wang, Y. COVID-19 patients' clinical characteristics, discharge rate, and fatality rate of meta-analysis. *J. Med. Virol.* **2020**, *92*, 577–583. [CrossRef]

21. Moccia, M.; Brescia Morra, V.; Lanzillo, R.; Loperto, I.; Giordana, R.; Fumo, M.; Petruzzo, M.; Capasso, N.; Triassi, M.; Sormani, M.; et al. Multiple sclerosis in the Campania Region (South Italy): Algorithm validation and 2015-2017 prevalence. *Int. J. Environ. Res. Public Health* **2020**, *17*, 3388. [CrossRef] [PubMed]

22. IHME COVID-19 Health Service Utilization Forecasting Team; Murray, C.J.L. Forecasting COVID-19 impact on hospital bed-days, ICU-days, ventilator-days and deaths by US state in the next 4 months. *MedRxiv* **2020**. [CrossRef]

23. ISTAT. Primi Risultati Dell'indagine di Sieroprevalenza sul SARS-CoV-2. 2020. Available online: http://www.salute.gov.it/portale/news/p3_2_1_1_1.jsp?lingua=italiano&menu=notizie&p=dalministero&id=4998 (accessed on 16 December 2020).

24. Bryan, A.; Pepper, G.; Wener, M.H.; Fink, S.L.; Morishima, C.; Chaudhary, A.; Jerome, K.R.; Mathias, P.C.; Greninger, A.L. Performance Characteristics of the Abbott Architect SARS-CoV-2 IgG Assay and Seroprevalence in Boise, Idaho. *J. Clin. Microbiol.* **2020**, *58*. [CrossRef] [PubMed]

25. Sood, N.; Simon, P.; Ebner, P.; Eichner, D.; Reynolds, J.; Bendavid, E.; Bhattacharya, J. Seroprevalence of SARS-CoV-2-Specific Antibodies Among Adults in Los Angeles County, California, on April 10–11, 2020. *JAMA* **2020**, *13*, 98–99. [CrossRef]

26. Korth, J.; Wilde, B.; Dolff, S.; Anastasiou, O.E.; Krawczyk, A.; Jahn, M.; Cordes, S.; Ross, B.; Esser, S.; Lindemann, M.; et al. SARS-CoV-2-specific antibody detection in healthcare workers in Germany with direct contact to COVID-19 patients. *J. Clin. Virol.* **2020**, *128*, 104437. [CrossRef]

27. Behrens, G.M.N.; Cossmann, A.; Stankov, M.V.; Witte, T.; Ernst, D.; Happle, C.; Jablonka, A. Perceived versus proven SARS-CoV-2-specific immune responses in health-care professionals. *Infection* **2020**, *48*, 631–634. [CrossRef]

28. Wijnands, J.M.A.; Zhu, F.; Kingwell, E.; Fisk, J.D.; Evans, C.; Marrie, R.A.; Zhao, Y.; Tremlett, H. Disease-modifying drugs for multiple sclerosis and infection risk: A cohort study. *J. Neurol. Neurosurg. Psychiatry* **2018**, *89*, 1050–1056. [CrossRef]

29. Sormani, M.P.; Study, I. Correspondence An Italian programme for COVID-19 infection. *Lancet Glob. Health* **2020**, *4422*, 30147. [CrossRef]

30. Montero-Escribano, P.; Matías-Guiu, J.; Gómez-Iglesias, P.; Porta-Etessam, J.; Pytel, V.; Matias-Guiu, J.A. Anti-CD20 and COVID-19 in multiple sclerosis and related disorders: A case series of 60 patients from Madrid, Spain. *Mult. Scler. Relat. Disord.* **2020**, *42*, 102185. [CrossRef]

31. De Angelis, M.; Petracca, M.; Lanzillo, R.; Brescia Morra, V.; Moccia, M. Mild or no COVID-19 symptoms in cladribine-treated multiple sclerosis: Two cases and implications for clinical practice. *Mult. Scler. Relat. Disord.* **2020**, *45*, 102452. [CrossRef]

32. Evangelou, N.; Garjani, A.; DasNair, R.; Hunter, R.; Tuite-Dalton, K.A.; Craig, E.M.; Rodgers, W.J.; Coles, A.; Dobson, R.; Duddy, M.; et al. Self-diagnosed COVID-19 in people with multiple sclerosis: A community-based cohort of the UK MS Register. *J. Neurol. Neurosurg. Psychiatry* **2020**. [CrossRef]

33. Loonstra, F.C.; Hoitsma, E.; van Kempen, Z.L.E.; Killestein, J.; Mostert, J.P. COVID-19 in multiple sclerosis: The Dutch experience. *Mult. Scler.* **2020**, *26*, 1256–1260. [CrossRef] [PubMed]

34. Louapre, C.; Collongues, N.; Stankoff, B.; Giannesini, C.; Papeix, C.; Bensa, C.; Deschamps, R.; Créange, A.; Wahab, A.; Pelletier, J.; et al. Clinical Characteristics and Outcomes in Patients with Coronavirus Disease 2019 and Multiple Sclerosis. *JAMA Neurol.* **2020**, *77*, 1079–1088. [CrossRef] [PubMed]

35. Fan, M.; Qiu, W.; Bu, B.; Xu, Y.; Yang, H.; Huang, D.; Lau, A.Y.; Guo, J.; Zhang, M.-N.; Zhang, X.; et al. Risk of COVID-19 infection in MS and neuromyelitis optica spectrum disorders. *Neurol. Neuroimmunol. Neuroinflamm.* **2020**, *7*, e787. [CrossRef] [PubMed]

36. Li, Y.; Yao, L.; Li, J.; Chen, L.; Song, Y.; Cai, Z.; Yang, C. Stability issues of RT-PCR testing of SARS-CoV-2 for hospitalized patients clinically diagnosed with COVID-19. *J. Med. Virol.* **2020**, *92*, 903–908. [CrossRef] [PubMed]

37. Du, Z.; Zhu, F.; Guo, F.; Yang, B.; Wang, T. Detection of antibodies against SARS-CoV-2 in patients with COVID-19. *J. Med. Virol.* **2020**, *92*, 1735–1738. [CrossRef]

38. Epstein, D.J.; Dunn, J.; Deresinski, S. Infectious complications of multiple sclerosis therapies: Implications for screening, prophylaxis, and management. *Open Forum Infect. Dis.* **2018**, *5*, ofy174. [CrossRef]

3

Spinal Cord Involvement in MS and Other Demyelinating Diseases

Mariano Marrodan, María I. Gaitán and Jorge Correale *

Neurology Department, Fleni, C1428AQK Buenos Aires, Argentina; mmarrodan@fleni.org.ar (M.M.); migaitan@fleni.org.ar (M.I.G.)

* Correspondence: jcorreale@fleni.org.ar or jorge.correale@gmail.com;

Abstract: Diagnostic accuracy is poor in demyelinating myelopathies, and therefore a challenge for neurologists in daily practice, mainly because of the multiple underlying pathophysiologic mechanisms involved in each subtype. A systematic diagnostic approach combining data from the clinical setting and presentation with magnetic resonance imaging (MRI) lesion patterns, cerebrospinal fluid (CSF) findings, and autoantibody markers can help to better distinguish between subtypes. In this review, we describe spinal cord involvement, and summarize clinical findings, MRI and diagnostic characteristics, as well as treatment options and prognostic implications in different demyelinating disorders including: multiple sclerosis (MS), neuromyelitis optica spectrum disorder, acute disseminated encephalomyelitis, anti-myelin oligodendrocyte glycoprotein antibody-associated disease, and glial fibrillary acidic protein IgG-associated disease. Thorough understanding of individual case etiology is crucial, not only to provide valuable prognostic information on whether the disorder is likely to relapse, but also to make therapeutic decision-making easier and reduce treatment failures which may lead to new relapses and long-term disability. Identifying patients with monophasic disease who may only require acute management, symptomatic treatment, and subsequent rehabilitation, rather than immunosuppression, is also important.

Keywords: myelitis; spinal cord; multiple sclerosis; neuromyelitis optica; acute disseminated encephalomyelitis; myelin oligodendrocyte glycoprotein; glial fibrillary acidic protein

1. Introduction

Diagnostic accuracy in myelopathies is poor and therefore a challenge for neurologists in daily practice, mainly due to the multiple underlying pathophysiologic mechanisms observed in this group of disorders. In an initial approach, temporal profile (time to symptom nadir) contributes to differentiate vascular or traumatic causes from those of metabolic, neoplastic, and infectious or inflammatory etiology. To further assist in the identification of patients with acute vascular myelopathies for whom specific treatment strategies may be indicated, patients whose symptoms reach maximal severity in <4 h from onset are currently presumed to have an ischemic pathology unless proven otherwise [1]. By contrast, inflammatory processes affecting the spinal cord produce symptoms in a subacute manner, typically over hours or days. However, despite extensive patient work-up, a significant number of myelopathy cases are ultimately considered idiopathic [2]. Unfortunately, the term inflammatory myelitis is still applied to a complex and heterogeneous subgroup of post-infectious, rheumatologic, granulomatous, paraneoplastic, and demyelinating diseases, commonly affecting the spinal cord in which substantial overlap in clinical and imaging findings subsists. Identifying relapsing forms of disease has prognostic implications and can guide preventive treatment. Failure to indicate appropriate treatments may lead to new relapses and long-term disability. In contrast, patients in whom monophasic disease is suspected may only require acute management, symptomatic treatment, and subsequent rehabilitation rather than immunosuppression. In the case of demyelinating disorders, although multiple sclerosis (MS) is the main cause of inflammatory myelitis, other important differential diagnoses need to be ruled out to select the best treatment strategy in individual patients [3,4]. Thorough understanding of individual case etiology is therefore crucial, not only for correct treatment, but also to determine patient outcome.

In this review, we describe the epidemiologic characteristics, pathophysiology, clinical and (magnetic resonance imaging) MRI findings, treatment options and prognostic implications in MS and other demyelinating disorders including: neuromyelitis optica spectrum disorder (NMOSD), acute disseminated encephalomyelitis (ADEM), anti-myelin oligodendrocyte glycoprotein (MOG)-antibodies (ab) associated disease, and glial fibrillary acidic protein (GFAP)-IgG associated disease, to provide guidance in the diagnosis of these conditions.

A Pubmed search was conducted for articles published between 2000 and 2020, that included the terms: "acute disseminated encephalomyelitis; "demyelinating diseases"; "glial fibrillary acidic protein"; "multiple sclerosis"; "myelin oligodendrocyte glycoprotein"; "myelitis"; "neuromyelitis optica"; and "spinal cord diseases". Only those originally in English were considered. Earlier publications were identified from references cited in the articles reviewed.

2. Multiple Sclerosis

MS is a chronic inflammatory disease of the CNS leading to demyelination, neurodegeneration, and gliosis. It is by far the most common demyelinating disease, affecting over 2 million people worldwide [5]. Although its etiology remains elusive, environmental factors and susceptibility genes are now known to be involved in the pathogenesis [6]. Results from immunological, genetic, and histopathology studies of patients with MS support the concept that autoimmunity plays a major role in the disease [7]. In the majority of cases, the disease follows a relapsing remitting course (RRMS) from onset, which may later convert into a secondary progressive form (SPMS). Less often, patients show continued progression from disease debut (primary progressive MS, PPMS) [8].

Spinal cord abnormalities are common in MS and include a variety of pathological processes, such as demyelination, neuroaxonal loss and gliosis. Ultimately these result in motor weakness with accompanying difficulties in deambulation, spasticity, sensory disturbances, as well as bladder and bowel dysfunction [9]. Relapsing remitting MS can cause acute myelitis presenting with sensory loss, gait impairment, and incoordination, generally worsening over days to weeks, followed by stabilization or recovery [10]. During progressive phases of the disease however, especially in PPMS, slowly increasing or stuttering gait impairment due to demyelinating myelopathy is the most frequent presentation [11]. Once gait impairment has developed, cumulative disability increase will depend on patient age, clinical, and radiological disease activity and degree of spinal cord atrophy [12–15].

Histopathology findings in the spinal cord are characterized by significant decrease in axonal density in normal-appearing white matter (NAWM); perivascular T-cell infiltrates are rare, but robust, and diffuse inflammation is observed both in normal-appearing parenchyma and particularly in the meninges. Extent of diffuse axonal loss in NAWM correlates with both MHC class II$^+$ microglia cell density in NAWM, and significant increase in T cell density in the meninges. Interestingly, close interaction has been observed between T cells and MHC class II$^+$ macrophages in spinal cord meninges from MS patients, suggesting the meninges may form an immunological niche in which T lymphocytes become activated and proliferate in response to antigen presentation [16]. In support of this concept, similar findings have previously been described in experimental autoimmune encephalomyelitis [17], raising the possibility that activated meningeal T cells, through release of soluble factors such as IFN-γ, could instruct parenchymal macrophages/microglia to engage in neurotoxic activation programs [18].

Although spinal cord involvement has been difficult both to characterize and to quantify because current clinical and MRI parameters lack sensitivity and specificity [19], the spinal cord was one of four anatomical locations incorporated in a revision to McDonald diagnostic criteria for MS in 2017, to document spatial dissemination in patients presenting clinical isolated syndrome (CIS) suggestive of

MS. Likewise, new or gadolinium-enhancing spinal cord lesions can be used to document chronological progression [20].

Poor correlation between spinal cord injury load and clinical disability may be due to several different factors. Spinal cord MRI is more challenging than brain imaging in patients with MS. The spine is extremely thin and commonly subjected to ghosting artifacts (due to breathing, swallowing, and/or pulsation of blood and cerebrospinal fluid (CSF)) [21]. The amount of bone and fat may also produce significant artifacts, greater than those observed in brain imaging. Conventional, sagittal proton density (PD) and T2-weighted scans, with spatial resolution of $3 \times 1 \times 1$ mm, should be considered the reference standard to detect MS spinal cord lesions [22,23]. Short-tau inversion recovery (STIR) sequences seem to be more sensitive to lesion detection than T2-weighted sequences and may be used to substitute PD sequences [24]. Contrast-enhanced T1-weighted images are recommended if T2 lesions are detected.

Conventional spine MRI has low sensitivity and specificity in relation to the pathological changes observed in MS [25]. Use of sagittal sections alone may underestimate lesion numbers [25]. Axial imaging may detect more lesions than sagittal imaging [26], especially smaller ones in the spinal cord periphery [27] and 2D or 3D T2-weighted sequences should be included in MRI protocols [21]. Axial multiple-echo recombined gradient echo (MERGE) seems to provide greater sensitivity for cord lesion detection and may represent a good alternative [28]. Ultimately, combined use of sagittal and axial images can facilitate identification and location of spinal lesions (Figure 1A–F) [26].

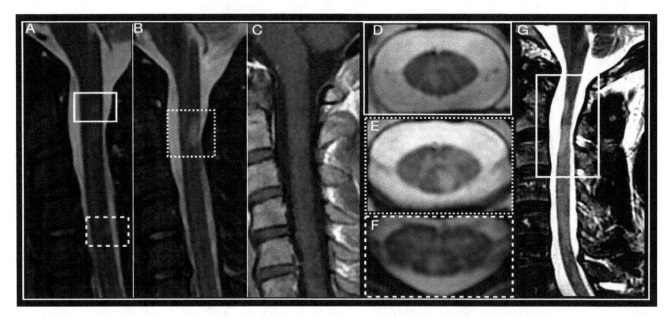

Figure 1. Multiple Sclerosis myelitis. (**A–F**) 32-year-old woman diagnosed with relapsing remitting course (RRMS) 2 years earlier, EDSS 0. (**A,B**) Sagittal short-tau inversion recovery (STIR) showing small, focal, chronic, peripheral lesions. (**C**) Sagittal post-contrast T1 weighted, absence of enhancement, T2 lesions are isointense. (**D–F**) axial T2 multiple-echo recombined gradient echo (MERGE). (**D**) right paramedian posterior lesion corresponds to lesion framed by a box in (**A**). (**E**) left paramedian posterior lesion corresponds to lesion framed by a dotted box in (**A**). (**F**) posterior lesion corresponds to lesion framed by a dotted line in (**A**). (**G**) 46-year-old man diagnosed with primary progressive multiple sclerosis (PPMS) in 2011, EDSS 6. Sagittal T2-weighted, framed area shows multiple sclerosis (MS) lesions and spinal cord atrophy.

Often more than one demyelinating plaque is present in spinal cord MRIs from patients with MS. The cervical spine (53–59%) is the most common location, followed by the thoracic region (20–47%) [10]. Lesions usually present as hyperintense on T2-weighted and isointense on T1-weighted sequences. Gadolinium enhancement is variable and depends mainly on acquisition timing, with acute lesions usually enhancing during 4–8 weeks [29,30]. Most MS lesions are small in size, wedge-shaped in axial and ovoid-shaped in sagittal views, and predominantly found in ascending sensory (i.e., posterior column), and descending motor (i.e., corticospinal) spinal cord tracts, because of the high myelin concentration within these fascicules [31]. Rarely, they may extend to involve central grey matter, occupying over half the cross-sectional area of the cord. Small focal lesions may coalesce to form more extensive ones, involving three or more segments, particularly in cases of progressive MS. High-resolution axial MRI demonstrates these images actually result from the confluence of multiple discrete lesions [25,32].

Spinal cord lesions, when present, are particularly helpful to discriminate MS from its radiological mimics, which include conditions such as migraine and cerebrovascular disorders. They can also present together with multifocal T2 lesions in brain white matter [33].

In addition to their diagnostic value, spine lesions contribute prognostic information in MS. Asymptomatic lesions are present in approximately 35% of patients with radiological isolated syndrome [34], in one-third of patients with CIS [35], and 83% of patients with early RRMS [36]. Interestingly, the number of asymptomatic lesions found in patients with CIS has been linked to risk of a second clinical event at 2 and 5 years [37,38], making spine MRI advisable in CIS patient workup. However, detection of asymptomatic spinal cord lesions during follow-up of RRMS patients was less common than detection of asymptomatic lesions in the brain, suggesting spinal cord MRI may be less useful than brain MRI for monitoring patients with RRMS [39]. Some authors have observed that greater number of spinal cord lesions at MS time of diagnosis and lesional topography at time of relapse were associated with increased relapse rates and higher risk of developing secondary progressive MS [10,11,39].

Spinal cord atrophy (Figure 1G) present in early stages of the disease may correlate with degree of disability and predict long term outcome [38,40]. Measuring changes in cross-sectional area at the cervical level yields the most reproducible results and shows closest correlation to clinical findings [41,42]. Grey matter atrophy on the other hand correlates more strongly with degree of physical disability than other MRI parameters of brain and cord atrophy [43–45]. Notably, a significant association between reduced cervical cord sectional diameter and disability progression has been demonstrated in different studies, independent of brain atrophy [46–48]. Cord atrophy has also been associated with reduction in retinal nerve layer thickness [48], suggesting it is probably part of a global pathological process and not just determined by local damage.

Rate of atrophy is more accelerated in the spinal cord than in the brain (1.5–2.2% per year vs. 0.5–1% per year) [49,50], and in patients with SPMS than in patients with CIS or RRMS. In RRMS, cord atrophy presents primarily in the posterior spinal cord, while in SPMS, atrophy is generalized [49]. Interestingly, regional atrophy does not seem to be influenced by focal lesion presence [51–53]. A recent study reported that a 1% increase in the annual rate of spinal cord volume loss was associated with a 28% risk of disability progression in the subsequent year [50]. Unfortunately, widespread use of this parameter has so far been limited by poor reproducibility and lack of sensitivity to small changes in the cord cross-sectional area. Since the rate of spinal atrophy over time appears to be associated with disability progression, atrophy has been considered a secondary outcome measure in phase 3 clinical trials of progressive MS [50,51]. When it was later analyzed more thoroughly, results were inconclusive [54–56]. This may have been due to lack of treatment efficacy, inadequate patient selection, poor reproducibility of cord atrophy quantification, or low sensitivity of MRI techniques used to detect small changes in cord cross-sectional area [30]. Eventually, spinal cord atrophy could also be considered a primary outcome in phase 2 clinical trials of progressive MS. However, this will require adequate patient selection and more precise MR imaging techniques for exact assessment.

It should be noted that neuronal loss in MS is not limited to white matter only, post mortem studies have also shown extensive neuronal loss in gray matter of the spinal cord as well, generating considerable interest in detection of gray matter abnormalities in MS [57]. The use of a combination of axial fast-field echo (FFE) and phase-sensitive inversion recovery (PSIR) sequences has been proposed to identify gray matter abnormalities in the upper cervical spinal cord [58]. However, further studies are still necessary to verify the sensitivity of this technique. Although both double inversion recovery (DIR) and PSIR can help distinguish focal gray matter lesions from normal-appearing tissue on sagittal views [59,60], these are often confounded by artifacts [61,62]. Use of 3T and higher field-strength (4.7 T) scanners as well as dedicated imaging sequences have increased MRI sensitivity for MS-associated gray matter lesion detection in the spinal cord [63,64]. Nevertheless, greater knowledge of spinal cord lesion pathogenesis, as well as its relationship to disability progression, still need to be established to better define the role of spinal cord assessment in MS diagnosis and follow-up [30].

More sensitive and better standardized methods are needed to assess clinical manifestations related to spinal cord atrophy over time, as well as monitor disease course and response to therapy. Promising MRI techniques to study the spinal cord include myelin water imaging, magnetization transfer imaging, diffusion tensor imaging, and magnetic resonance spectroscopy. At present however, use of these modalities is mostly restricted to research. Automated image-acquisition techniques, increased precision, and reduced quantification variability over time still need to be developed, and application in the clinical setting will likely be limited to select sites with experience using advanced imaging techniques.

Several studies have demonstrated that residual deficits persist after MS relapses affecting the spinal cord, contributing to stepwise progression of disability. For this reason, prompt and adequate treatment of relapses is key, although optimal regimens have to be better defined [65,66]. Unfortunately, despite significant advances in disease-modifying treatment, management of acute MS relapses with intravenous or oral corticosteroids has remained largely unchanged for the past 20 years [67].

Since the first prospective trial demonstrated superiority of high-dose intravenous methylprednisolone use (IVMPS; up to 1000 mg daily) over placebo, acute MS relapses are initially treated with IVMPS during three to five days [68]. Although faster recovery of relapses has been documented, clinical improvement is insufficient in approximately 25% of patients after the first course of IVMPS [69]. Aside from increasing steroid treatment dose and prolonging treatment (up to 2000 mg daily for five additional days), use of plasma exchange (PLEX) has also been considered an alternative option [70]. One recent study in a group of patients receiving PLEX within 6 weeks of a relapse showed not only significantly better response rates than those of patients receiving extended IVMPS treatment, but also lower risk deterioration 3 months after discharge [71,72]. For long-term treatment of MS, the last 2 decades have seen the development of numerous drugs aimed at correcting the different pathogenic mechanisms proposed in multiple sclerosis, most of which have been compounds targeting immune system dysfunction. Several clinical trials are currently ongoing, some using neuroprotective therapies to halt progression, others aimed at reversing neurological disability, at least in part, by repairing damaged brain and spinal cord tissue. Discussion of particular disease-modifying therapies for MS is beyond the scope of this manuscript, however, several comprehensive reviews on the subject have recently been published [73–76].

3. Acute Disseminated Encephalomyelitis

Acute disseminated encephalomyelitis (ADEM) is an autoimmune demyelinating disorder of the CNS, commonly affecting brain and spinal cord white matter, although deep grey matter nuclei (e.g., thalamus and basal ganglia) may also be involved [77,78]. ADEM is more common in children (mean age 5 to 8 years), but can occur at any age [79] with an estimated annual incidence of 0.23 to 0.40/100,000 children [80–82]. Although no clear gender predominance has been identified, slight male preponderance has been described in some pediatric ADEM cohorts [79]. Most pediatric ADEM cases appear to be preceded by symptoms of viral or bacterial infection, usually of the upper-respiratory tract. Vaccination has also been reported to precede ADEM, although at much lower rates [83]. Some cases have been linked to specific vaccines produced in neural tissue cultures (rabies and Japanese B encephalitis). However, a marked drop in post vaccination ADEM has occurred since CNS tissue culture-derived production was replaced by recombinant protein-based vaccines. Nevertheless in up to 26% of patients, no triggering event can be observed [84].

Histopathology findings in ADEM show perivenular inflammatory infiltrates consisting of T cells and macrophages, associated with perivenular demyelination and relative preservation of axons in most cases. In hemorrhagic variants, demyelination is often more widespread through the CNS, with important neutrophilic infiltrates [79].

The pathogenesis of ADEM is still unclear. Two main hypotheses have been proposed. One, the molecular mimicry hypothesis, suggests partial structural or amino-acid sequence homology may exist between certain pathogens or vaccines and host CNS myelin antigens, which in turn may activate myelin-reactive T cells, thereby eliciting a CNS-specific autoimmune response [85]. The second hypothesis proposes CNS infection may directly prompt a secondary inflammatory cascade, leading to blood-brain barrier rupture, exposure of CNS-antigens, and breakdown of tolerance resulting in an autoimmune attack driven mainly by T cells [86].

Criteria for ADEM diagnosis, established in 2013 by the International Multiple Sclerosis Study Group (IPMSSG), require the following to be present: (1) an initial polyfocal clinical CNS event of presumed inflammatory demyelinating cause; (2) encephalopathy (alteration in consciousness or behavior unexplained by fever, systemic illness, or post ictal symptoms); (3) brain MRI abnormalities consistent with demyelination during the acute phase (first 3 months); (4) no new clinical or MRI findings 3 months or more after onset [87].

Depending on the series, spinal cord involvement has been described in 20% to 54% of ADEM patients, predominantly affecting the thoracic region [88]. Coincident brain and spinal cord lesions are more common; isolated spinal cord ADEM is exceptional [89] and typically extends over multiple segments, cause cord swelling, and showing variable enhancement in the acute phase. In most ADEM patients, partial or complete resolution of MRI abnormalities occurs within a few months of treatment [84,90]. Interestingly, ADEM patients with anti-MOG antibodies show large, more widespread brain lesions with ill-defined borders and longitudinally extensive spinal cord lesions on MRI [91]. Lesions involving more than two segments are more frequent in adults than in children (50% vs. 27%, respectively) [92].

No specific studies on CSF have been conducted in ADEM. Pleocytosis is typically mild, with a high percentage of lymphocytes and monocytes [92,93] and increased protein levels (up to 1.1 g/L) in 23% to 62% of pediatric patients [94–96]. OCBs are only present in 0% to 29% of cases [79]. However, they are usually transient as opposed to those observed in MS.

Although ADEM usually has a monophasic course, multiphasic forms have been reported in 10–31% of patients [84,97], making differential diagnosis with MS more difficult in these cases. Multiphasic forms are defined as new encephalopathic events consistent with ADEM, separated by a 3-month interval from the initial illness but not followed by any further event [98]. Relapsing disease following ADEM occurring beyond a second encephalopathic event is no longer consistent with multiphasic ADEM, but rather indicates a chronic disorder such as MS, NMOSD, or ADEM-optic neuritis [98,99], and should prompt testing for anti-MOG ab. It is worth highlighting that progression from ADEM to MS is relatively low, estimated at 0% to 17% in studies with follow-up periods lasting several years [88].

Clinical presentation and outcome of ADEM in adults differs from that of children. Disease course is worse in adults, with more than one-third of patients requiring admission to an ICU, and duration of hospitalization can be twice as long. Outcome is also less favorable, complete motor recovery is observed in only 15% of adults compared to 58% of children and more adult patients die, although no difference in the occurrence of relapses or conversion to MS has been reported [92,100]. Poorer outcomes in adults cannot be explained by differences in clinical presentation (preceding factors, symptoms, blood and CSF parameters or radiological features are all similar). Perhaps reduced plasticity in ageing CNS tissue is the cause, rather than a difference in pathophysiology from onset [92].

No randomized-controlled studies have been conducted on ADEM treatment. Despite the lack of conclusive evidence, a widely accepted regimen in use today is administration of IV methylprednisolone (30 mg/kg/day in children or 1000 mg/day in adults) for 5 days, followed by oral taper with dexamethasone at a starting dose of 1–2 mg/kg/day, for 4–6 weeks [101,102]. Plasma exchange is recommended for therapy-refractory patients with fulminant disease [103,104]. Beyond treatment of the initial event, it is important to have a plan for long term follow-up to exclude a multiphasic disorder, which would warrant further diagnostic evaluation and a different therapeutic approach.

4. Neuromyelitis Optica Spectrum-Disorder

Neuromyelitis optica (NMO) is an inflammatory disorder, traditionally considered monophasic, although relapsing cases have been described in which patients present optic neuritis and transverse myelitis [105]. NMO had been considered a variant of MS until an autoantibody against the water channel protein aquaporin-4 (AQP4), expressed abundantly on astrocyte end-feet, called AQP4-IgG (also called NMO-IgG), was discovered in patients with NMO, and found to be absent in patients with MS [106,107]. Incorporation of AQP4-IgG serology to revised NMO diagnostic criteria broadened the clinical and radiological spectrum of NMO [108]. The term NMO spectrum disorders (NMOSD) was introduced to include AQP4-IgG seropositive patients with limited forms of NMO, and at risk of future attacks, as well as patients with cerebral, diencephalic, and brainstem lesions, or coexisting autoimmune disease (e.g., systemic lupus erythematosus [SLE] or Sjögren syndrome [SS]) [109]. Accordingly, NMOSD was recognized as a humoral disease entity distinct from MS, and diagnostic criteria were revised in 2015 unifying the terms NMO and NMOSD [110].

Evidence supporting a pathogenic role of AQP4-IgG comes from different sources. Complement- as well as ab-dependent cytotoxicity [101,102] has been associated to AQP4-IgG, which when administered along with complement and/or pathogenic T cells, promotes development of NMOSD-like CNS lesions in rodents [111,112]. Inflammatory damage is characterized by astrocyte loss and deposition of both immunoglobulins and complement, followed by neutrophil, monocyte, phagocyte and eosinophil infiltration [113]. Importantly, AQP4 distribution coincides with deposition patterns of IgG, IgM, and products of complement activation present in active NMO tissue [114,115], and MRI lesions of patients with NMO overlap with sites of high AQP4 expression [116]. AQP4-IgG is believed to determine internalization of the glutamate transporter EAAT2, limiting glutamate uptake from the extracellular space into astrocytes, also resulting in oligodendrocyte damage and myelin loss [117]. Although most strongly expressed in the CNS, AQP4 is also present in the collecting duct of the kidney, parietal cells of the stomach, as well as in airways, salivary glands, and skeletal muscle [118]. However, peripheral organ damage does not typically occur, probably due to the presence of complement inhibitory proteins in these secondary target organs [119].

Despite caveats in knowledge on NMOSD epidemiology, prevalence has been estimated depending on the study population at 0.1–4.4 cases/100,000 individuals, and annual incidence at 0.20–4.0 per 1,000,000 [120,121]. Initial clinical manifestations occur at around 40 years of age, although children and the elderly account for 18% of cases. Female/male predominance is around 9:1, but not in children, where equal gender distribution has been observed [32,122].

According to the most recent diagnostic criteria, core clinical characteristics can involve 1 of 6 CNS regions, namely: optic nerve, spinal cord, area postrema of the dorsal medulla, brainstem, diencephalon, or cerebrum [110]. Clinical presentation particularly suggestive of NMOSD diagnosis includes: bilateral ON involving the optic chiasm with poor recovery compared to MS-ON, complete spinal cord syndrome determining paroxysmal spasms, and area postrema clinical syndrome characterized by intractable hiccups, or nausea and vomiting. No single clinical characteristic is pathognomonic of NMOSD, however [110]. In AQP4-IgG seronegative patients, diagnostic criteria are more rigorous. Patients must present at least 2 of the core clinical characteristics, and at least one of these must be: ON, longitudinally extensive transverse myelitis (LETM), or area postrema syndrome.

Given the focus of this review, in the following sections, only aspects related to NMOSD-related to spinal cord involvement will be addressed.

Acute transverse myelitis symptoms in NMOSD patients (motor, sensitive, and frequently sphincter) are usually severe and bilateral, and recovery is incomplete compared to MS. Although overlap of clinical characteristics in MS and NMOSD myelitis does occur, symptom magnitude and disease history frequently contribute to establish differential diagnosis [30,32,120], as do certain MRI findings. LETM is the most specific neuroimaging characteristic found in NMOSD, and is uncommon in MS (Figure 2) [108]. Mirroring severe underlying tissue damage, lesions are generally hyperintense on T2-weighted, and hypointense on T1-weighted sequences [30]. Extending over three or more complete vertebral segments, they tend to localize in the center of the cord, because of the abundant AQP4 channel expression in grey matter. Lesions will usually occupy over 50% of the cross-sectional surface area of the spine, representing a complete, rather than incomplete, form of transverse myelitis which is more characteristic in MS. However, they also may be lateral, anterior, or posterior over the length of the lesion and be accompanied by cord swelling. The latter, when present, can generate concern over presence of a spinal cord tumor [123]. Chronic necrosis caused by NMOSD can in some cases result in spinal cord cavitation and cystic myelomalacia. Small areas of strong hyperintensity, higher than that of the surrounding cerebrospinal fluid (CSF), so-called bright spotty lesions, may be observed and could be useful to distinguish NMOSD from MS [124]. Acute NMO lesions extensively enhance following IV gadolinium administration. Lens-shaped ring-enhancement is detected in up to 32% of NMOSD patients [29,125,126]. Rostral extension of cervical lesions to the area postrema is another characteristic of NMOSD and can be helpful to distinguish it from other causes of longitudinal extensive myelopathy such as sarcoidosis, spondylotic myelopathy with enhancement, dural arteriovenous fistula, spinal cord infarct, and paraneoplastic myelopathy [127]. Although LETM is the most frequent form, 7–14% of NMO-myelitis involve <3 vertebral segments. However, short forms of NMO-myelitis are followed by LETM in ninety percent of cases. Short cord lesions should be suspected in patients with tonic spasm, coexistence of autoimmune disease, grey matter involvement and absence of OCB. As in MS, in 7–14% of cases, variation in presentation will be linked to time at which MRI scans are obtained [128–130]. Lesions limited to less than three segments will be detected at the beginning of disease or during remission [131]. In contrast, patients with longstanding disease may present short but coalescing lesions suggesting a LETM pattern [22]. Presence of a longitudinally extensive segment of cord atrophy is another characteristic finding in support of prior NMOSD myelitis [131].

Although in NMOSD the relationship between spinal cord atrophy, disease activity and disability is not fully known, two observations deserve mention. First, NMOSD patients predominately show spinal cord atrophy with only mild brain atrophy, while MS patients demonstrate more brain atrophy, especially in gray matter, suggesting a different underlying pathogenic mechanism [132]. Second, spinal cord atrophy can occur in patients without a clinical history of myelitis or visible spinal cord lesions on MRI, suggesting cord atrophy may be due to a diffuse underlying process. Alternatively, or perhaps in co-contributory fashion, patients may have experienced transient or subclinical inflammatory events not evident on conventional MRI [133].

Serum AQP4-IgG assay is the most useful test for NMOSD diagnosis. Based on criteria proposed by the International Panel for NMOSD, approximately 73–90% of patients with NMOSD express AQP4-IgG [134,135]. A cell-based assay (CBA) is recommended whenever possible because of its higher sensitivity (76.7%) and very low false-positive rate (0.1%) [136,137]. Indirect immunofluorescence assays and ELISA have less sensitivity (63–64% each), and can yield false-positive results (0.5–1.3% for ELISA) particularly at low titers [135,137]. Ultimately, 10–27% of patients with typical clinical and radiological features of NMOSD will not have detectable AQP4-IgG despite use of the best available assay. Lack of a diagnostic biomarker makes management of these patients more challenging especially of patients with monophasic disease [121,136]. Notably, using CBA, approximately 15–40% of AQP4-IgG seronegative NMOSD patients have been reported to have detectable antibodies against myelin oligodendrocyte glycoprotein (MOG) [137,138]. Aside from causing optico-spinal disease resembling NMOSD, anti-MOG antibodies have been identified in patients with clinical characteristics unlike those of patients with AQP4-IgG [32,137,139] (see below), suggesting a different underlying pathogenesis. Occasionally, patients without detectable serum AQP4-IgG are later found to be positive, possibly related to assay timing (antibody levels increase during exacerbations), or to impact of immunosuppressive treatment.

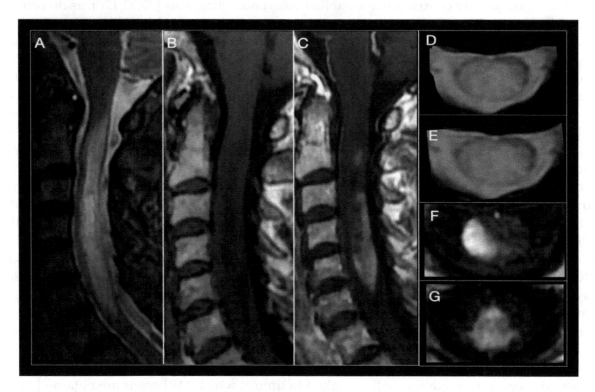

Figure 2. Neuromyelitis optica (NMO) myelitis. Images from a 58-year-old woman with acute longitudinally extensive myelitis (C1–C7). (**A**) Sagittal STIR showing an extensive lesion, involving more than 3 segments, that widens the cervical spinal cord. (**B**) Sagittal T1-weighted sequences show an extensive T1-hypointense lesion. (**C**) T1-weighted images after contrast administration, extensive enhancement of cervical lesion. (**D,E**) Axial T2-MERGE hyperintense area that involves more than half the diameter of the spinal cord. (**E,F**) Axial T1-weighted, intense contrast enhancement of lateral (**E**) and central-posterior (**F,G**) areas.

Serum AQP4-IgG concentration is much higher than that found in CSF. The hypothesis behind this is that most AQP4-IgG is produced in peripheral lymphoid tissues and that a favorable serum/CSF antibody gradient is needed for penetration into the CNS, a concept supported by the fact that commercial CBA and flow cytometry detection of AQP4-IgG is more sensitive in serum than in CSF. Serum is therefore the optimal specimen for AQP4-IgG testing [140].

Some patients with NMOSD produce other autoantibodies in addition to AQP4-IgG, as occurs in patients with SLE or SS [118]. Since LETM has also been described in patients with these conditions, the possibility exists that NMOSD symptoms arise secondary to SLE or SS. Limited existing data in this regard shows that in such patients, AQP4-IgG detection rates are similar to those observed in patients with NMOSD without associated rheumatic disease, suggesting LETM in NMOSD is not secondary to SLE or SS, and these patients suffer from two independent, coexisting autoimmune diseases [118,141–143].

CSF pleocytosis (>50 cells/μL) or presence of neutrophils or eosinophils during NMOSD attacks may help to distinguish NMOSD from MS [123,137].CSF OCBs are usually absent, although they may sometimes be transiently detectable during an attack [123,144].Given the high morbidity associated with NMOSD exacerbations, the goals of pharmacotherapy are to aggressively treat acute attacks, (including the initial episode) and prevent future relapses, minimizing CNS damage and long-term disability [145,146]. Different pathophysiologic mechanisms are known to characterize MS and NMOSD, a finding at least partially demonstrated by the fact that exacerbations can be precipitated by fingolimod, IFNβ and natalizumab, treatments that are effective in MS. Aside from the need for accurate diagnosis, evaluation of occult infection or metabolic disturbances should be carried out to identify pseudo-relapses Although there are no randomized controlled trials in large cohorts examining treatment of acute relapses, NMOSD exacerbations are typically treated with 1 g of IVMP for 3–5 consecutive days [147,148]. Severe NMOSD relapses or patients who do not respond to treatment with IVMP may benefit from plasma exchange (PLEX) [72,147–149]; which targets specific antibodies, complement and several pro-inflammatory proteins [150] Early (≤5 days), aggressive treatment with PLEX is linked to better outcome [151]. Interestingly, positive results of PLEX are obtained both in seropositive as well as seronegative NMOSD patients [152–154]. In order to avoid relapses, different immunosuppressive strategies are used in daily neurological practice including: oral corticosteroids, mycophenolate mofetil or azathioprine (both oral purine analog anti-metabolites), rituximab (IV anti-CD20 monoclonal antibody) and tocilizumab (anti-IL-6 receptor monoclonal antibody [146,147]. However, none of these agents have been specifically approved for NMOSD treatment, and off-label use has arisen based almost entirely on results from uncontrolled observational studies [146,147]. Recently, three new monoclonal antibodies with different mechanisms of action and routes of administration have shown efficacy in NMOSD patients: eculizumab (anti-complement protein C5) [155], inebilizumab (anti-CD19) [156], and satralizumab (anti-IL-6R) [157], significantly reducing risk of new relapses compared to placebo, particularly in AQP4-ab-positive patients, with clinical stabilization or improvement in most cases. All these drugs demonstrated good safety and tolerability profiles with limited side effects. Future evaluation in real-life studies will be needed though, to estimate annual relapse rates and compare results to those of older drugs.

5. Myelin Oligodendrocyte Glycoprotein Antibody-Associated Disease

Myelin oligodendrocyte glycoprotein, a member of the immunoglobulin superfamily, is exclusively expressed on the surface of oligodendrocytes and on the outermost lamellae of myelin sheaths in the CNS. Given its structure and location it could potentially function as a cell surface receptor, or cell adhesion molecule. Furthermore, its extracellular location makes it a target for autoimmune ab- and cell-mediated responses, in inflammatory demyelinating diseases. Interesting results from animal studies on MOG ab-associated demyelination lead to this antibody being considered a marker for MS [158,159]. However, subsequent studies in large populations of MS patients found seropositivity prevalence in this condition was similar to that detected in other inflammatory neurological diseases, as well as to levels in control subjects, generating skepticism over whether these ab could be considered a true biomarker of MS [160–162]. Seminal studies using murine anti-MOG ab have highlighted the fact that ab target epitopes of native MOG are biologically relevant in their conformational state, rather than in linearized or denatured MOG. Therefore, CBA, which maintains the native conformational form of the extracellular portion of MOG, is the most recommended technique to study ab levels.

There is current international consensus that anti-MOG ab are important in both pediatric and adult demyelination. Different research groups have identified seropositive MOG ab populations in children with ADEM, particularly in recurrent forms of the disease [163–166]. Other studies later confirmed presence of MOG ab in 25% to 30% of AQP4 seronegative NMOSD patients with recurrent ON. Substantial differences between both diseases in histopathology, as well as in vivo and vitro studies demonstrating a direct pathogenic role for MOG-IgG, suggest it represents a separate individual entity. Anti-MOG ab are already present at disease onset, both in serum and CSF, in some patients, persisting also during remission in the majority of patients, which argues against anti-MOG ab presence as a secondary epiphenomenon [167–170]. Notably, serum anti-MOG ab detection is more sensitive than CSF assay.

Since these observations, an increasing number of patients with diverse phenotypes related to these antibodies have been described. A comparison of patients with MOG ab disease to AQP4 NMOSD cases showed the former were younger [68,169–171], did not show significant female predominance [172], and were more commonly Caucasians; whereas AQP4-seropositive NMOSD was found predominantly in non-Caucasian populations [173,174].

The most commonly reported presentation of anti-MOG ab-associated disease is ON, which can be bilateral and recurrent in up to 61% of cases. Interesting, imaging of the optic nerve frequently shows peri-optic nerve sheath contrast enhancement, extending into the surrounding soft tissue, a radiological characteristic not observed in MS or AQP4 positive patients [175,176].

Approximately half the patients with MOG ab-associated disease present episodes involving the spinal cord [177,178]. The most common symptoms include paraparesis, and sensory and sphincter dysfunction. On MRI, LETM is frequent and short myelitis less common. Any segment of the spinal cord can be affected, although lesions are more frequent in the thoracolumbar and/or conus medullaris regions, as opposed to the more common cervicothoracic involvement observed in AQP4 ab positive and MS myelitis cases [178,179]. Anti-MOG ab associated myelitis is hyperintense on T2-weighted and iso-hypointense on T1-weighted sequences, showing contrast enhancement during acute phases in up to 70% of cases [172]; Figures 3 and 4. MOG ab-related disease does not commonly result in cord necrosis or cavitations as observed in AQP4-mediated cases [134,175,178]. Due to the predilection for conus localization, bladder, bowel, and erectile dysfunction is observed in approximately 70% of patients [167]. In comparison to AQP4-IgG$^+$ NMOSD, MOG ab disease myelitis appears to more focal and with better clinical outcome, although poor outcome with permanent disability has been described for both conditions [156]. Notably, anti-MOG ab serum titers follow disease activity levels, with significantly higher concentration during acute attacks than remission, further supporting the concept of their pathogenic role [172].

Although ON and myelitis are the two most frequent forms of presentation of anti-MOG ab disease, coexistence of brain, brainstem, or cerebellar involvement is frequent, and may even be extensive. Nausea, vomiting, and respiratory disturbances are some of the symptoms that can be present in cases of brainstem involvement [177].

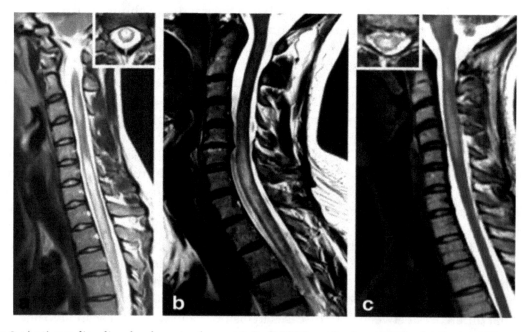

Figure 3. Anti-myelin oligodendrocyte glycoprotein (MOG) antibody myelitis. (**a**) Sagittal T2-weighted spinal MRI performed at disease onset revealed a large longitudinal centrally-located lesion extending over the entire spinal cord, as well as swelling of the cord. (**b**) Longitudinally extensive central spinal cord T2 lesion in another patient. (**c**) T2-hyperintense lesions extending from the pontomedullary junction throughout the cervical cord to C5, in a third patient. Insets in (**a**) and C show axial sections of the thoracic cord at lesion level [172].

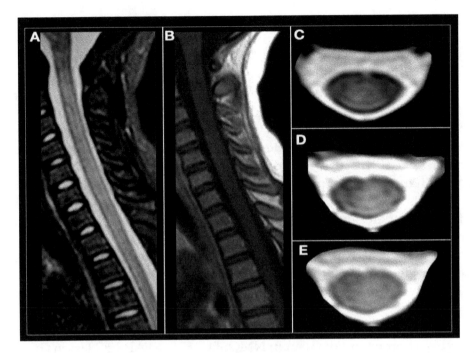

Figure 4. Anti-MOG antibody myelitis. A 12-year-old girl with relapse in the cervical spine. (**A**) sagittal STIR, subtle and diffuse hyperintensity of the cervical spinal cord. (**B**) Sagittal T1-weighted, spinal cord is isointense without contrast enhancement. (**C–E**) axial T2-weighted images showing subtle and diffuse spinal cord hyperintensity (Courtesy Dr. Angeles Schteinschnaider).

Different study groups have developed MRI diagnostic criteria to differentiate MS, from NMOSD and from anti-MOG ab-associated disease, showing 91% sensitivity distinguishing MS from AQP4+ NMOSD, and 95% from anti-MOG ab-associated disease [173,179]. More recently, the criteria were subtly modified to include spinal cord in the analysis, increasing sensitivity to 100% and specificity to 79%, reflecting the crucial importance of spinal cord findings in anti-MOG-ab disease. Interestingly, this radiological criterion was particularly useful in patients with ON, a clinical presentation common to all three diseases [180].

Patients with anti-MOG ab-associated disease were initially described as experiencing a monophasic disease [91,140,178]. However, recent studies found a high proportion of patients presenting relapsing disease [173,181]. Anti-MOG ab-positive patients exhibited better motor and visual outcome compared to AQP4-IgG positive patients after the first episode [170,181].

Anti-MOG ab are present in approximately 40% of children with ADEM. In this group, most patients develop LETM, and similar to patients without anti-MOG ab, show large, ill-defined, bilateral lesions in the brain, which typically resolve completely, in correlation with improved clinical outcome [165,177].

MOG ab-positive patients show rapid response to steroids and plasma exchange [177], but tend to relapse quickly after steroid withdrawal or cessation [182,183]. Therefore, slow steroid taper is recommended to minimize chances of early relapses. In adult patients, persistent seropositivity following initial treatment and clinical resolution is one of the main reasons to consider long term immunosuppression with steroid-sparing agents including mycophenolate, azathioprine or rituximab [135,169,170,184–186]. The significance of this finding is less clear in pediatric patients with ADEM and persistence of serum anti-MOG abs.

6. Glial Fibrillary Acid Protein Antibody-Associated Myelitis

A novel autoimmune CNS disorder characterized by the presence of antibodies specific for glial fibrillary acidic protein (GFAP) has recently been described. In the largest series published to date, median symptom onset age was around 40 years, with similar incidence in both women and men [187,188]. All patients with GFAP-IgGs reacted against the mature (α) GFAP isoform, with only a few patients showing immunoreactivity against the immature (ϵ) isoform [188]. GFAP is a cytoplasmic protein not accessible to IgG in intact cells, therefore, it is possible that immune cells also contribute to the tissue damage observed in this condition, for example GFAP peptide-specific CD8$^+$ T lymphocytes [189]. Eventually other immune cells sensitive to steroids, such as microglia and macrophages, can also play a role in the disease, acting directly, or through the release of molecules modulating the immune response such as cytokines or chemokines [187,190–192].

Clinical phenotype of GFAP-IgG astrocytopathy is heterogeneous and still poorly defined. The predominant clinical syndrome includes meningitis, encephalitis, and myelitis, or all three (meningoencephalomyelitis) with or without optic disc edema [188,193,194].

Myelitis occurs in up to 68% of patients with GFAP-IgG. However, its presentation as isolated clinical manifestation is infrequent. Despite the fact that autoimmune GFAP astrocytopathy and NMOSD-related myelitis share some clinical features, certain differences are worth mentioning [195]. Influenza-like prodromal symptoms and bowel/bladder dysfunction are common features in GFAP-IgG myelitis, while numbness and weakness followed by tonic spasms, frequent NMOSD symptoms, are rare. Notably, sensory level and Lhermitte's phenomenon are usually absent in GFAP-IgG myelitis, which is found in the cervical or thoracic spinal cord, in central location, usually involving at least three vertebral segments [195]. Lesions are hyperintense on T2-weighted sequences and may show a thin and linear pattern of contrast enhancement along the course of the central canal, different to the patchy or ring-like contrast uptake seen in NMOSD [187]. GFAP-IgG lesions have poorly-defined margins and less cord swelling compared to AQP4-IgG myelitis [195]. Short myelitis has also been reported in association with brain symptoms [187,194,195].

Notably, brain MRI findings significantly contribute to discriminate GFAP-IgG from other pathologies. A striking pattern of linear radial periventricular contrast enhancement is highly specific for GFAP-IgG-associated disease. Similar radial enhancement patterns have been described in the cerebellum in a lower percentage of patients [184,185,193].

Anti-GFAP abs can be detected in serum in 45% of patients, but sensitivity increases to 92% when ab are assayed in CSF [187]. Up to 50% of cases coexist with N-methyl-D-aspartate receptor (NMDAr) antibodies or anti-AQP4 ab, and up to 34% of patients may present concomitant neoplasms, with ovarian teratoma as the most prevalent [187]. These associations explain the diverse phenotypes reported [187,188,194]. Marked elevation of white cells and protein are common findings in CSF, and intrathecal oligoclonal bands may be present in 50% of patients [187].

Most reported GFAP-IgG cases show improvement in clinical, radiological, and CSF abnormalities after receiving high-dose intravenous methylprednisolone for 3–5 days [184,192]. Although nonresponsive-patients have been described, need for plasma exchange is significantly less frequent compared to patients with NMOSD [193,195,196]. In one study, 50% of patients with long-term follow-up (>24 months) had a relapsing course, 27% had a monophasic course and 23% had progressive disease in spite of adequate treatment. Clinical relapses were frequently associated with recurrent gadolinium enhancement on MRI and elevated CSF white cell count, with further remission observed after restarting steroids [187].

GFAP-IgG is unlikely to be directly pathogenic, as GFAP is an intracellular protein. However, it could be an excellent biomarker, identifying a neoplasm early on, leading to prompt and efficient treatment and prevention of long-term disability in GFAP-IgG myelitis cases.

7. Conclusions

Overall, demyelinating myelopathies belong to a complex and heterogeneous group of diseases, in which differential diagnosis can be difficult (Table 1). Clinical features, time-course, CSF characteristics, specific serum assays, and brain and spinal cord MRI findings all contribute to determine diagnosis, select the best treatment option and establish prognosis for each subtype. Early treatment with IV steroids and PLEX is accepted in all etiologies, but more specific treatment strategies may subsequently be adopted based on final diagnosis.

Table 1. Main features in demyelinating myelopathies of different etiology.

	MS	ADEM	NMOSD	MOG-IgG Disease	GFAP-IgG Disease
Estimated F:M ratio	3:1	1:1	9:1	1.3:1	1:1
Age * (yrs)	30	6	37	33	40
Myelitis clinical features	Sensory loss, gait impairment, weakness, sphincter involvement	Transverse myelitis	Transverse myelitis	Paraparesis, sensory symptoms and sphincter involvement	Sensory symptoms, sphincter disfunction
Clinical course	Relapsing (85%) or progressive (15%)	Typically monophasic (69-90%)	Relapsing (90%)	Monophasic (58%) or relapsing (42%)	Relapsing (50%), monophasic (27%) or progressive (23%)
Serology findings	Not relevant	Not relevant	Serum AQP4-IgG. coexistence with other systemic disease antibodies (ANA, SSA or SSB).	Serum MOG-IgG	Anti-GFAP ab + in serum or CSF (Serum Anti-AQP4-IgG and/or anti-NMDAr ab coexistence,
Presence of OCB	80-95%	0% to 29% (usually transient)	Up to 30% (usually transient)	Up to 12%	Up to 50%
CSF	Generally normal or mild inflammatory changes	Mild pleocytosis and increased proteins up to 62%	Pleocytosis (neutrophils and eosinophils can be found) and mild elevated proteins	Normal or slightly inflammatory changes	Marked elevation of white blood cells and elevated protein levels
Brain MRI	Dawson fingers, lesions perpendicular to ventricles Cortical/yuxtacortical lesions Perivenular Nodular or ring/open-ring enhancing lesions Unilateral short optic nerve enhancement	Subcortical or deep gray matter bilateral, sometimes poorly-defined Simultaneous enhancement with gadolinium	Periependimal lesions Tumefactive lesions Involvement of corticospinal tract Marked enhancement, 'cloud like' Bilateral, long optic nerve enhancement	Non-specific supratentorial subcortical or small deep white matter foci. Occasionally T2 lesions in brainstem, and infratentorial regions Anterior bilateral ON with perineural optic nerved enhancement	Linear radial periventricular contrast enhancement pattern
Spinal cord MRI	Small, peripheral, posterolateral lesions Less than 3 segments Gadolinium enhancement during acute phase	LETM or multiple short segment myelitis Edematous lesions and gadolinium enhancement in acute phase	Central LETM Edematous Necrosis or cavitation Gadolinium enhancement in acute phase	LETM or short myelitis, frequent conus medullaris involvement Linear gadolinium enhancement of the ependymal canal	LETM Central lesions

Ab: antibodies, ADEM: acute disseminated encephalomyelitis, AQP4: Aquaporin 4, F: female, GFAP: glial fibrillary acid protein, LETM: longitudinally extensive transverse myelitis, M: male, MOG: myelin oligodendrocyte glycoprotein, MRI: magnetic resonance imaging, MS: multiple sclerosis, NMDAr: N-Methyl-D-aspartate receptor, NMOSD: neuromyelitis optica spectrum disorder, OCB: oligoclonal bands. * estimated media.

Author Contributions: M.M. contributed to draft the original manuscript, design the figures, revise the draft and provide important intellectual contributions. M.I.G. contributed to draft the original manuscript, design the figures, revise the draft and provide important intellectual contributions. J.C. contributed to the conception and design of the manuscript, draft the original manuscript, revise the draft, provide important intellectual contributions, and supervised the writing of the manuscript. All authors have read and agreed to the published version of the manuscript.

Acknowledgments: We thank Angeles Schteinschnaider for providing Figure 4 and Ismael L. Calandri for providing the graphical abstract.

References

1. Barreras, P.; Fitzgerald, K.C.; Mealy, M.A.; Jimenez, J.A.; Becker, D.; Newsome, S.D.; Levy, M.; Gailloud, P.; Pardo, C.A. Clinical biomarkers differentiate myelitis from vascular and other causes of myelopathy. *Neurology* **2018**, *90*, E12–E21. [CrossRef] [PubMed]

2. Transverse Myelitis Consortium Working Group. Proposed diagnostic criteria and nosology of acute transverse myelitis. *Neurology* **2002**, *59*, 499–505. [CrossRef] [PubMed]

3. de Seze, J.; Lanctin, C.; Lebrun, C.; Malikova, I.; Papeix, C.; Wiertlewski, S.; Pelletier, J.; Gout, O.; Clerc, C.; Moreau, C.; et al. Idiopathic acute transverse myelitis: Application of the recent diagnostic criteria. *Neurology* **2005**, *65*, 1950–1953. [CrossRef] [PubMed]

4. Jacob, A.; Weinshenker, B.G. An approach to the diagnosis of acute transverse myelitis. *Semin. Neurol.* **2008**, *28*, 105–120. [CrossRef] [PubMed]

5. GBD 2015 Neurological Disorders Collaborator Group. Global, regional, and national burden of neurological disorders during 1990–2015: A systematic analysis for the Global Burden of Disease Study 2015. *Lancet Neurol.* **2017**, *16*, 877–897. [CrossRef]

6. Dendrou, C.A.; Fugger, L.; Friese, M.A. Immunopathology of multiple sclerosis. *Nat. Rev. Immunol.* **2015**, *15*, 545–558. [CrossRef] [PubMed]

7. McFarland, H.F.; Martin, R. Multiple sclerosis: A complicated picture of autoimmunity. *Nat. Immunol.* **2007**, *8*, 913–919. [CrossRef]

8. Lublin, F.D.; Reingold, S.C.; Cohen, J.A.; Cutter, G.R.; Sørensen, P.S.; Thompson, A.J.; Wolinsky, J.S.; Balcer, L.J.; Banwell, B.; Barkhof, F.; et al. Defining the clinical course of multiple sclerosis: The 2013 revisions. *Neurology* **2014**, *83*, 278–286. [CrossRef]

9. Compston, A.; Mc Donald, I.; Noseworthy, J.; Lassmann, H.; Miller, D.; Smith, K.; Wekerle, H.; Confavreux, C. *McAlpine's Multiple Sclerosis*, 4th ed.; Churchill-Livingstone: London, UK, 2005.

10. Cordonnier, C.; De Seze, J.; Breteau, G.; Ferriby, D.; Michelin, E.; Stojkovic, T.; Pruvo, J.P.; Vermersch, P. Prospective study of patients presenting with acute partial transverse myelopathy. *J. Neurol.* **2003**, *250*, 1447–1452. [CrossRef]

11. Kantarci, O.H. Phases and Phenotypes of Multiple Sclerosis. *Continuum (Minneap Minn)* **2019**, *25*, 636–654. [CrossRef]

12. Ingle, G.T.; Sastre-Garriga, J.; Miller, D.H.; Thomson, A.J. Is inflammation important in early PPMS? A longitudinal MRI study. *J. Neurol. Neurosurg. Psychiatry* **2005**, *76*, 1255–1258. [CrossRef] [PubMed]

13. Koch, M.W.; Greenfield, J.; Javizian, O.; Deighton, S.; Wall, W.; Metz, L.M. The natural history of early versus late disability accumulation in primary progressive M.S. *J. Neurol. Neurosurg. Psychiatry* **2015**, *86*, 615–621. [CrossRef] [PubMed]

14. Vukusic, S.; Confavreux, C. Primary and secondary progressive multiple sclerosis. *J. Neurol. Sci.* **2003**, *206*, 153–155. [CrossRef]

15. Marrodan, M.; Bensi, C.; Pappolla, A.; Rojas, J.I.; Gaitán, M.I.; Ysrraelit, M.C.; Negrotto, L.; Fiol, M.P.; Patrucco, L.; Cristiano, E. Disease activity impacts disability progression in primary progressive multiple sclerosis. *Mult. Scler. Relat. Disord.* **2020**, *39*, 101892. [CrossRef] [PubMed]

16. Androdias, G.; Reynolds, R.; Chanal, M.; Ritleng, C.; Confavreux, C.; Nataf, S. Meningeal T cells associate with diffuse axonal loss in multiple sclerosis spinal cords. *Ann. Neurol.* **2010**, *68*, 465–476. [CrossRef] [PubMed]

17. Cross, A.H.; McCarron, R.; McFarlin, D.E.; Raine, C.S. Adoptively transferred acute and chronic relapsing autoimmune encephalomyelitis in the PL/J mouse and observations on altered pathology by intercurrent virus infection. *Lab. Investig.* **1987**, *57*, 499–512.

18. Schwartz, M.; Butovsky, O.; Brück, W.; Hanisch, U.K. Microglial phenotype: Is the commitment reversible? *Trends Neurosci.* **2006**, *29*, 68–74. [CrossRef]

19. Krieger, S.C.; Lublin, F.D. Location, location, location. *Mult. Scler. J.* **2018**, *24*, 1396–1398. [CrossRef]

20. Thompson, A.J.; Banwell, B.L.; Barkhof, F.; Carroll, W.M.; Coetzee, T.; Comi, G.; Correale, J.; Fazekas, F.; Filippi, M.; Freedman, M.S.; et al. Diagnosis of multiple sclerosis: 2017 revisions of the McDonald criteria. *Lancet Neurol.* **2018**, *17*, 162–173. [CrossRef]

21. Lycklama, G.; Thompson, A.; Filippi, M.; Miller, D.; Polman, C.; Fazekas, F.; Barkhof, F. Spinal-cord MRI in multiple sclerosis. *Lancet Neurol.* **2003**, *2*, 555–562. [CrossRef]

22. Lycklama, À.; Nijeholt, G.J.; Castelijns, J.A.; Weerts, J.; Adèr, H.; van Waesberghe, J.H.; Polman, C.; Barkhof, F. Sagittal MR of multiple sclerosis in the spinal cord: Fast versus conventional spin-echo imaging. *Am. J. Neuroradiol.* **1998**, *19*, 355–360.

23. Gass, A.; Rocca, M.A.; Agosta, F.; Ciccarelli, O.; Chard, D.; Valsasina, P.; Brooks, J.C.; Bischof, A.; Eisele, P.; Kappos, L.; et al. MRI monitoring of pathological changes in the spinal cord in patients with multiple sclerosis. *Lancet Neurol.* **2015**, *14*, 443–454. [CrossRef]

24. Rovira, Á.; Wattjes, M.P.; Tintoré, M.; Tur, C.; Yousry, T.A.; Sormani, M.P.; De Stefano, N.; Filippi, M.; Auger, C.; Rocca, M.A.; et al. Evidence-based guidelines: MAGNIMS consensus guidelines on the use of MRI in multiple sclerosis—Clinical implementation in the diagnostic process. *Nat. Rev. Neurol.* **2015**, *11*, 471–482. [CrossRef]

25. Bergers, E.; Bot, J.C.J.; De Groot, C.J.A.; Polman, C.H.; Lycklama, G.J.; Nijeholt, Á.; Castelijns, J.A.; van der Valk, P.; Barkhof, F. Axonal damage in the spinal cord of MS patients occurs largely independent of T2 MRI lesions. *Neurology* **2002**, *59*, 1766–1771. [CrossRef]

26. Weier, K.; Mazraeh, J.; Naegelin, Y.; Thoeni, A.; Hirsch, J.G.; Fabbro, T.; Bruni, N.; Duyar, H.; Bendfeldt, K.; Radue, E.W. Biplanar MRI for the assessment of the spinal cord in multiple sclerosis. *Mult. Scler. J.* **2012**, *18*, 1560–1569. [CrossRef] [PubMed]

27. Breckwoldt, M.O.; Gradl, J.; Hähnel, S.; Hielscher, T.; Wildemann, B.; Diem, R.; Platten, M.; Wick, W.; Heiland, S.; Bendszus, M. Increasing the sensitivity of MRI for the detection of multiple sclerosis lesions by long axial coverage of the spinal cord: A prospective study in 119 patients. *J. Neurol.* **2017**, *264*, 341–349. [CrossRef]

28. Martin, N.; Malfair, D.; Zhao, Y.; Li, D.; Traboulsee, A.; Lang, F.; Vertinsky, A.T. Comparison of MERGE and axial T2-weighted fast spin-echo sequences for detection of multiple sclerosis lesions in the cervical spinal cord. *Am. J. Roentgenol.* **2012**, *199*, 157–162. [CrossRef] [PubMed]

29. Zalewski, N.L.; Morris, P.P.; Weinshenker, B.G.; Lucchinetti, C.F.; Guo, Y.; Pittock, S.J.; Krecke, K.N.; Kaufmann, T.J.; Wingerchuk, D.M.; Kumar, N.; et al. Ring-enhancing spinal cord lesions in neuromyelitis optica spectrum disorders. *J. Neurol. Neurosurg. Psychiatry* **2017**, *88*, 218–225. [CrossRef] [PubMed]

30. Ciccarelli, O.; Cohen, J.A.; Reingold, S.C.; Weinshenker, B.G. Spinal cord involvement in multiple sclerosis and neuromyelitis optica spectrum disorders. *Lancet Neurol.* **2019**, *18*, 185–197. [CrossRef]

31. de Seze, J. Acute myelopathies: Clinical, laboratory and outcome profiles in 79 cases. *Brain* **2001**, *124*, 1509–1521. [CrossRef]

32. Kitley, J.L.; Leite, M.I.; George, J.S.; Palace, J.A. The differential diagnosis of longitudinally extensive transverse myelitis. *Mult. Scler. J.* **2012**, *18*, 271–285. [CrossRef] [PubMed]

33. Geraldes, R.; Ciccarelli, O.; Barkhof, F.; De Stefano, N.; Enzinger, C.; Filippi, M.; Hofer, M.; Paul, F.; Preziosa, P.; Rovira, A.; et al. The current role of MRI in differentiating multiple sclerosis from its imaging mimics. *Nat. Rev. Neurol.* **2018**, *14*, 199–213. [CrossRef] [PubMed]

34. Kantarci, O.H.; Lebrun, C.; Siva, A.; Keegan, M.B.; Azevedo, C.J.; Inglese, M.; Tintoré, M.; Newton, B.D.; Durand-Dubief, F.; Amato, M.P.; et al. Primary Progressive Multiple Sclerosis Evolving from Radiologically Isolated Syndrome. *Ann. Neurol.* **2016**, *79*, 288–294. [CrossRef]

35. O'Riordan, J.I.; Thompson, A.J.; Kingsley, D.P.E.; MacManus, D.G.; Kendall, B.E.; Rudge, P.; McDonald, W.I.; Miller, D.H. The prognostic value of brain MRI in clinically isolated syndromes of the CNS. A 10-year follow-up. *Brain* **1998**, *121*, 495–503. [CrossRef] [PubMed]

36. Bot, J.C.J.; Barkhof, F.; Polman, C.H.; Lycklama, Á.; Nijeholt, G.J.; de Groot, V.; Bergers, E.; Ader, H.J.; Castelijns, J.A. Spinal cord abnormalities in recently diagnosed MS patients: Added value of spinal MRI examination. *Neurology* **2004**, *62*, 226–233. [CrossRef] [PubMed]

37. Arrambide, G.; Tintore, M.; Auger, C.; Río, J.; Castilló, J.; Vidal-Jordana, A.; Galán, I.; Nos, C.; Comabella, M.; Mitjana, R.; et al. Lesion topographies in multiple sclerosis diagnosis: A reappraisal. *Neurology* **2017**, *89*, 2351–2356. [CrossRef] [PubMed]

38. Brownlee, W.J.; Altmann, D.R.; Alves Da Mota, P.; Swanton, J.K.; Miszkiel, K.A.; Wheeler-Kingshott, C.G.; Ciccarelli, O.; Miller, D.H. Association of asymptomatic spinal cord lesions and atrophy with disability 5 years after a clinically isolated syndrome. *Mult. Scler. J.* **2017**, *23*, 665–674. [CrossRef] [PubMed]

39. Zecca, C.; Disanto, G.; Sormani, M.P.; Riccitelli, G.C.; Cianfoni, A.; Del Grande, F.; Pravatà, E.; Gobbi, C. Relevance of asymptomatic spinal MRI lesions in patients with multiple sclerosis. *Mult. Scler. J.* **2016**, *22*, 782–791. [CrossRef]

40. Vukusic, S.; Confavreux, C. Prognostic factors for progression of disability in the secondary progressive phase of multiple sclerosis. *J. Neurol. Sci.* **2003**, *206*, 135–137. [CrossRef]

41. Biberacher, V.; Boucard, C.C.; Schmidt, P.; Engl, C.; Buck, D.; Berthele, A.; Hoshi, M.M.; Zimmer, C.; Hemmer, B.; Mühlau, M. Atrophy and structural variability of the upper cervical cord in early multiple sclerosis. *Mult. Scler. J.* **2015**, *21*, 875–884. [CrossRef]

42. Casserly, C.; Seyman, E.E.; Alcaide-Leon, P.; Guenette, M.; Lyons, C.; Sankar, S.; Svendrovski, A.; Baral, S.; Oh, J. Spinal Cord Atrophy in Multiple Sclerosis: A Systematic Review and Meta-Analysis. *J. Neuroimaging* **2018**, *28*, 556–586. [CrossRef] [PubMed]

43. Schlaeger, R.; Papinutto, N.; Zhu, A.H.; Lobach, I.V.; Bevan, C.J.; Bucci, M.; Castellano, A.; Gelfand, J.M.; Graves, J.S.; Green, A.J.; et al. Association Between Thoracic Spinal Cord Gray Matter Atrophy and Disability in Multiple Sclerosis. *JAMA Neurol.* **2015**, *72*, 897–904. [CrossRef] [PubMed]

44. Agosta, F.; Pagani, E.; Caputo, D.; Fillippi, M. Associations between cervical cord gray matter damage and disability in patients with multiple sclerosis. *Arch. Neurol.* **2007**, *64*, 1302–1305. [CrossRef] [PubMed]

45. Schlaeger, R.; Papinutto, N.; Panara, V.; Bevan, C.; Lobach, I.V.; Bucci, M.; Caverzasi, E.; Gelfand, J.M.; Green, A.J.; Jordan, K.M.; et al. Spinal cord gray matter atrophy correlates with multiple sclerosis disability. *Ann. Neurol.* **2014**, *76*, 568–580. [CrossRef]

46. Tsagkas, C.; Magon, S.; Gaetano, L.; Pezold, S.; Naegelin, Y.; Amann, M.; Stippich, C.; Cattin, P.; Wuerfel, J.; Bieri, O.; et al. Spinal cord volume loss: A marker of disease progression in multiple sclerosis. *Neurology* **2018**, *91*, e349–e358. [CrossRef]

47. Kearney, H.; Rocca, M.A.; Valsasina, P.; Balk, L.; Sastre-Garriga, J.; Reinhardt, J.; Ruggieri, J.; Rovira, A.; Stippich, C.; Kappos, L.; et al. Magnetic resonance imaging correlates of physical disability in relapse onset multiple sclerosis of long disease duration. *Mult. Scler. J.* **2014**, *20*, 72–80. [CrossRef]

48. Oh, J.; Sotirchos, E.S.; Saidha, S.; Whetstone, A.; Chen, M.; Newsome, S.D.; Zackowski, K.; Balcer, L.J.; Frohman, E.; Prince, J.; et al. Relationships between quantitative spinal cord MRI and retinal layers in multiple sclerosis. *Neurology* **2015**, *84*, 720–728. [CrossRef]

49. Valsasina, P.; Agosta, F.; Absinta, M.; Sala, S.; Caputo, D.; Filippi, M. Cervical cord functional MRI changes in relapse-onset MS patients. *J. Neurol. Neurosurg. Psychiatry* **2010**, *81*, 405–408. [CrossRef]

50. Lukas, C.; Knol, D.L.; Sombekke, M.H.; Bellenberg, B.; Hahn, H.K.; Popescu, V.; Weier, K.; Radue, E.W.; Gass, A.; Kappos, L.; et al. Cervical spinal cord volume loss is related to clinical disability progression in multiple sclerosis. *J. Neurol. Neurosurg. Psychiatry* **2015**, *86*, 410–418. [CrossRef]

51. Rocca, M.A.; Valsasina, P.; Damjanovic, D.; Horsfield, M.A.; Mesaros, S.; Stosic-Opincal, T.; Drulovic, J.; Filippi, M. Voxel-wise mapping of cervical cord damage in multiple sclerosis patients with different clinical phenotypes. *J. Neurol. Neurosurg. Psychiatry* **2013**, *84*, 35–41. [CrossRef]

52. Lin, X.; Blumhardt, L.D.; Constantinescu, C.S. The relationship of brain and cervical cord volume to disability in clinical subtypes of multiple sclerosis: A three-dimensional MRI study. *Acta Neurol. Scand.* **2003**, *108*, 401–406. [CrossRef] [PubMed]

53. Gilmore, C.P.; Deluca, G.C.; Bö, L.; Owens, T.; Lowe, J.; Esiri, M.M.; Evangelou, N. Spinal cord neuronal pathology in multiple sclerosis. *Brain Pathol.* **2009**, *19*, 642–649. [CrossRef] [PubMed]

54. Montalban, X.; Sastre-Garriga, J.; Filippi, M.; Khaleeli, Z.; Téllez, N.; Vellinga, M.M.; Tur, C.; Brochet, B.; Barkhof, F.; Rovaris, M.; et al. Primary progressive multiple sclerosis diagnostic criteria: A reappraisal. *Mult. Scler.* **2009**, *15*, 1459–1465. [CrossRef] [PubMed]

55. Kapoor, R.; Furby, J.; Hayton, T.; Smith, K.J.; Altmann, D.R.; Brenner, R.; Chataway, J.; Hughes, R.A.; Miller, D.H. Lamotrigine for neuroprotection in secondary progressive multiple sclerosis: A randomised, double-blind, placebo-controlled, parallel-group trial. *Lancet Neurol.* **2010**, *9*, 681–688. [CrossRef]

56. Cawley, N.; Tur, C.; Prados, F.; Plantone, D.; Kearney, H.; Abdel-Aziz, K.; Ourselin, S.; Wheeler-Kingshott, C.A.G.; Miller, D.H.; Thompson, A.J.; et al. Spinal cord atrophy as a primary outcome measure in phase II trials of progressive multiple sclerosis. *Mult. Scler. J.* **2018**, *24*, 932–941. [CrossRef]

57. Evangelou, N.; DeLuca, G.C.; Owens, T.; Esiri, M.M. Pathological study of spinal cord atrophy in multiple sclerosis suggests limited role of local lesions. *Brain* **2005**, *128*, 29–34. [CrossRef]

58. Kearney, H.; Miszkiel, K.A.; Yiannakas, M.C.; Ciccarelli, O.; Miller, D.H. A pilot MRI study of white and grey matter involvement by multiple sclerosis spinal cord lesions. *Mult. Scler. Relat. Disord.* **2013**, *2*, 103–108. [CrossRef]

59. Philpott, C.; Brotchie, P. Comparison of MRI sequences for evaluation of multiple sclerosis of the cervical spinal cord at 3 T. *Eur. J. Radiol.* **2011**, *80*, 780–785. [CrossRef]

60. Calabrese, M.; De Stefano, N.; Atzori, M.; Bernardi, V.; Mattisi, I.; Barachino, L.; Rinaldi, L.; Morra, A.; McAuliffe, M.M.; Perini, P.; et al. Detection of cortical inflammatory lesions by double inversion recovery magnetic resonance imaging in patients with multiple sclerosis. *Arch. Neurol.* **2007**, *64*, 1416–1422. [CrossRef]

61. Bot, J.C.; Barkhof, F.; Lycklama à Nijeholt, G.J.; Bergers, E.; Polman, C.H.; Adèr, H.J.; Castelijns, J.A. Comparison of a conventional cardiac-triggered dual spin-echo and a fast STIR sequence in detection of spinal cord lesions in multiple sclerosis. *Eur. Radiol.* **2000**, *10*, 753–758. [CrossRef]

62. Sethi, V.; Yousry, T.A.; Muhlert, N.; Ron, M.; Golay, X.; Wheeler-Kingshott, C.; Miller, D.H.; Chard, D.T. Improved detection of cortical MS lesions with phase-sensitive inversion recovery MRI. *J. Neurol. Neurosurg. Psychiatry* **2012**, *83*, 877–882. [CrossRef] [PubMed]

63. Nair, G.; Absinta, M.; Reich, D.S. Optimized T1-MPRAGE sequence for better visualization of spinal cord multiple sclerosis lesions at 3T. *AJNR Am. J. Neuroradiol.* **2013**, *34*, 2215–2222. [CrossRef] [PubMed]

64. Gilmore, C.P.; Bö, L.; Owens, T.; Lowe, J.; Esiri, M.M.; Evangelou, N. Spinal cord gray matter demyelination in multiple sclerosis-a novel pattern of residual plaque morphology. *Brain Pathol.* **2006**, *16*, 202–208. [CrossRef] [PubMed]

65. Lublin, F.D.; Baier, M.; Cutter, G. Effect of relapses on development of residual deficit in multiple sclerosis. *Neurology* **2003**, *61*, 1528–1532. [CrossRef] [PubMed]

66. Koch-Henriksen, N.; Thygesen, L.C.; Sørensen, P.S.; Migyari, M. Worsening of disability caused by relapses in multiple sclerosis: A different approach. *Mult. Scler. Relat. Disord.* **2019**, *32*, 1–8. [CrossRef] [PubMed]

67. Berkovich, R.R. Acute Multiple Sclerosis Relapse. *Continuum (Minneap Minn)* **2016**, *22*, 799–814. [CrossRef]

68. Goodin, D.S. Glucocorticoid treatment of multiple sclerosis. *Handb. Clin. Neurol.* **2014**, *122*, 455–464.

69. Stoppe, M.; Busch, M.; Krizek, L.; Then Bergh, F. Outcome of MS relapses in the era of disease-modifying therapy. *BMC Neurol.* **2017**, *17*, 151. [CrossRef]

70. Schröder, A.; Linker, R.A.; Gold, R. Plasmapheresis for neurological disorders. *Expert Rev. Neurother.* **2009**, *9*, 1331–1339. [CrossRef]

71. Pfeuffer, S.; Rolfes, L.; Bormann, E.; Sauerland, C.; Ruck, T.; Schilling, M.; Melzer, N.; Brand, M.; Pul, R.; Kleinschnitz, C.; et al. Comparing Plasma Exchange to Escalated Methyl Prednisolone in Refractory Multiple Sclerosis Relapses. *J. Clin. Med.* **2019**, *9*, 35. [CrossRef]

72. Keegan, M.; Pineda, A.A.; McClelland, R.L.; Darby, C.H.; Rodriguez, M.; Weinshenker, B.G. Plasma exchange for severe attacks of CNS demyelination: Predictors of response. *Neurology* **2002**, *58*, 143–148. [CrossRef] [PubMed]

73. Derfuss, T.; Mehling, M.; Papadopoulou, A.; Bar-Or, A.; Cohen, J.A.; Kappos, L. Advances in oral immunomodulating therapies in relapsing multiple sclerosis. *Lancet Neurol.* **2020**, *19*, 336–347. [CrossRef]

74. Ontaneda, D.; Tallantyre, E.; Kalincik, T.; Planchon, S.M.; Evangelou, N. Early highly effective versus escalation treatment approaches in relapsing multiple sclerosis. *Lancet Neurol.* **2019**, *18*, 973–980. [CrossRef]

75. Reich, D.S.; Lucchinetti, C.F.; Calabresi, P.A. Multiple sclerosis. *N. Engl. J. Med.* **2018**, *378*, 169–180. [CrossRef] [PubMed]

76. Correale, J.; Gaitán, M.I.; Ysrraelit, M.C.; Fiol, M.P. Progressive multiple sclerosis: From pathogenic mechanisms to treatment. *Brain* **2017**, *140*, 527–546. [CrossRef]

77. Young, N.P.; Weinshenker, B.G.; Lucchinetti, C.F. Acute disseminated encephalomyelitis: Current understanding and controversies. *Semin. Neurol.* **2008**, *28*, 84–94. [CrossRef]

78. Tenembaum, S.; Chitnis, T.; Ness, J.; Hahn, J.S.; International Pediatric MS Study Group. Acute disseminated encephalomyelitis. *Neurology* **2007**, *68*, S23–S36. [CrossRef]

79. Tenembaum, S.N. Acute disseminated encephalomyelitis. *Handb. Clin. Neurol.* **2013**, *112*, 1253–1262.

80. de Mol, C.L.; Wong, Y.Y.M.; van Pelt, E.D.; Ketelslegers, I.A.; Bakker, D.P.; Boon, M.; Braun, K.P.J.; van Dijk, K.G.J.; Eikelenboom, M.J.; Engelen, M.; et al. Incidence and outcome of acquired demyelinating syndromes in Dutch children: Update of a nationwide and prospective study. *J. Neurol.* **2018**, *265*, 1310–1319. [CrossRef]

81. Yamaguchi, Y.; Torisu, H.; Kira, R.; Ishizaki, Y.; Sakai, Y.; Sanefuji, M.; Ichiyama, T.; Oka, A.; Kishi, T.; Kimura, S.; et al. A nationwide survey of pediatric acquired demyelinating syndromes in Japan. *Neurology* **2016**, *87*, 2006–2015. [CrossRef]

82. Xiong, C.H.; Yan, Y.; Liao, Z.; Peng, S.H.; Wen, H.R.; Zhang, Y.X.; Chen, S.H.; Li, J.; Chen, H.Y.; Feng, X.W.; et al. Epidemiological characteristics of acute disseminated encephalomyelitis in Nanchang, China: A retrospective study. *BMC Public Health* **2014**, *14*, 111. [CrossRef] [PubMed]

83. Karussis, D.; Petrou, P. The spectrum of post-vaccination inflammatory CNS demyelinating syndromes. *Autoimmun. Rev.* **2014**, *13*, 215–224. [CrossRef] [PubMed]

84. Tenembaum, S.; Chamoles, N.; Fejerman, N. Acute disseminated encephalomyelitis: A long-term follow-up study of 84 pediatric patients. *Neurology* **2002**, *59*, 1224–1231. [CrossRef] [PubMed]

85. Fujinami, R.S.; Oldstone, M.B. Amino acid homology between the encephalitogenic site of myelin basic protein and virus: Mechanism for autoimmunity. *Science* **1985**, *230*, 1043–1045. [CrossRef]

86. Smyk, D.S.; Alexander, A.K.; Walker, M.; Walker, M. Acute disseminated encephalomyelitis progressing to multiple sclerosis: Are infectious triggers involved? *Immunol. Res.* **2014**, *60*, 16–22. [CrossRef]

87. Krupp, L.B.; Tardieu, M.; Amato, M.P.; Banwell, B.; Chitnis, T.; Dale, R.C.; Ghezzi, A.; Hintzen, R.; Kornberg, A.; Poh, D.; et al. International Pediatric Multiple Sclerosis Study Group criteria for pediatric multiple sclerosis and immune-mediated central nervous system demyelinating disorders: Revisions to the 2007 definitions. *Mult. Scler. J.* **2013**, *19*, 1261–1267. [CrossRef]

88. Cole, J.; Evans, E.; Mwangi, M.; Mar, S. Acute Disseminated Encephalomyelitis in Children: An Updated Review Based on Current Diagnostic Criteria. *Pediatr. Neurol.* **2019**, *100*, 26–34. [CrossRef]

89. Flanagan, E.P. Autoimmune myelopathies. *Handb. Clin. Neurol.* **2016**, *133*, 327–351.

90. Callen, D.J.A.; Shroff, M.M.; Branson, H.M.; Li, D.K.; Lotze, T.; Stephens, D.; Banwell, B.L. Role of MRI in the differentiation of ADEM from MS in children. *Neurology* **2009**, *72*, 968–973. [CrossRef]

91. Baumann, M.; Sahin, K.; Lechner, C.; Wendel, E.M.; Lechner, C.; Behring, B.; Blaschek, A.; Diepold, K.; Eisenkölbl, A.; Fluss, J.; et al. Clinical and neuroradiological differences of paediatric acute disseminating encephalomyelitis with and without antibodies to the myelin oligodendrocyte glycoprotein. *J. Neurol. Neurosurg. Psychiatry* **2015**, *86*, 265–272. [CrossRef]

92. Ketelslegers, I.A.; Visser, I.; Neuteboom, R.F.; Boon, M.; Catsman-Berrevoets, C.E.; Hintzen, R.Q. Disease course and outcome of acute disseminated encephalomyelitis is more severe in adults than in children. *Mult. Scler. J.* **2011**, *17*, 441–448. [CrossRef] [PubMed]

93. Leake, J.A.D.; Albani, S.; Kao, A.S.; Senac, M.O.; Billman, G.F.; Nespeca, M.P.; Paulino, A.D.; Quintela, E.R.; Sawyer, M.H.; Bradley, J.S. Acute disseminated encephalomyelitis in childhood: Epidemiologic, clinical and laboratory features. *Pediatr. Infect. Dis. J.* **2004**, *23*, 756–764. [CrossRef] [PubMed]

94. Hung, P.C.; Wang, H.S.; Chou, M.L.; Lin, K.L.; Hsieh, M.Y.; Wong, A.M.C. Acute disseminated encephalomyelitis in children: A single institution experience of 28 patients. *Neuropediatrics* **2012**, *43*, 64–71. [CrossRef] [PubMed]

95. Pavone, P.; Pettoello-Mantovano, M.; Le Pira, A.; Giardino, I.; Pulvirenti, A.; Giugno, R.; Parano, E.; Polizzi, A.; Distefano, A.; Ferro, A.; et al. Acute disseminated encephalomyelitis: A long-term prospective study and meta-analysis. *Neuropediatrics* **2010**, *41*, 246–255. [CrossRef]

96. Erol, I.; Ozkale, Y.; Alkan, O.; Alehan, F. Acute disseminated encephalomyelitis in children and adolescents: A single center experience. *Pediatr. Neurol.* **2013**, *49*, 266–273. [CrossRef]

97. Mikaeloff, Y.; Caridade, G.; Husson, B.; Suissa, S.; Tardieu, M.; Neuropediatric KIDSEP Study Group of the French Neuropediatric Society. Acute disseminated encephalomyelitis cohort study: Prognostic factors for relapse. *Eur. J. Paediatr. Neurol.* **2007**, *11*, 90–95. [CrossRef]

98. Pohl, D.; Alper, G.; Van Haren, K.; Kornberg, A.J.; Lucchinetti, C.F.; Tenembaum, S.; Belman, A.L. Acute disseminated encephalomyelitis: Updates on an inflammatory CNS syndrome. *Neurology* **2016**, *87*, S38–S45. [CrossRef]

99. Verhey, L.H.; Branson, H.M.; Shroff, M.M.; Callen, D.J.; Sled, J.G.; Narayanan, S.; Sadovnick, A.D.; Bar-Or, A.; Arnold, D.L.; Marrie, R.A.; et al. MRI parameters for prediction of multiple sclerosis diagnosis in children with acute CNS demyelination: A prospective national cohort study. *Lancet Neurol.* **2011**, *10*, 1065–1073. [CrossRef]

100. Lin, C.H.; Jeng, J.S.; Hsieh, S.T.; Yip, P.K.; Wu, R.M. Acute disseminated encephalomyelitis: A follow-up study in Taiwan. *J. Neurol. Neurosurg. Psychiatry* **2007**, *78*, 162–167. [CrossRef]

101. Waldman, A.; Gorman, M.; Rensel, M.; Austin, T.E.; Hertz, D.P.; Kuntz, N.L. Network of Pediatric Multiple Sclerosis Centers of Excellence of the National Multiple Sclerosis Society. Management of Pediatric Central Nervous System Demyelinating Disorders: Consensus of United States Neurologists. *J. Child. Neurol.* **2011**, *26*, 675–682. [CrossRef]

102. Dale, R.C. Acute disseminated encephalomyelitis, multiphasic disseminated encephalomyelitis and multiple sclerosis in children. *Brain* **2000**, *123*, 2407–2422. [CrossRef] [PubMed]

103. Khurana, D.S.; Melvin, J.J.; Kothare, S.V.; Valencia, I.; Hardison, H.H.; Yum, S.; Faerber, E.N.; Legido, A. Acute disseminated encephalomyelitis in children: Discordant neurologic and neuroimaging abnormalities and response to plasmapheresis. *Pediatrics* **2005**, *116*, 431–436. [CrossRef] [PubMed]

104. Pohl, D.; Tenembaum, S. Treatment of acute disseminated encephalomyelitis. *Curr. Treat. Options Neurol.* **2012**, *14*, 264–275. [CrossRef] [PubMed]

105. Jarius, S.; Wildemann, B. The history of neuromyelitis optica. *J. Neuroinflamm.* **2013**, *10*, 8. [CrossRef] [PubMed]

106. Lennon, P.V.A.; Wingerchuk, D.M.; Kryzer, T.J.; Pittock, S.J.; Lucchinetti, C.F.; Fujihara, K.; Nakashima, I.; Weinshenker, B.G. A serum autoantibody marker of neuromyelitis optica: Distinction from multiple sclerosis. *Lancet* **2004**, *364*, 2106–2112. [CrossRef]

107. Lennon, V.A.; Kryzer, T.J.; Pittock, S.J.; Verkman, A.S.; Hinson, S.R. IgG marker of optic-spinal multiple sclerosis binds to the aquaporin-4 water channel. *J. Exp. Med.* **2005**, *202*, 473–477. [CrossRef]

108. Wingerchuk, D.M.; Lennon, V.A.; Pittock, S.J.; Lucchinetti, C.F.; Weinshenker, B.G. Revised diagnostic criteria for neuromyelitis optica. *Neurology* **2006**, *66*, 1485–1489. [CrossRef]

109. Wingerchuk, D.M.; Lennon, V.A.; Lucchinetti, C.F.; Pittock, S.J.; Weinshenker, B.G. The spectrum of neuromyelitis optica. *Lancet Neurol.* **2007**, *6*, 805–815. [CrossRef]

110. Wingerchuk, D.M.; Banwell, B.; Bennett, J.L.; Cabre, P.; Carroll, W.; Chitnis, T.; de Seze, J.; Fujihara, K.; Greenberg, B.; Jacob, A.; et al. International consensus diagnostic criteria for neuromyelitis optica spectrum disorders. *Neurology* **2015**, *85*, 177–189. [CrossRef]

111. Saadoun, S.; Waters, P.; Bell, B.A.; Vincent, A.; Verkman, A.S.; Papadopoulos, M.C. Intra-cerebral injection of neuromyelitis optica immunoglobulin G and human complement produces neuromyelitis optica lesions in mice. *Brain* **2010**, *133*, 349–361. [CrossRef]

112. Ratelade, J.; Asavapanumas, N.; Ritchie, A.M.; Wemlinger, S.; Bennett, J.L.; Verkman, A.S. Involvement of antibody-dependent cell-mediated cytotoxicity in inflammatory demyelination in a mouse model of neuromyelitis optica. *Acta Neuropathol.* **2013**, *126*, 699–709. [CrossRef] [PubMed]

113. Bradl, M.; Misu, T.; Takahashi, T.; Watanabe, M.; Mader, S.; Reindl, M.; Adzemovic, M.; Bauer, J.; Berger, T.; Fujihara, K.; et al. Neuromyelitis optica: Pathogenicity of patient immunoglobulin in vivo. *Ann. Neurol.* **2009**, *66*, 630–643. [CrossRef] [PubMed]

114. Chang, V.T.W.; Chang, H.M. Review: Recent advances in the understanding of the pathophysiology of neuromyelitis optica spectrum disorder. *Neuropathol. Appl. Neurobiol.* **2020**, *46*, 199–218. [CrossRef] [PubMed]

115. Lucchinetti, C.F.; Mandler, R.N.; McGavern, D.; Bruck, W.; Gleich, G.; Ransohoff, R.M.; Trebst, C.; Weinshenker, B.; Wingerchuk, D.; Parisi, J.E.; et al. A role for humoral mechanisms in the pathogenesis of Devic's neuromyelitis optica. *Brain* **2002**, *125 Pt 7*, 1450–1461. [CrossRef]

116. Misu, T.; Fujihara, K.; Kakita, A.; Konno, H.; Nakamura, M.; Watanabe, S.; Takahashi, T.; Nakashima, I.; Takahashi, H.; Itoyama, Y. Loss of aquaporin 4 in lesions of neuromyelitis optica: Distinction from multiple sclerosis. *Brain* **2007**, *130*, 1224–1234. [CrossRef]

117. Pittock, S.J.; Lennon, V.A.; Krecke, K.; Wingerchuk, D.M.; Lucchinetti, C.F.; Weinshenker, B.G. Brain abnormalities in neuromyelitis optica. *Arch. Neurol.* **2006**, *63*, 390–396. [CrossRef]

118. Hinson, S.R.; Roemer, S.F.; Lucchinetti, C.F.; Fryer, J.P.; Kryzer, T.J.; Chamberlain, J.L.; Howe, C.L.; Pittock, S.J.; Lennon, V.A. Aquaporin-4-binding autoantibodies in patients with neuromyelitis optica impair glutamate transport by down- Regulating EAAT2. *J. Exp. Med.* **2008**, *205*, 2473–2481. [CrossRef]

119. Papadopoulos, M.; Verkman, A.S. Aquaporin 4 and neuromyelitis optica. *Lancet Neurol.* **2009**, *53*, 820–833. [CrossRef]

120. Rosenthal, J.F.; Hoffman, B.M.; Tyor, W.R. CNS inflammatory demyelinating disorders: MS, NMOSD and MOG antibody associated disease. *J. Investig. Med.* **2020**, *68*, 321–330. [CrossRef]

121. Jarius, S.; Ruprecht, K.; Wildemann, B.; Kuempfel, T.; Ringelstein, M.; Geis, C.; Kleiter, I.; Kleinschnitz, C.; Berthele, A.; Brettschneider, J.; et al. Contrasting disease patterns in seropositive and seronegative neuromyelitis optica: A multicentre study of 175 patients. *J. Neuroinflamm.* **2012**, *9*, 14. [CrossRef]

122. Ghezzi, A.; Bergamaschi, R.; Martinelli, V.; Trojano, M.; Tola, M.R.; Merelli, E.; Mancardi, L.; Gallo, P.; Filippi, M.; Zaffaroni, M.; et al. Clinical characteristics, course and prognosis of relapsing Devic's Neuromyelitis Optica. *J. Neurol.* **2004**, *251*, 47–52. [CrossRef] [PubMed]

123. Wingerchuk, D.M.; Hogancamp, W.F.; O'Brien, P.C.; Weinshenker, BG. The clinical course of neuromyelitis optica (Devic's syndrome). *Neurology* **1999**, *53*, 1107–1114. [CrossRef] [PubMed]

124. Yonezu, T.; Ito, S.; Mori, M.; Ogawa, Y.; Makino, T.; Uzawa, A.; Kuwabara, S. Bright spotty lesions on spinal magnetic resonance imaging differentiate neuromyelitis optica from multiple sclerosis. *Mult. Scler. J.* **2014**, *20*, 331–337. [CrossRef] [PubMed]

125. Flanagan, E.P.; Kaufmann, T.J.; Krecke, K.N.; Aksamit, A.J.; Pittock, S.J.; Keegan, B.M.; Giannini, C.; Weinshenker, B.G. Discriminating long myelitis of neuromyelitis optica from sarcoidosis. *Ann. Neurol.* **2016**, *79*, 437–447. [CrossRef] [PubMed]

126. Iorio, R.; Damato, V.; Mirabella, M.; Evoli, A.; Marti, A.; Plantone, D.; Frisullo, G.; Batocchi, A.P. Distinctive clinical and neuroimaging characteristics of longitudinally extensive transverse myelitis associated with aquaporin-4 autoantibodies. *J. Neurol.* **2013**, *260*, 2396–2402. [CrossRef]

127. Flanagan, E.P.; Weinshenker, B.G.; Krecke, K.N.; Lennon, V.A.; Lucchinetti, C.F.; McKeon, A.; Wingerchuk, D.M.; Shuster, E.A.; Jiao, Y.; Horta, E.S.; et al. Short myelitis lesions in aquaporin-4-IgG-positive neuromyelitis optica spectrum disorders. *JAMA Neurol.* **2015**, *72*, 81–87. [CrossRef]

128. Kim, S.H.; Huh, S.Y.; Kim, W.; Park, M.S.; Ahn, S.E.; Cho, J.Y.; Kim, B.J.; Kim, H.J. Clinical characteristics and outcome of multiple sclerosis in Korea: Does multiple sclerosis in Korea really differ from that in the Caucasian populations? *Mult. Scler. J.* **2013**, *19*, 1493–1498. [CrossRef]

129. Scott, T.F. Nosology of idiopathic transverse myelitis syndromes. *Acta Neurol. Scand.* **2007**, *115*, 371–376. [CrossRef]

130. Asgari, N.; Skejoe, H.P.B.; Lillevang, S.T.; Steenstrup, T.; Stenager, E.; Kyvik, K.O. Modifications of longitudinally extensive transverse myelitis and brainstem lesions in the course of neuromyelitis optica (NMO): A population-based, descriptive study. *BMC Neurol.* **2013**, *13*, 33. [CrossRef]

131. Hamid, S.H.M.; Elsone, L.; Mutch, K.; Solomon, T.; Jacob, A. The impact of 2015 neuromyelitis optica spectrum disorders criteria on diagnostic rates. *Mult. Scler. J.* **2017**, *23*, 228–233. [CrossRef]

132. Liu, Y.; Fu, Y.; Schoonheim, M.M.; Zhang, N.; Fan, M.; Su, L.; Shen, Y.; Yan, Y.; Yang, L.; Wang, Q.; et al. Structural MRI substrates of cognitive impairment in neuromyelitis optica. *Neurology* **2015**, *85*, 1491–1499. [CrossRef] [PubMed]

133. Ventura, R.E.; Kister, I.; Chung, S.; Babb, J.S.; Shepherd, T.M. Cervical spinal cord atrophy in NMOSD without a history of myelitis or MRI-visible lesions. *Neurol. Neuroimmunol. Neuroinflamm.* **2016**, *3*, e224. [CrossRef] [PubMed]

134. Hyun, J.W.; Jeong, I.H.; Joung, A.; Kim, S.H.; Kim, H.J. Evaluation of the 2015 diagnostic criteria for neuromyelitis optica spectrum disorder. *Neurology* **2016**, *86*, 1772–1779. [CrossRef] [PubMed]

135. Marignier, R.; Bernard-Valnet, R.; Giraudon, P.; Collongues, N.; Papeix, C.; Zéphir, H.; Cavillon, G.; Rogemond, V.; Casey, R.; Frangoulis, B.; et al. Aquaporin-4 antibody-negative neuromyelitis optica: Distinct assay sensitivity-dependent entity. *Neurology* **2013**, *80*, 2194–2200. [CrossRef]

136. Pittock, S.J.; Lennon, V.A.; Bakshi, N.; Shen, S.; McKeon, A.; Quach, H.; Briggs, F.B.S.; Bernstein, A.L.; Schaefer, C.A.; Barcellos, L.F. Seroprevalence of aquaporin-4-IgG in a northern California population representative cohort of multiple sclerosis. *JAMA Neurol.* **2014**, *71*, 1433–1436. [CrossRef]

137. Jarius, S.; Wildemann, B.; Paul, F. Neuromyelitis optica: Clinical features, immunopathogenesis and treatment. *Clin. Exp. Immunol.* **2014**, *176*, 149–164. [CrossRef]

138. van Pelt, E.D.; Wong, Y.Y.M.; Ketelslegers, I.A.; Hamann, D.; Hintzen, R.Q. Neuromyelitis optica spectrum disorders: Comparison of clinical and magnetic resonance imaging characteristics of AQP4-IgG versus MOG-IgG seropositive cases in the Netherlands. *Eur. J. Neurol.* **2016**, *23*, 580–587. [CrossRef]

139. Hamid, S.H.M.; Whittam, D.; Mutch, K.; Linaker, S.; Solomon, T.; Das, K.; Bhojak, M.; Jacob, A. What proportion of AQP4-IgG-negative NMO spectrum disorder patients are MOG-IgG positive? A cross sectional study of 132 patients. *J. Neurol.* **2017**, *264*, 2088–2094. [CrossRef]

140. Höftberger, R.; Sepulveda, M.; Armangue, T.; Blanco, Y.; Rostásy, K.; Cobo Calvo, A.; Olascoaga, J.; Ramió-Torrentà, L.; Reindl, M.; Benito-León, J.; et al. Antibodies to MOG and AQP4 in adults with neuromyelitis optica and suspected limited forms of the disease. *Mult. Scler. J.* **2015**, *21*, 866–874. [CrossRef]

141. Majed, M.; Fryer, J.P.; McKeon, A.; Lennon, V.A.; Pittock, S.J. Clinical utility of testing AQP4-IgG in CSF: Guidance for physicians. *Neurol. Neuroimmunol. NeuroInflamm.* **2016**, *3*, e231. [CrossRef]

142. Javed, A.; Balabanov, R.; Arnason, B.G.W.; Kelly, T.J.; Sweiss, N.J.; Pytel, P.; Walsh, R.; Blair, E.A.; Stemer, A.; Lazzaro, M.; et al. Minor salivary gland inflammation in Devic's disease and longitudinally extensive myelitis. *Mult. Scler. J.* **2008**, *14*, 809–814. [CrossRef] [PubMed]

143. Wandinger, K.P.; Stangel, M.; Witte, T.; Venables, P.; Charles, P.; Jarius, S.; Wildemann, B.; Probst, C.; Iking-Konert, C.; Schneider, M. Autoantibodies against aquaporin-4 in patients with neuropsychiatric systemic lupus erythematosus and primary Sjögren's syndrome. *Arthritis Rheumatol.* **2010**, *62*, 1198–1200. [CrossRef] [PubMed]

144. Jarius, S.; Paul, F.; Franciotta, D.; Ruprecht, K.; Ringelstein, M.; Bergamaschi, R.; Rommer, P.; Kleiter, I.; Stich, O.; Reuss, R.; et al. Cerebrospinal fluid findings in aquaporin-4 antibody positive neuromyelitis optica: Results from 211 lumbar punctures. *J. Neurol. Sci.* **2011**, *306*, 82–90. [CrossRef] [PubMed]

145. Weinshenker, B.G.; Wingerchuk, D.M. Neuromyelitis Spectrum Disorders. *Mayo Clin. Proc.* **2017**, *92*, 663–679. [CrossRef]

146. Kessler, R.A.; Mealy, M.A.; Levy, M. Treatment of Neuromyelitis Optica Spectrum Disorder: Acute, Preventive, and Symptomatic. *Curr. Treat. Options Neurol.* **2016**, *18*, 2. [CrossRef]

147. Trebst, C.; Jarius, S.; Berthele, A.; Paul, F.; Schippling, S.; Wildemann, B.; Borisow, N.; Kleiter, I.; Aktas, O.; Kümpfel, T.; et al. Update on the diagnosis and treatment of neuromyelitis optica: Recommendations of the Neuromyelitis Optica Study Group (NEMOS). *J. Neurol.* **2014**, *261*, 1–16. [CrossRef]

148. Palace, J.; Leite, I.; Jacob, A. A practical guide to the treatment of neuromyelitis optica. *Pract. Neurol.* **2012**, *12*, 209–214. [CrossRef]

149. Magaña, S.M.; Keegan, B.M.; Weinshenker, B.G.; Erickson, B.J.; Pittock, S.J.; Lennon, V.A.; Rodriguez, M.; Thomsen, K.; Weigand, S.; Mandrekar, J.; et al. Beneficial Plasma Exchange Response in CNS Inflammatory Demyelination. *Arch. Neurol.* **2012**, *68*, 870–878. [CrossRef]

150. Reeves, H.M.; Winters, J.L. The mechanisms of action of plasma exchange. *Br. J. Haematol.* **2014**, *164*, 342–351. [CrossRef]

151. Bonnan, M.; Valentino, R.; Debeugny, S.; Merle, H.; Fergé, J.L.; Mehdaoui, H.; Cabre, P. Short delay to initiate plasma exchange is the strongest predictor of outcome in severe attacks of NMO spectrum disorders. *J. Neurol. Neurosurg. Psychiatry* **2018**, *89*, 346–351. [CrossRef]

152. Lim, Y.M.; Pyun, S.Y.; Kang, B.H.; Kim, J.; Kim, K.K. Factors associated with the effectiveness of plasma exchange for the treatment of NMO-IgG-positive neuromyelitis optica spectrum disorders. *Mult. Scler. J.* **2013**, *19*, 1216–1218. [CrossRef] [PubMed]

153. Bonnan, M.; Valentino, R.; Olindo, S.; Mehdaoui, H.; Smadja, D.; Cabre, P. Plasma exchange in severe spinal attacks associated with neuromyelitis optica spectrum disorder. *Mult. Scler. J.* **2009**, *15*, 487–492. [CrossRef] [PubMed]

154. Watanabe, S.; Nakashima, I.; Misu, T.; Miyazawa, I.; Shiga, Y.; Fujihara, K.; Itoyama, Y. Therapeutic efficacy of plasma exchange in NMO-IgG-positive patients with neuromyelitis optica. *Mult. Scler. J.* **2007**, *13*, 128–132. [CrossRef] [PubMed]

155. Pittock, S.J.; Berthele, A.; Fujihara, K.; Kim, H.J.; Levy, M.; Palace, J.; Nakashima, I.; Terzi, M.; Totolyan, N.; Viswanathan, S.; et al. Eculizumab in aquaporin-4-positive neuromyelitis optica spectrum disorder. *N. Engl. J. Med.* **2019**, *381*, 614–625. [CrossRef]

156. Cree, B.A.C.; Bennett, J.L.; Kim, H.J.; Weinshenker, B.G.; Pittock, S.J.; Wingerchuk, D.M.; Fujihara, K.; Paul, F.; Cutter, G.R.; Marignier, R.; et al. Inebilizumab for the treatment of neuromyelitis optica spectrum disorder (N-MOmentum): A double-blind, randomised placebo-controlled phase 2/3 trial. *Lancet* **2019**, *394*, 1352–1363. [CrossRef]

157. Yamamura, T.; Kleiter, I.; Fujihara, K.; Palace, J.; Greenberg, B.; Zakrzewska-Pniewska, B.; Patti, F.; Tsai, C.P.; Saiz, A.; Yamazaki, H.; et al. Trial of satralizumab in neuromyelitis optica spectrum disorder. *N. Engl. J. Med.* **2019**, *381*, 2114–2124. [CrossRef]

158. Reindl, M.; Linington, C.; Brehm, U.; Egg, R.; Dilitz, E.; Deisenhammer, F.; Poewe, W.; Berger, T. Antibodies against the myelin oligodendrocyte glycoprotein and the myelin basic protein in multiple sclerosis and other neurological diseases: A comparative study. *Brain* **1999**, *122*, 2047–2056. [CrossRef]

159. Berger, T.; Rubner, P.; Schautzer, F.; Egg, R.; Ulmer, H.; Mayringer, I.; Dilitz, E.; Deisenhammer, F.; Reindl, M. Antimyelin antibodies as a predictor of clinically definite multiple sclerosis after a first demyelinating event. *N. Engl. J. Med.* **2003**, *349*, 139–145. [CrossRef]

160. Berger, T.; Reindl, M. Lack of association between antimyelin antibodies and progression to multiple sclerosis. *N. Engl. J. Med.* **2007**, *356*, 1888–1889.

161. Lampasona, V.; Franciotta, D.; Furlan, R.; Zanaboni, S.; Fazio, R.; Bonifacio, E.; Comi, G.; Martino, G. Similar low frequency of anti-MOG IgG and IgM in MS patients and healthy subjects. *Neurology* **2004**, *62*, 2092–2094. [CrossRef]

162. Lim, E.T.; Berger, T.; Reindl, M.; Dalton, C.M.; Fernando, K.; Keir, G.; Thompson, E.J.; Miller, D.H.; Giovannoni, G. Anti-myelin antibodies do not allow earlier diagnosis of multiple sclerosis. *Mult. Scler. J.* **2005**, *11*, 492–494. [CrossRef] [PubMed]

163. Hennes, E.M.; Baumann, M.; Schanda, K.; Anlar, B.; Bajer-Kornek, B.; Blaschek, A.; Brantner-Inthaler, S.; Diepold, K.; Eisenkölbl, A.; Gotwald, T.; et al. Prognostic relevance of MOG antibodies in children with an acquired demyelinating syndrome. *Neurology* **2017**, *89*, 900–908. [CrossRef] [PubMed]

164. Brilot, F.; Dale, R.C.; Selter, R.C.; Grummel, V.; Kalluri, S.R.; Aslam, M.; Busch, V.; Zhou, D.; Cepok, S.; Hemmer, B. Antibodies to native myelin oligodendrocyte glycoprotein in children with inflammatory demyelinating central nervous system disease. *Ann. Neurol.* **2009**, *66*, 833–842. [CrossRef] [PubMed]

165. Huppke, P.; Rostasy, K.; Karenfort, M.; Huppke, B.; Seidl, R.; Leiz, S.; Reindl, M.; Gärtner, J. Acute disseminated encephalomyelitis followed by recurrent or monophasic optic neuritis in pediatric patients. *Mult. Scler. J.* **2013**, *19*, 941–946. [CrossRef]

166. O'Connor, K.C.; McLaughlin, K.A.; De Jager, P.L.; Chitnis, T.; Bettelli, E.; Xu, C.; Robinson, W.H.; Cherry, S.V.; Bar-Or, A.; Banwell, B.; et al. Self-antigen tetramers discriminate between myelin autoantibodies to native or denatured protein. *Nat. Med.* **2007**, *13*, 211–217. [CrossRef]

167. Jarius, S.; Ruprecht, K.; Kleiter, I.; Borisow, N.; Asgari, N.; Pitarokoili, K.; Pache, F.; Stich, O.; Beume, L.A.; Hümmert, M.W.; et al. MOG-IgG in NMO and related disorders: A multicenter study of 50 patients. Part 1, Frequency, syndrome specificity, influence of disease activity, long-term course, association with AQP4-IgG, and origin. *J. Neuroinflamm.* **2016**, *13*, 279. [CrossRef]

168. Rostasy, K.; Mader, S.; Schanda, K.; Huppke, P.; Gärtner, J.; Kraus, V.; Karenfort, M.; Tibussek, D.; Blaschek, A.; Bajer-Kornek, B.; et al. Anti-myelin oligodendrocyte glycoprotein antibodies in pediatric patients with optic neuritis. *Arch. Neurol.* **2012**, *69*, 752–756. [CrossRef]

169. Mader, S.; Gredler, V.; Schanda, K.; Rostasy, K.; Dujmovic, I.; Pfaller, K.; Lutterotti, A.; Jarius, S.; Di Pauli, F.; Kuenz, B.; et al. Complement activating antibodies to myelin oligodendrocyte glycoprotein in neuromyelitis optica and related disorders. *J. Neuroinflamm.* **2011**, *8*, 184. [CrossRef]

170. Hyun, J.W.; Woodhall, M.R.; Kim, S.H.; Jeong, I.H.; Kong, B.; Kim, G.; Kim, Y.; Park, M.S.; Irani, S.R.; Waters, P.; et al. Longitudinal analysis of myelin oligodendrocyte glycoprotein antibodies in CNS inflammatory diseases. *J. Neurol. Neurosurg. Psychiatry* **2017**, *88*, 811–817. [CrossRef]

171. Ramanathan, S.; Mohammad, S.; Tantsis, E.; Nguyen, T.K.; Merheb, V.; Fung, V.S.C.; White, O.B.; Broadley, S.; Lechner-Scott, J.; Vucic, S.; et al. Clinical course, therapeutic responses and outcomes in relapsing MOG antibody-associated demyelination. *J. Neurol. Neurosurg. Psychiatry* **2018**, *89*, 127–137. [CrossRef]

172. Jarius, S.; Ruprecht, K.; Kleiter, I.; Borisow, N.; Asgari, N.; Pitarokoili, K.; Pache, F.; Stich, O.; Beume, L.A.; Hümmert, M.W.; et al. MOG-IgG in NMO and related disorders: A multicenter study of 50 patients. Part 2, Epidemiology, clinical presentation, radiological and laboratory features, treatment responses, and long-term outcome. *J. Neuroinflamm.* **2016**, *13*, 280. [CrossRef] [PubMed]

173. Sepúlveda, M.; Armangué, T.; Sola-Valls, N.; Arrambide, G.; Meca-Lallana, J.E.; Oreja-Guevara, C.; Mendibe, M.; Alvarez de Arcaya, A.; Aladro, Y.; Casanova, B.; et al. Neuromyelitis optica spectrum disorders: Comparison according to the phenotype and serostatus. *Neurol. Neuroimmunol. NeuroInflamm.* **2016**, *3*, e225. [CrossRef] [PubMed]

174. Jurynczyk, M.; Geraldes, R.; Probert, F.; Woodhall, M.R.; Waters, P.; Tackley, G.; DeLuca, G.; Chandratre, S.; Leite, M.I.; Vincent, A.; et al. Distinct brain imaging characteristics of autoantibody-mediated CNS conditions and multiple sclerosis. *Brain* **2017**, *140*, 617–627. [CrossRef] [PubMed]

175. Kim, H.J.; Paul, F.; Lana-Peixoto, M.A.; Tenembaum, S.; Asgari, N.; Palace, J.; Klawiter, E.C.; Sato, D.K.; de Seze, J.; Wuerfel, J.; et al. MRI characteristics of neuromyelitis optica spectrum disorder: An international update. *Neurology* **2015**, *84*, 1165–1173. [CrossRef]

176. Kim, S.M.; Woodhall, M.R.; Kim, J.S.; Kim, S.J.; Park, K.S.; Vincent, A.; Lee, K.W.; Waters, P. Antibodies to MOG in adults with inflammatory demyelinating disease of the CNS. *Neurol. Neuroimmunol. NeuroInflamm.* **2015**, *2*, e163. [CrossRef]

177. Jarius, S.; Kleiter, I.; Ruprecht, K.; Asgari, N.; Pitarokoili, K.; Borisow, N.; Hümmert, M.W.; Trebst, C.; Pache, F.; Winkelmann, A.; et al. MOG-IgG in NMO and related disorders: A multicenter study of 50 patients. Part 3, Brainstem involvement—Frequency, presentation and outcome. *J. Neuroinflamm.* **2016**, *13*, 281. [CrossRef]

178. Kitley, J.; Waters, P.; Woodhall, M.; Leite, M.I.; Murchison, A.; George, J.; Küker, W.; Chandratre, S.; Vincent, A.; Palace, J. Neuromyelitis optica spectrum disorders with aquaporin-4 and myelin-oligodendrocyte glycoprotein antibodies a comparative study. *JAMA Neurol.* **2014**, *71*, 276–283. [CrossRef]

179. Sato, D.K.; Callegaro, D.; Lana-Peixoto, M.A.; Waters, P.J.; de Haidar Jorge, F.M.; Takahashi, T.; Nakashima, I.; Apostolos-Pereira, S.L.; Talim, N.; Simm, R.F.; et al. Distinction between MOG antibody positive and AQP4 antibody-positive NMO spectrum disorders. *Neurology* **2014**, *82*, 474–481. [CrossRef]

180. Matthews, L.; Marasco, R.; Jenkinson, M.; Küker, W.; Luppe, S.; Leite, M.I.; Giorgio, A.; De Stefano, N.; Robertson, N.; Johansen-Berg, H.; et al. Distinction of seropositive NMO spectrum disorder and MS brain lesion distribution. *Neurology* **2013**, *80*, 1330–1337. [CrossRef]

181. Bensi, C.; Marrodan, M.; González, A.; Chertcoff, A.; Osa Sanz, E.; Chaves, H.; Schteinschnaider, A.; Correale, J.; Farez, M.F. Brain and spinal cord lesion criteria distinguishes AQP4-positive neuromyelitis optica and MOG-positive disease from multiple sclerosis. *Mult. Scler. Relat. Disord.* **2018**, *25*, 246–250. [CrossRef]

182. Cobo-Calvo, A.; Ruiz, A.; Maillart, E.; Audoin, B.; Zephir, H.; Bourre, B.; Ciron, J.; Collongues, N.; Brassat, D.; Cotton, F.; et al. Clinical spectrum and prognostic value of CNS MOG autoimmunity in adults: The MOGADOR study. *Neurology* **2018**, *90*, e1858–e1869. [CrossRef] [PubMed]

183. Chalmoukou, K.; Alexopoulos, H.; Akrivou, S.; Stathopoulos, P.; Reindl, M.; Dalakas, M.C. Anti-MOG antibodies are frequently associated with steroid-sensitive recurrent optic neuritis. *Neurol. Neuroimmunol. Neuroinflamm.* **2015**, *2*, e131. [CrossRef] [PubMed]

184. Kitley, J.; Woodhall, M.; Waters, P.; Leite, M.I.; Devenney, E.; Craig, J.; Palace, J.; Vincent, A. Myelin-oligodendrocyte glycoprotein antibodies in adults with a neuromyelitis optica phenotype. *Neurology* **2012**, *79*, 1273–1277. [CrossRef] [PubMed]

185. Kim, S.H.; Kim, W.; Li, X.F.; Jung, I.J.; Kim, H.J. Repeated treatment with rituximab based on the assessment of peripheral circulating memory B cells in patients with relapsing neuromyelitis optica over 2 years. *Arch. Neurol.* **2011**, *68*, 1412–1420. [CrossRef] [PubMed]

186. Montcuquet, A.; Collongues, N.; Papeix, C.; Zephir, H.; Audoin, B.; Laplaud, D.; Bourre, B.; Brochet, B.; Camdessanche, J.P.; Labauge, P.; et al. Effectiveness of mycophenolate mofetil as first-line therapy in AQP4-IgG, MOG-IgG, and seronegative neuromyelitis optica spectrum disorders. *Mult. Scler. J.* **2017**, *23*, 1377–1384. [CrossRef]

187. Flanagan, E.P.; Hinson, S.R.; Lennon, V.A.; Fang, B.; Aksamit, A.J.; Morris, A.P.; Basal, E.; Honorat, J.A.; Alfugham, N.N.; Linnoila, J.J.; et al. GFAP-IgG as Biomarker of Autoimmune Astrocytopathy: Analysis of 102 Patients. *Ann. Neurol.* **2017**, *81*, 298–309. [CrossRef]

188. Fang, B.; McKeon, A.; Hinson, S.R.; Kryzer, T.J.; Pittock, S.J.; Aksamit, A.J.; Lennon, V.A. Autoimmune glial fibrillary acidic protein astrocytopathy: A novel meningoencephalomyelitis. *JAMA Neurol.* **2016**, *73*, 1297–1307. [CrossRef]

189. Sasaki, K.; Bean, A.; Shah, S.; Schutten, E.; Huseby, P.G.; Peters, B.; Shen, Z.T.; Vanguri, V.; Liggitt, D.; Huseby, E.S. Relapsing–Remitting Central Nervous System Autoimmunity Mediated by GFAP-Specific CD8 T Cells. *J. Immunol.* **2014**, *192*, 3029–3042. [CrossRef]

190. Schweingruber, N.; Fischer, H.J.; Fischer, L.; van den Brandt, J.; Karabinskaya, A.; Labi, V.; Villunger, A.; Kretzschmar, B.; Huppke, P.; Simons, M.; et al. Chemokine-mediated redirection of T cells constitutes a critical mechanism of glucocorticoid therapy in autoimmune CNS responses. *Acta Neuropathol.* **2014**, *127*, 713–729. [CrossRef]

191. Sofroniew, M.V. Multiple roles for astrocytes as effectors of cytokines and inflammatory mediators. *Neuroscientist* **2014**, *20*, 160–172. [CrossRef]

192. Ramamoorthy, S.; Cidlowski, J.A. Corticosteroids: Mechanisms of Action in Health and Disease. *Rheum. Dis. Clin. N. Am.* **2016**, *42*, 15–31. [CrossRef] [PubMed]

193. Kunchok, A.; Zekeridou, A.; McKeon, A. Autoimmune glial fibrillary acidic protein astrocytopathy. *Curr. Opin. Neurol.* **2019**, *32*, 452–458. [CrossRef] [PubMed]

194. Iorio, R.; Damato, V.; Evoli, A.M.; Guessi, M.; Gaudino, S.; Di Lazzaro, V.; Spagni, G.; Sluijs, J.A.; Hol, E.M. Clinical and immunological characteristics of the spectrum of GFAP autoimmunity: A case series of 22 patients. *J. Neurol. Neurosurg. Psychiatry* **2018**, *89*, 138–146. [CrossRef] [PubMed]

195. Sechi, E.; Morris, P.P.; Mckeon, A.; Pittock, S.J.; Hinson, S.R.; Winshenker, B.G.; Aksamit, A.J.; Krecke, K.N.; Kaufmann, T.J.; Jolliffe, E.A.; et al. Glial fibrillary acidic protein IgG related myelitis: Characterisation and comparison with aquaporin-4-IgG myelitis. *J. Neurol. Neurosurg. Psychiatry* **2019**, *90*, 488–490. [CrossRef] [PubMed]

196. Shan, F.; Long, Y.; Qiu, W. Autoimmune Glial Fibrillary Acidic Protein Astrocytopathy: A Review of the Literature. *Front. Immunol.* **2018**, *9*, 2802. [CrossRef] [PubMed]

4

Mechanisms of Neurodegeneration and Axonal Dysfunction in Progressive Multiple Sclerosis

Jorge Correale *, Mariano Marrodan and María Célica Ysrraelit

Department of Neurology, FLENI, Buenos Aires 1428, Argentina; mmarrodan@fleni.org.ar (M.M.); mcysrraelit@fleni.org.ar (M.C.Y.)
* Correspondence: jcorreale@fleni.org.ar or jorge.correale@gmail.com;

Abstract: Multiple Sclerosis (MS) is a major cause of neurological disability, which increases predominantly during disease progression as a result of cortical and grey matter structures involvement. The gradual accumulation of disability characteristic of the disease seems to also result from a different set of mechanisms, including in particular immune reactions confined to the Central Nervous System such as: (a) B-cell dysregulation, (b) CD8$^+$ T cells causing demyelination or axonal/neuronal damage, and (c) microglial cell activation associated with neuritic transection found in cortical demyelinating lesions. Other potential drivers of neurodegeneration are generation of oxygen and nitrogen reactive species, and mitochondrial damage, inducing impaired energy production, and intra-axonal accumulation of Ca^{2+}, which in turn activates a variety of catabolic enzymes ultimately leading to progressive proteolytic degradation of cytoskeleton proteins. Loss of axon energy provided by oligodendrocytes determines further axonal degeneration and neuronal loss. Clearly, these different mechanisms are not mutually exclusive and could act in combination. Given the multifactorial pathophysiology of progressive MS, many potential therapeutic targets could be investigated in the future. This remains however, an objective that has yet to be undertaken.

Keywords: autoimmunity; axon; cortex; demyelination; mitochondria; multiple sclerosis; myelin; neurodegeneration; oligodendrocyte; progressive multiple sclerosis

1. Introduction

Multiple Sclerosis (MS) is a chronic inflammatory disease of the Central Nervous System (CNS) leading to demyelination and diffuse neurodegeneration in both brain and spinal cord grey and white matter of the brain and spinal cord [1,2]. Although its etiology remains elusive results from immunological, genetic, and histopathology studies of patients with MS support the concept that autoimmunity plays a major role in disease pathogenesis [1,3]. Disease course can be highly variable, however most patients present recurring clinical symptoms from onset followed by total or partial recovery, the classic relapsing–remitting form of the disease (RRMS). After 10–15 years the pattern becomes progressive in up to 50% of untreated patients, and symptoms slowly progress over a period of many years. This stage is defined as secondary progressive MS (SPMS). Fifteen percent of MS patients can present a progressive from onset, and is named primary progressive MS (PPMS) [4]. Actually, it is not known to whether PPMS is a different form of MS or is simply SPMS, without identifiable clinical relapses.

The most characteristic brain tissue injury in MS is primary demyelination with partial preservation of axons [2]. In general, actively demyelinating plaques in RRMS involves the movement of immune cells from the periphery into the CNS, which is associated with disruption of the blood-brain-barrier (BBB). In contrast, progressive disease involves the development of compartmentalized pathological processes within the brain mediated mainly by resident CNS cells. Evidence of this comes from MRI showing decreased gadolinium (Gd) enhancement in CNS lesions found in progressive MS patients, indicating reduced BBB breakdown and less movement of immune cells into the CNS. Several tissue pathology findings are associated with progressive MS. The most prominent is brain atrophy, caused chiefly by degeneration and chronic demyelination of axons, ultimately leading to neuronal loss [5]. Representing a major cause of irreversible neurological disability [6]. Although imaging and neuropathological studies have shown that both axonal degeneration and neuronal death are present in acute or active MS lesions [7], progression likely occurs once axonal loss exceeds CNS compensatory capacity. Whether inflammation and neurodegeneration are primary or secondary processes, and how they interact during the course of disease remains unclear. Another major pathological substrate of progressive MS is cortical demyelination. Grey matter demyelination is also observed in cerebellar cortex, the hippocampus, and in deep grey matter nuclei [8–11]. In addition to demyelination and oligodendrocyte loss, demyelinating cortical lesions show neuritic transection, neuronal death and reduced presynaptic terminal numbers [8,12]. In progressive MS lesions diffuse pathology is also present in normal appearing white and grey matter, reflected by diffuse axonal injury with profound microglia activation within a background of a global inflammation of the entire brain and the meninges [13]. Interestingly, MRI studies suggest that cortical atrophy may be more closely related to diffuse neurodegeneration in the normal appearing white matter than to the extent of focal white-matter demyelination [14].

In recent decades, better understanding of mechanisms underlying RRMS has led to the development of different disease-modifying therapies, reducing both severity and frequency of new relapses through immune system modulation [15,16]. In contrast, therapeutic options available for progressive MS are comparatively disappointing, and remain a challenge. One possible reason may be lack of knowledge regarding the pathogenic mechanisms driving progressive MS. At present, abnormal tissue findings seen in progressive MS remain poorly represented in experimental animal models.

This review discusses present knowledge on grey matter involvement in progressive MS, as well as the putative mechanisms that can determine the processes of neurodegeneration and neuronal death.

2. Grey Matter Changes Observed in MS

2.1. Cortical Compromise in MS

Even though MS was considered early on to be a demyelinating disease of CNS white matter mediated by inflammation, the possibility has been raised in recent years that cortical and deep grey matter demyelination may exceed that of white-matter demyelination, with both postmortem and in vivo studies revealing presence of extensive lesions in grey matter (GM) structures [8,17,18]. Initially articles explained GM compromise as a phenomenon associated exclusively with prolonged disease duration and progressive forms. Recently, however, cortical and deep grey matter lesions in the thalamus, caudate, putamen and cerebellum cortex have been detected during early stages of disease independent of white-matter pathology [19–22]. Indeed, evidence establishing that grey matter involvement related to disease activity and more aggressive forms is growing [23]. In contrast to other neurodegenerative diseases, it is not known whether cortical atrophy in MS is a more diffuse process or develops instead following distinct anatomical patterns. Cortical regions of the frontal lobe, posterior cingulate, insula and temporal lobes (especially hippocampus) as well as of the cerebellum are by far the most frequent areas affected early on, causing disability progression and cognitive impairment [24]. Recently different patterns of cortical atrophy with or without concomitant white-matter lesions have been described in patients with long-lasting MS. Most of these show a non-random and symmetric distribution, as well as, stronger associations with clinical dysfunction than global cortical atrophy [25]. In CNS tissue samples obtained at autopsy, different cortical lesions have been detected [8,17] in around 60% of the cases, while more recent 7T MRI protocols estimate a frequency above 90% [8,17,26]. Three types of cortical lesions have been reported in MS brain tissue: leukocortical, intracortical and subpial [27]. Leukocortical lesions or type 1 lesions seems to start in the subcortical white matter and extend into the cortex to layers V and VI (Figure 1A,B). Cortical sectors of these lesions showed increased numbers of lymphocytes and microglia/monocytes compared to normal appearing cortex from the same brain or from aged-matched control brains, although numbers of these cells are substantially less abundant than those seen in subcortical white matter [8]. Leukocortical lesions have been detected in patients even during the earliest stages of MS. Intracortical lesions or type 2 lesions are located entirely within the cerebral cortex, are not in direct contact with subcortical white matter or pia mater, and are in general small and perivascular. Finally, subpial lesions or type 3 lesions represent the most abundant type of cortical lesions, and are most prominent during progressive stages. These lesions often show myelin loss in cortical layers I through IV spanning several gyri. On occasion, they can involve all six cortical layers, but rarely invade subcortical white matter, and are mostly associated with meningeal inflammation [17,28,29]. With the exception of loss of myelin, subpial lesions lack most of the other pathological signature findings described in white-matter lesions such as blood-brain-barrier breakdown, as well as immune cells infiltration, perivascular cuffs, astrogliosis, loss of oligodendrocyte progenitor cells, and complement activation. Active tissue damage is also associated with microglial activation [22,30]. However, no correlation has been observed between subpial and white-matter lesion loads [31,32], suggesting subpial demyelination occurs independently of white-matter demyelination. General consensus from autopsy studies would indicate subpial lesions are abundant in progressive stages of MS (both PPMS and SPMS) and rare in MS patients with acute disease or during early stages of RRMS.

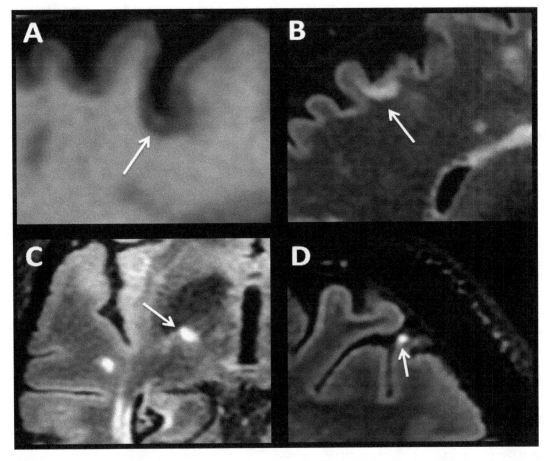

Figure 1. (**A**) Three-dimension sagittal T1-weighted. Hypointense cortical lesion (white arrow). (**B**) Three-dimension sagittal T2-Fluid Attenuated Inversion Recovery (FLAIR). Hyperintense leukocortical lesion (white arrow). (**C**) Axial FLAIR. Subcortical temporal demyelinating plaque and perithalamic internal capsule lesion (white arrow). (**D**) Post-contrast 3D sagittal FLAIR. Focal area of leptomeningeal enhancement (white arrow).

2.2. Deep Grey Matter (DGM) Structures Changes in MS

Although less well studied, DGM structures involvement is often present together with cortical atrophy, particularly of the thalamus. To date estimation of whole-brain volume has been used most often as a surrogate marker of atrophy in MS, because it is relatively easy to measure. However, there is growing evidence that grey matter volume loss may be more pronounced than that of white matter and be more strongly linked to long-term disability [33,34]. The thalamus may be particularly susceptible to neurodegeneration through different mechanisms, of which two are particularly prominent. First, demyelinating lesions can occur in the thalamus and in perithalamic regions (Figure 1C). Indeed, DGM demyelination can be frequently observed in postmortem MS brain, particularly in the caudate, and in the medial and anterior thalamic nuclei [11]. Histopathologic characterization of the thalamic lesions recapitulates the spectrum of active, chronically demyelinated, lesions observed in the white matter. Similar to changes found in cortical grey matter at autopsy, parenchymal infiltration by T and B cells is limited when compared to levels observed in classic active white-matter lesions. Second, recent work has shown clear patterns of grey matter atrophy in patients with MS that are focused in regions that are strongly connected with diverse neuronal networks [25]. Because DGM structures are extensively connected to cortical grey matter regions, atrophy could also be due to a retrograde event resulting from axonal transection in white-matter tracts projecting from the thalamus, or secondary to trans-synaptic deafferentation of thalamic neurons [11,35]. Interestingly, recent studies have shown that volume loss in DGM over time is faster than in other brain regions across all clinical phenotypes, and drives disability [21,36,37]. Together these studies provide strong evidence that thalamic volume and DGM volume more broadly, are dramatically affected in MS.

3. Mechanisms of Neurodegeneration

Different theories have been put forward to explain how progressive MS is triggered. One suggestion is that although brain damage is driven by inflammatory processes similar to those observed during RRMS, during progressive disease stages, a microenvironment is created within the CNS favoring homing and retention of inflammatory cells, ultimately making disease-modifying therapies ineffective [38]. A second possibility is that MS starts out as an inflammatory disease, but after several years a neurodegenerative process independent of inflammatory responses becomes the key mechanism behind disease progression [39]. Finally, MS could be a neurodegenerative disease, with inflammation occurring as a secondary response, amplifying progressive states [40,41]. Clearly, these different mechanisms are not mutually exclusive and could occur in combination. Therefore, in MS neurodegeneration and ultimately progression of disease and chronic disability develop as a result of many different molecular mechanisms. These have been summarized in Table 1.

Table 1. Mechanisms proposed to explain Multiple Sclerosis progression.

Immunological Mechanisms and Effectors	Mechanisms of Neurodegeneration and Axonal Dysfunction
B Cells	**Mitochondrial Injury**
Antibody production, Ag presentation, ectopic formation of follicle-like structures	Impaired activity of respiratory chain complexes (I, III and IV)
Induction of compartmentalized population driving CNS injury, independent of peripheral immune activity.	Alterations in mitochondrial molecular motors mtDNA deletions
Secretion of IL-6, TNF-α, IL-10, and IL-35: Complement activation and T cell functions	Energy deficiency: failure of Na^+/K^+ ATPase, reverse activity of NCX, and excess of intra-axonal Ca^{2+}.
EBV-infected B-cell Induce CD8-mediated immune responses against brain tissue	Amplify oxidative stress. Mediates histotoxic hypoxia, which magnifies energy deficiency
CD8$^+$ cytotoxic T lymphocytes	**Release of Fe^{3+}**
Release of TNF-α: neuronal cell death via p55 receptor; IFN-γ: increased Glutamate neurotoxicity and Ca^{2+} influx; secretion of perforin and granzyme: cellular membrane damage, associated to Na^+ and Ca^{2+} influx	Iron accumulates with aging. The release of Fe^{3+} from damaged OGD amplifies oxidative injury

Table 1. *Cont.*

Immunological Mechanisms and Effectors	Mechanisms of Neurodegeneration and Axonal Dysfunction
Astrocytes *	**Anomalous Distribution of Ion Channels**
Secretion of pro-inflammatory cytokines (IL-1, IL-6, TNF-α), chemokines (CCL-2, CCL-5, IP-10, CXCL-12, IL-8) and BAFF. Blood-brain-barrier breakthrough: action on endothelial cells and tight junctions Activation of microglia: secretion of CXCL-10/CXR3, GM-CSF, M-CSF and TGF-β. Production of Lactosylceramide: induces secretion of CCL2 and GM-CSF Production of ROS, RNS, NO and ONOO-limited Glutamate transporters, increasing Glutamate excitotoxicity Reactive astrogliosis: inhibition of remyelination and axonal regeneration by over-secretion of FGF-2, CSPGs and EPH. Upregulation of purinergic receptors: increased responsiveness to ATP, formation of membrane pores and increased of Ca^{2+} influx Cellular senescence: low level of chronic inflammation, altered Ca^{2+} homeostasis	Redistribution of Na$^+$ channels (Na$_v$, 1.2, 1.6 and 1.8) along the denuded axon: increased energy demand. Activation of VGCC, ASIC1 and TRPM4 contributes to excess of intra-axonal Ca^{2+} Glutamate excitotoxicity mediates massive influx of Ca^{2+} into neurons Excess of intra-axonal Ca^{2+} stimulates catabolic enzyme systems: leading to proteolytic degradation of cytoskeletal proteins
Microglia *	**Loss of Myelin-Derived Trophic Support and Deficit in Axonal Transport**
Decreased expression of immunosuppressive factors: fractalkine-CX3CR1, and CD200-CD200R. Secretion of pro-inflammatory cytokines: IL-1, IL-6, TNF-α, IFN-γ. Ag presentation of CD4$^+$ T cells via Major Histocompatibility Complex (MHC) Class II Oxidative burst: production of ROS and RNS Acquisition of aging phenotype: expression of AGE and RAGE	Alteration of a single myelin protein synthesis (PLP, MGA, or CNP) can cause axonal dysfunction Deficit in axonal transport can reduced expression of kinesins (anterograde transport) and dyneins (retrograde transport)

* Only deleterious mechanisms are presented. Ag: antigen; AGE: Advanced glycation end products; ASIC1: acid-sensing ion channel; BAFF: B-cell-activating factor; CNP: 2′3′ cyclic-nucleotide 3′ phosphodiesterase; CNS: Central Nervous System; CSPGs: chondroitin sulphate proteoglycans; EBV: Epstein–Barr virus; EPH: ephrins; FGF-2: fibroblast growth factor 2; GM-CSF: granulocyte-macrophage-colony stimulating factor; MAG: myelin-associated glycoprotein; M-CSF: macrophage-colony stimulating factor; mtDNA: mitochondrial DNA; NCX: sodium calcium exchanger; NO: nitric oxide; OGD: oligodendrocytes; ONOO$^-$: peroxynitrite; PLP: proteolipid-protein; RAGE: AGE receptor; RNS: reactive nitrogen species; ROS: reactive oxygen species; TRPM4: transient potential receptor melastatin 4; VGCC: Voltage-gated Ca^{2+} channel.

4. Inflammatory Events

Evidence from animal models and immunological studies in MS patients suggests that peripheral immune response targeting the CNS drives the disease process during early phases, whereas immune reactions confined to the CNS dominate later phases of progression [42,43]. The composition of the inflammatory infiltrate within the CNS results from the combination of peripheral immune cells influx, and resident cell activation, particularly of microglial cells, which can change their intrinsic "resting" state in response to prolonged inflammation. Among potential candidates driving inflammation during progressive MS, the role of B cells appears to be prominent. B-cell functions that could be of relevance in progressive MS include: antibody production, increased secretion of pro-inflammatory cytokines, deficient production of regulatory cytokines which impact complement activation and T cell function, as well as antigen presentation and ectopic formation of follicle-like structures [44,45]. Ectopic follicle-like structures are pathological tissue formations resembling tertiary lymph nodes, found in the subarachnoid space of leptomeninges close to inflamed blood vessels (Figure 1D), and also present in other chronic inflammatory diseases [46,47]. They can be induced by follicular T- helper cells cytokine networks acting as positive (i.e., IL-21, and IL-22) and negative (i.e., IL-27) regulators, as well by changes in the stromal networks in connective tissue [48,49]. Composition of these pathologic structures is characterized by aggregates of T and B cells often showing T/B segregation, and development of high endothelial venules, and follicular dendritic cell networks [19,46]. They are capable of sustaining in situ antibody diversification, isotype switching, B-cell differentiation and oligoclonal expansion similar to ectopic germinal centers, which can also support the production of autoreactive plasma cells at the site of local inflammation [48]. These structures co-localize with grey matter lesions and parenchymal infiltrates [50], and are present during different stages of development, ranging from simple T and B-cell clusters to highly organized follicles encapsulated by reticulin lining [51]. Once follicle-like develop, lymphoid chemokines CCL19, CCL21, CXCL12, and CXCL13 are critical for their perpetuation and function, controlling homing recruitment, maturation and antigenic selection of B cells [52], which in turn sustain a high level of humoral response within the CNS independent of peripheral inflammation. This is of particular relevance during progressive MS, when the BBB is intact and contribution to disease activity from entry of peripheral immune cells into the brain is negligible. Antibodies against both myelin antigens and to non-myelin antigens such as neurofascin, neurofilaments and the glial potassium channel KIR 4. 1 has been shown to play an important role in axonal and neuronal damage through complement cascade activation [53–55]. In progressive MS cortical demyelination, neurodegeneration and atrophy show positive correlation with diffuse inflammatory infiltrates and lymphoid-follicle structures in leptomeninges, indicating activation of these structures contribute to cortical pathology [2,19,23]. As in other chronic inflammatory diseases follicle-like structures occur in around 40% of SPMS cases [45,56], but are uncommon in PPMS cases. However, it is not known whether follicle-like structures are a typical feature of different disease subtypes from the beginning, or develop as a result of persistent tissue damage and antigen release [20,49]. Notably, meningeal inflammation in SPMS is associated with damage of glial limitans, and a gradient of neuronal loss, which is greater in superficial cortical layers (I-III) nearer the pial surface than in inner cortical layers [23]. These findings suggest cytotoxic factors diffusing from the infiltrated meninges may play a major role in subpial cortical lesions development. Indeed, presence of follicle-like structures in patients with SPMS has been associated with a more severe clinical course, shorter disease duration and earlier death [28,57,58]. Despite this evidence, some studies have reported no substantial perivascular infiltration in pure intracortical lesions found postmortem in patients with longstanding progressive MS [8,17]. These contradictory findings could be due to a reduced sample size, or to insufficient inflammatory activity in the tissue analyzed. Of note, questions remaining regarding neurodegenerative and immunological mechanisms underlying PPMS and SPMS pathology are different. In both cases diffuse meningeal inflammation and cortical neuronal pathology may be significant contributors to clinical progression, suggesting similar pathogenic mechanisms, irrespective of a prior relapsing–remitting course, or the presence of follicle-like structures [59]. Differences observed between both forms of the disease are more quantitative than qualitative in nature [60]. Because serological and epidemiological studies have found an association between B-lymphotropic Epstein–Barr virus (EBV) infection and MS [61], it has been hypothesized that EBV infection of CNS- infiltrating B cells may drive MS pathology [62]. Analysis of postmortem brain tissue from MS patients with different forms of disease, have shown that accumulation of EBV-infected B cells/plasma cells in the meninges and perivascular compartment of white-matter lesions is common and that numbers of EBV-harboring cells correlates with the degree of brain inflammation. Absence of EBV in brain-infiltrating B cells in other inflammatory neurological diseases indicates that homing of EBV-infected B cells to the CNS is specific to MS and not a general phenomenon driven by inflammation [63]. Colonization of cortical lesions has been associated with EBV-encoded small nuclear mRNA (EBER) transcripts in B cells and plasma cells, predominantly expressed during the latent phase of viral infection. Expression of the latency proteins EBNA2 and LMP1, which provide proliferative and prosurvival signals to B cells, in active white-matter lesions and in the meninges in most MS cases, as well as the presence of foci of B-cell proliferation in the MS brain tissue, support a mechanism of EBV-driven B-cell expansion. Ectopic follicle-like structures contained numerous LMP1[+], but no EBNA2[+] cells. Meanwhile lytic proteins BZLF1 and BERF1 were found restricted to plasma cells located in active cortical lesions, indicating these structures represent main sites of viral reactivation [63]. Because cells expressing EBNA2 and LMP1 are usually not found in blood, their presence in brain suggests complete disruption of EBV regulation [64]. However, other authors report absence of CNS EBV infection in MS [65]. Interestingly, early lytic EBV antigens elicited CD8-mediated immune responses, triggering strong cytotoxic effects in brain tissue [66]. Indeed, the most active cortical MS lesions are often crowded with CD8[+] T cells, and contain few B cells o plasma cells, suggesting cortical inflammation correlate with reduction in both B and plasma cell numbers [67]. These observations suggest that EBV reactivation combined with a strong cytotoxic antiviral response mediated by CD8[+] T cells may drive acute inflammation in both white and grey matter, as well as within the meningeal compartment. CD8[+] T cells can also recognize specific antigens present on oligodendrocytes, neurons or axons. Once activated, they may be partly responsible for demyelination or axonal/neuronal damage in MS [68–70]. Most CD8[+] T lymphocytes recovered from MS lesions belonged to a few clones [71]. Samples obtained from patients studied longitudinally have shown that certain CD8[+] T cell clones found in MS patients may persisted over many years in CSF and/or CNS tissue [5,72]. In sharp contrast, the repertoire of CD4[+] T cells recovered from the CNS in MS patients is heterogeneous [5,71,72]. Overall, these findings reinforce the concept that CD8[+] T lymphocytes present in the CNS of MS patients are not just bystander cells but are engaged in active immune responses [73]. Axonal damage in white-matter lesions correlates with the number of both CD8[+] T cells [74] and of activated microglia/macrophages [75] and resident CNS cells which show intense MHC I expression in all types of inflammatory lesions [76]. These observations collectively suggest that in white-matter lesions, CD8[+] T cells contribute as effector cells causing oligodendrocyte as well as axonal damage. However, there is still controversy over the underlying mechanisms, through which cytotoxic CD8[+] T lymphocytes harm axons and neurons in MS. Cytotoxic CD8[+] T lymphocytes release cytokines, such as IFN-γ, and TNF-α, as well as perforin, and granzymes A and B [70,77,78]. IFN-γ for instance, can increase glutamate neurotoxicity and Ca^{2+} influx into neurons through modulation of the IFN-γ/AMPA Glutamate receptor complex [78]. TNF-α on the other hand triggers cell death via the p55 receptor present on neurons [79]. Perforin and granzymes directly damage the cell membrane, causing Na^+ and Ca^{2+} influx, ultimately leading to energy breakdown and consequent activation of lytic cell enzymes (see below). Granzymes disrupted calcium homeostasis by increasing resting levels, and enhancing IP3-mediated endoplasmic reticulum calcium release. Elevated concentrations of Ca^{2+} are sufficient to activate calcium-dependent death effectors, including caspases [80]. Although perforin did enhance GrB-mediated neurotoxicity, recombinant GrB can itself induce neurotoxicity, independently of perforin [80]. Likewise, interactions between Fas antigen on CD8[+] cytotoxic T lymphocytes and Fas ligand on neurons triggers Ca^{2+} release from intracellular storage sites resulting in additional activation of the intracellular caspase cascade causing further axonal/neuronal damage [81].

The role of cytotoxic CD4[+] T cells in progressive MS has not always been highlighted. However, recent studies demonstrated an increase of this T cell population in late/chronic Experimental Autoimmune Encephalomyelits (EAE) lesions as compared with acute lesions. Moreover, proportions of cytotoxic CD4[+] T cells were further enriched in the CSF from SPMS patients as compared with corresponding blood samples [82]. These cells arise from repeated antigenic stimulation, after which they lose the co-stimulatory molecule CD28, presenting a cytotoxic phenotype, comparable with NK and CD8[+] T cells [83]. In addition, CD4[+]CD28[-] T cells lose their sensitivity to apoptosis induction [84], and are resistant to the suppressive actions of regulatory T cells [85]. Expansion of CD4[+]CD28[-] T cells is associated with several autoimmune and chronic inflammatory conditions, including MS [86,87], whereas in healthy individuals they are almost undetectable [88]. They have been identified not just in the circulation of patients with chronic inflammatory diseases, but also in target tissues. In MS CD4[+]CD28[-] T cells are capable of migrating to the CNS mainly through the fractalkine (CX3CL1-CX3CR1) system. It comes as no surprise that patients who have high numbers of these cells have more severe disease and poor prognosis. Indeed, recently baseline percentage of CD4[+]CD28[-] T cells was associated with multimodal evoked potential (EP), indicating a link between these cells and disease severity. In addition, the baseline CD4[+]CD28[-] T cells percentage had a prognostic value since it was associated with EP after 3 years and with EP and Expanded Disability Status Scale (EDSS) after 5 years [89]. Notably, in patients with chronic inflammatory disorders it has been shown that CD4$^+$CD28$^-$ T cells have oligoclonal antigen receptors [90], produce high levels of inflammatory cytokines such as IFN-γ, and GM-CSF, and express cytotoxic molecules (e.g., NKG2D, perforin and Granzyme B), features similar to innate-like T cells, which together could lead to neuronal and axonal loss similar as described by CD8$^+$ T cell [68,83]. It remains unclear to date which are the antigens or cues that trigger and/or drive the expansion of CD4$^+$CD28$^-$ T cells and what stage they acquire cytotoxic activity that contributes to tissue damage and consequent disease progression in MS.

Active demyelination and neurodegeneration have also been linked to microglial activation in early lesions [91]. While in the surveillance state, microglia monitor brain parenchyma detecting danger signals. This state seems to be maintained through a number of interactions with neurons. For example, interactions have been described between CD200-CD200R, CD47-CD172a, and fractalkine-CX3CR1 interactions. As a consequence of brain injury or disease these interactions are lost and resident microglia change their phenotype developing an "activated" state. This change can be induced through several mechanisms including: production of pro-inflammatory cytokines released by Th1 or Th17 T cells, presence of microbial pathogens (PAMPs) recognized by Toll-like receptors (TLRs) or leucine-rich repeat containing receptors (NLRs), release of intracellular components from necrotic or apoptotic cells, as well as presence of heat shock proteins, misfolded proteins (DAMPs) or components of the complement cascade [92]. Microglial activation is not restricted to lesions, but is also diffusely present in normal appearing white and grey matter [13]. In normal appearing white matter (NAWM) for example clustering of activated microglia, so-called microglial nodules, are abundant in areas adjacent to plaques, particularly in patients with progressive MS [93]. Notably, microglia nodules have been associated with damaged axons expressing amyloid precursor protein (APP) accumulation, and changes in neurofilament phosphorylation in the periplaque white matter. Furthermore, direct spatial association has been observed between microglial nodules and axons undergoing Wallerian degeneration [94]. These findings indicate microglial activation is associated with signs of neuronal damage and tissue atrophy strongly suggesting microglial cells contribute to CNS damage in progressive MS.

Damage induced by microglial cells in MS is mediated through different mechanisms (Figure 2A), including secretion of pro-inflammatory cytokines such as IL-1, IL-6, TNF-α, and IFN-γ, phagocytic activity and presentation of antigens to CD4$^+$ T cells via MHC Class II molecules [95,96]. Pro-inflammatory cytokines can also induce mitochondrial injury both in neurons and glial cells. In addition, reactive oxygen and nitrogen species (ROS/RNS), produced by microglial cells, cause direct damage to neuron through loss of cytochrome C oxidase (COX1), as well as mitochondrial respiratory chain complex IV activity, leading to mitochondrial dysfunction (see below) [97]. Importantly, release of Fe^{2+} into the extracellular space from injured oligodendrocytes may amplify oxidative damage by generating highly toxic hydroxyl (OH) radicals, from H$_2$O$_2$. Fe^{2+} uptake by activated microglia determines their fragmentation and degeneration, leading to a second wave of Fe^{2+} release, which can increase susceptibility of surrounding tissues to free radicals-driven axonal and neuronal destruction [98].

Interestingly, cortical demyelinated lesions lack inflammatory lymphocyte or macrophage infiltrates in progressive MS and does not show complement deposition. The majority of phagocytic cells are ramified microglia in close apposition to neurites and neuronal cell bodies [8]. Activated microglia also possesses a puzzling array of neuroprotective functions, including debris phagocytosis and clearance, growth factors production and neuronal-circuit shaping [95]. Distinguish neuroprotective from pro-inflammatory phenotypes remains a challenge when interpreting microglial function.

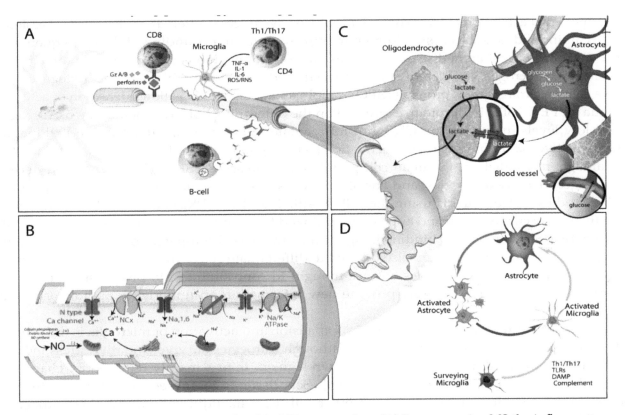

Figure 2. Possible mechanisms involved in MS progression. (**A**) In progressive MS the inflammatory phenomena eventually leading to axonal degeneration and loss are compartmentalized within the CNS. Cellular components are represented by cells that come from the periphery (T and B lymphocytes), as well as by resident CNS cells (microglia cells and astrocytes). B cells can form ectopic follicle-like structures resembling tertiary lymph nodes, producing antibodies against myelin and non-myelin antigens, shown to play an important role in axonal and neuronal damage through complement cascade activation. In turn, CD8+ lymphocytes can recognize specific axonal antigens and produce tissue damage through secretion of perforin or granzymes A and B. Autoreactive CD4+ Th1 and Th17 lymphocytes can activate microglial cells, which in turn produce pro-inflammatory cytokines (IL-1, IL-6, TNF-α) or oxygen or nitrogen free radicals (ROS/RNS) causing axonal damage and neuronal loss through a bystander mechanism. (**B**) Following demyelination, energy requirements increase due to disruption of paranodal myelin loops. Reduction in neuronal ATP production may lead to failure of the Na^+/K^+ pump failure, generating a sustained sodium current, which drives reverse sodium/calcium exchange and accumulation of intra-axonal calcium. This, in turn activates degradative enzymes, including proteases, phospholipases, and calpains, resulting in further neuronal and/or axonal damage as well as impaired ATP production. (**C**) Axonal damage could be cause by poor trophic support. Oligodendrocytes capture glucose from circulation, breaking it down glucose to form pyruvate or lactate, which can enter axons, and be imported by mitochondria for ATP synthesis. An alternative source of energy for axons comes from glycogen stored in astrocytes, which can be transformed into glucose and later into pyruvate or lactate, depending on oxygen availability. (**D**) Several mechanisms cause surveillance microglia activation including Th1 or Th17 T cells; presence of microbial pathogens (PAMPs) recognized by Toll-like receptors (TLRs) or leucin-rich repeat containing receptors (NLRs); release of intracellular components from necrotic or apoptotic cells; presence of heat shock proteins, misfolded proteins (DAMPs), or components of the complement cascade. Once activated they in induce activation and proliferation of astrocytes, leading to astrogliosis.

As previously mentioned, postmortem tissue studies have shown increased microglial numbers and increased activation are associated with variable degrees of axonal/neuritic injury, demyelination, and neuronal loss in cortical grey matter during progressive stages of MS. However, it is as yet unclear how early during the course of MS these degenerative events begin. Future longitudinal in vivo studies linking microglial activation to local cortical atrophy or dysfunction levels as well as to progression of disability in individual subjects should help to improve our understanding of the consequences of cortical pathology at different disease stages. In this context, in vivo positron emission tomography (PET) images of microglia, could clarify the role of activated microglia in MS-related neurodegeneration. Use of a selective translocator protein (TSPO) radioligand 11C-PK11195 allows detection of activated microglia on PET. TSPO is a protein, expressed on the outer mitochondrial membrane of microglial cells, at low levels in the healthy CNS, but up-regulated upon microglial activation [99] making TSPO a sensitive "real-time" marker of activation [100,101]. In non-neoplastic injury to CNS without BBB damage, microglial are the main cell population expressing TSPO. However, blood-derived macrophages, reactive astrocytes, and endothelial cells in the vasculature express TSPO [100,102]. Imaging studies in MS patients using the TSPO radioligand 11C-PK11195 have shown microglial cells activation occurs early on and appears to be linked to disability and brain atrophy [103]. In the NAWM of SPMS patients TSPO binding is significantly increased compared to age-matched healthy controls [102,104]. PET imaging can also be used to differentiate active from inactive chronic lesions. Slowly expanding chronic active lesions are thought to contribute to MS progression. Detection of plaque kinetics in vivo will likely provide new information on underlying pathology driving progression [105].

As in other neurodegenerative disorders, expansion and activation of microglia is the primary mechanism behind astrocytosis (Figure 2D). Although astrocytes survive oxidative stress induced by inflammation and ROS/RNS, they still shown signs of injury, mainly reflected by changes in cell morphology and molecular expression [106]. Scar tissue is composed primarily of astrocytes, however in severe lesions, interaction with other cell types including oligodendrocyte progenitor cells, and fibromeningeal cells also occurs [107]. Several specific molecular and morphologic features have been observed in astrocytes during reactive astrogliosis both in human pathology and animal models [108], of which upregulation of Glial fibrillary acidic protein (GFAP), vimentin, nestin, and the less investigated synemin are hallmarks. Glial scars are evident in tissue from MS patients and mice with EAE and surround areas of demyelination [109]. The purpose of scar formation would appear to be isolation of damaged CNS areas, to prevent spread of tissue destruction. However, glial scar rigidity results in inhibition of both remyelination and axonal regeneration, both negative effects mediated through different mechanisms. Over-secretion of FGF-2 by astrocytes may be detrimental for remyelination, which in turn promotes oliogodendrocytes precursor cells (OPC) proliferation and survival, but prevents maturation [110]. Another molecule that appears to play an important role in preventing OPC maturation is the glycosaminoglycan hyaluronan, which is found throughout the extracellular matrix and CNS white matter [111]. Oligodendrocytes that co-localize with hyaluronan express an immature phenotype, and in vitro treatment of oligodendrocytes precursor cells with hyaluronan in vitro prevents maturation [112]. In addition, astrocytes in injured areas release inhibitory extracellular matrix molecules known as chondroitin sulphate proteoglycans (CSPGs) which can severely in injured areas, affect both cytoskeleton and membrane components of growth cone architecture [113]. CSPGs are a family of molecules characterized by a protein core to which highly sulphated glycosaminoglycan (GAG) chains are attached. Neurocan (secreted) and brevican (cell bound) are the major proteoglycans produced by astrocytes in vitro and both have been shown to inhibit axon growth, following CNS damage [114]. There is clear evidence that CSPGs are produced in excess by astrocytes when they become reactive and that CSPGs inhibitory activity depends on GAG content, as removal of GAG chains from the protein core suppresses CSPG- mediated inhibition [114]. Aside from CSPGs, other less studied inhibitory molecules expressed by astrocytes can suppress axonal growth. Ephrins (EPH) and their receptors for example are secreted by normal astrocytes and increased in MS lesions, inducing axonal growth cone collapse through activation of axon-bound EPH tyrosine-receptor kinase [115].

Likewise, astrocytes as part of the immune system could contribute to disease progression through several mechanisms. First, they can directly affect cell entry to the CNS, via de the BBB, by regulating expression of adhesion molecules, particularly vascular adhesion-molecule-1 (VCAM-1), and intercellular adhesion-molecule-1 (ICAM-1), that bind to lymphocyte receptors very late antigen-4 (VLA4), and lymphocyte function-associated antigen-1 (LFA-1), respectively [116,117]. Second, astrocytes secrete different chemokines such as CCL-2 (MCP-1), CCL5 (RANTES), IP-10 (CXCL10), CXCL12 (SDF-1) and IL-8 (CXCL8), which attract both peripheral immune cells (e.g., T cells, monocytes, and DCs), as well as resident CNS cells (microglia) to lesion sites [118]. In addition, astrocytes can secrete GM-CSF, M-CSF or TGF-β, which can regulate MHC Class II molecule expression by microglia and even their phagocytosis [119]. This could represent the primary mechanism through which astrocytes perpetuate immune-mediated demyelination and neurodegeneration. Recent investigations have demonstrated that in chronic phases of EAE, astrocyte depletion ameliorates disease severity. This deleterious effect of astrocytes on EAE is mediated by preferential expression of 4-galactosyltransferase 5 and 6 (B4GALT5 and B4GALT6) [120]. Notably, B4GALT6 is also expressed by reactive astrocytes in human MS lesions. These enzymes synthesize the signaling molecule lactosylceramide (LacCer), the CNS expression of which is significantly increased during progressive phases of EAE. LacCer promotes astrocyte activation in an autocrine manner [120,121], inducing GM-CSF and CCL2 genes, activating microglia and causing infiltration of monocytes from blood, respectively. Remarkably, inhibition or knockout of B4GALT6 in mice suppresses disease progression, local CNS innate immunity and neurodegeneration in EAE, and interferes with human astrocyte activation in vitro [120].

Third, B-cell-activating factor (BAFF), critical for both B-cell development and survival, as well as for immunoglobulin production, is constitutively expressed by astrocytes in normal CNS. BAFF expression in astrocytes is up-regulated in MS lesions and in EAE affected mice, suggesting astrocytes may contribute to drive B-cell-dependent autoimmunity [122], an important mechanism in disease progression as described above. Finally, an important function of innate immune cells is to act as antigen-presenting cells. However, although astrocytes express MHC Class I and Class II molecules in vitro capable of presenting myelin antigens, their ability to also express co-stimulatory molecules including CD40, CD80, and CD86 challenges this function, making their final effect unclear [123]. Nor is it clear to what degree astrocytes can perform phagocytosis, or process and present antigens, particularly under physiological conditions in vivo [124].

In addition to being part of the immune system, astrocytes contribute to MS progression through production of cytotoxic factors. In rodents, astrocytes stimulated with IL-17 or IFN-γ induce nitric oxide synthase (iNOS) [125]. Likewise, IL-1 as well as combined treatment with TGF-β plus IFN-γ increases the percentage of astrocyte secreted nitric oxide (NO), which is one of the most prominent damage-inducing molecules in neurodegeneration [126,127]. Simultaneously, NO stimulates glutamate release from astrocytes which further increase excitotoxicity [128]. Remarkably, the predominant contribution of NO to excitotoxicity depends on increased superoxide ion O_2^- production, which reacts with NO forming peroxynitrite ($ONOO^-$) resulting in neuronal necrosis or apoptosis, depending on its concentration [129]. Furthermore, $ONOO^-$ inactivates glutamate transporters in astrocytes, directly damaging myelin, oligodendrocytes, and axons [130]. Decreased uptake of glutamate by astrocyte transporters could also contribute to abnormal levels of extracellular glutamate, which are directly toxic to oligodendrocytes, axons and neurons [131]. Excitotoxicity is caused mainly by sustained activation of glutamate receptors and massive subsequent influx of Ca^{2+} into viable neurons, which in turn results in changes in microtubules and neurofilament phosphorylation, ultimately leading to axon cytoskeleton breakdown (see below) [132].

It is important to note astrocytes have a dual role, not only aiding axonal degeneration, but also creating a permissive environment promoting remyelination [133]. The actual impact of astrocytes on pathogenesis and repair of inflammation therefore, will be dependent on a number of factors, including timing after injury, type of lesion and surrounding microenvironment, as well as interaction with other cell types and factors influencing their activation [134].

5. Redistribution of Ion Channels and Axonal Damage

Because pathology findings and number of transected axons correlate with degree of inflammation in MS [7,135], great interest has been focused on neurotoxic products release by the innate immune system, in particular, ROS, RNS, and NO produced by macrophages, microglia, and astrocytes both in MS and EAE [136]. Mitochondria and mitochondrial DNA (mtDNA) are highly susceptible to oxidative injury. ROS and RNS generate mitochondrial enzymes deficit which can be either reversible or irreversible. In MS highly active lesions show diffuse mitochondrial damage, making energy failure the main mechanisms behind functional and structural loss [137]. During progressive MS mitochondrial injury emerges in grey matter, and neuronal cell bodies in deeper layers of the cortex show both impaired mitochondrial activity in the respiratory chain complexes as well as alterations in motor proteins responsible for mitochondria movement from the cell body to axons [96,138]. Axonal transport is essential for neuronal health, and has been implicated in different neurodegenerative conditions. Mitochondria, like other membranous organelles are transported along the axon by two major families of microtubule-based molecular motors, the kinesin family which mediates anterograde transport away from the cell body toward the axon terminal, and cytoplasmic dynein which drives retrograde transport from the distal axon toward the cell body [139]. Notably, in non-demyelinated cortex in progressive MS patients mitochondrial transport deficits, associated with kinesin decrease, preceded structural axons alterations, and morphological changes in mitochondria [140,141]. Additionally, progressive MS neurons in deeper cortical layers present mitochondrias with mtDNA deletions, indicative of an accelerated aging phenotype [138]. Consequences of mitochondrial abnormalities in neuronal cell bodies and axons are two-fold. First, mitochondrial dysfunction results in energy deficiency, which in mild forms will induce functional disturbances, in the absence of structural damage. However, when injury surpasses a certain threshold, energy deficiency will lead to axonal degeneration and cell death [142]. Once a neuronal system has lost it reserves capacity, it is less capable of spontaneous recovery and hence less prone to functional improvement. Second, mitochondrial injury may amplify oxidative stress through release of oxygen radicals, generated as a result of impaired respiratory chain function, establishing a vicious cycle of tissue destruction [143]. Following demyelination, redistribution of certain isoforms of Na^+ channels (Na_v 1.1 and Na_v 1.6) along the unmyelinated segment ensues, resulting in increased sodium influx. Early redistribution of Na^+ channels along denuded axons in white matter of MS plaques and EAE may allow continuation of action potentials in the context of MS recovery of clinical function [144,145]. Interestingly, Na_v 1.6, which generates persistent electrical current much larger than those of Na_v 1. 2 [146], is co-localized with Na^+/Ca^{2+} exchanger and with APP, a marker of axonal injury. Conversely, Na_v 1. 2 channels may serve an adaptive function with limited ability to sustain high-frequency conduction of action potentials and may contribute to slow depolarization, promoting ectopic firing patterns after demyelination [137]. Slow axonal transport of mitochondria as well as, mitochondrial damage may lead to failure of the Na^+/K^+ ATPase pump, generating a persistent sodium current. Na^+ accumulated in the axoplasm is replaced by Ca^{2+} through a reverse action of the Na^+/Ca^{2+} exchanger. Increased intra-axonal Ca^{2+} activate a variety of catabolic enzymes including proteases, phospholipases and calpains, ultimately leading to progressive proteolytic degradation of cytoskeletal proteins [147]; (Figure 2B). Moreover, intracellular Ca^{2+} increase results in changes in microtubules and neurofilaments (NF) phosphorylation, ultimately causing cytoskeleton breakdown [132]. Additional deleterious accumulation of Ca^{2+} in axons results from influx via L- and N-type Ca^{2+} channels [148], as well as release from intracellular stores in the axoplasmic reticulum. Abnormal axonal accumulation of Ca^{2+} may also result from glutamate neurotoxicity, which alters intracellular Ca^{2+} homeostasis through a mechanism mediated by axonal AMPA/kainate and metabotropic glutamate receptors, located in the intermodal region of the axons [149]. In addition to Na^+ channels, others ion channels show parallel adaptive changes to inflammatory stimuli by altering their distribution in neurons as an initial compensatory mechanism, to preserve conductance and axonal integrity. Redistribution of voltage-gated Ca^{2+} channels transient potential receptors melastatin 4 (TRPM4), and acid-sensing ion channels 1 (ASIC1) induce additional overload of Ca^{2+}, eliciting further deleterious effects on axons [142].

Abnormal accumulations of NF are a pathological hallmark of many human neurodegenerative disorders. Therefore, neurofilament light chain protein (NfL) together with the neurofilament medium (NfM) and heavy (NfH) subunits, are gaining increasing attention as candidate biomarkers of neuroaxonal injury because they are abundant structural scaffolding proteins of the cytoskeleton, with important roles in axon radial growth and stability, enabling effective nerve conduction velocity, as well as dendritic branching and growth [150]. They are exclusively expressed in neurons and reach abnormal levels as a result of axonal damage and eventual neuronal death. Under normal conditions NF are highly stable within axons and their turnover is low. Pathological processes that cause axonal damage release NF proteins into the CSF and peripheral blood, depending on the extent of damage. Initial studies in MS revealed that CSF levels of NfL were associated with the degree of disease activity and disability [151,152]. Furthermore, CSF levels of NfL, fall as a consequence of disease modifying therapies (DMT), suggesting that NfL can be used to monitor therapeutic efficacy [153–155]. However, despite these promising results in MS, a major barrier to widespread adoption of NfL assessment in MS research and clinical practice has been the need for CSF sampling, a problem overcome by use fourth-generation immunoassays, which allow evaluation of serum NfL levels [155]. High serum NfL levels have been associated with disability worsening and relapse status [155,156]. Patients under DMT have lower levels of serum NfL than untreated patients, indicating they are a marker of response to treatment [155]. Notably, a longitudinal study demonstrated patients with increased serum levels of NfL at baseline, independent of MRI variables, experience significantly more brain and spinal cord atrophy over 2 and 5 years of follow-up [156]. Collectively, these observations indicate serum NfL levels can be a useful marker of axonal damage, when applying adequate detection technique.

6. Loss of Myelin Trophism Induces Axonal Degeneration

Although myelin is traditionally viewed as a passive insulating structure, recent reports indicate it may exert a more dynamic role. It has become clear that myelin is metabolically active, allowing movement of macromolecules into the periaxonal space with important contributions to axonal health and neuronal survival. Indeed, once myelination is completed, a major task of oligodendrocytes is the provision of energy-rich substrates to axons required for fast axonal transport and propagation of action potentials. Furthermore, bi-directional signaling exists for efficient recruitment of resources, whereby the axons inform their myelinating cells of their metabolic needs proportionally to their activity. The myelin sheath and its subjacent axon should therefore be regarded as a functional unit coupled not only at the morphologic, but also at the metabolic level [157].

Animal studies have shown that oligodendrocytes exert a critical role in maintenance and long-term survival of axons and neurons. Mice mutant of the oligodendrocyte-specific *Plp1* gene, encoding PLP/DM20 a structural component of the myelin sheath, develop progressive axonal CNS degeneration at an older age. However, in this model PLP/DM20 absence has minimal impact on myelination [158]. Likewise, 2'3' cyclic-nucleotide 3' phosphodiesterase (CNP) knockout mice develop progressive axonopathy and die prematurely. Interestingly, these mice do not show demyelination at ages when axon degeneration is prominent [159,160]. This is surprising because there is strong evidence that CNP is expressed exclusively by oligodendrocytes. Although the pathology in both mutants is similar, mice deficient in both CNP and PLP develop a more severe axonal phenotype than either single mutant, indicating that each oligodendroglial protein serves a distinct role in supporting myelinated axon function [160]. Axonal pathology preceding axonal degeneration includes altered axonal transport and axonal ovoid formation. These findings are more prominent in paranodal regions, where myelin-axonal communication is most likely to occur, and are highly reminiscent of changes found in CNS tissue from MS patients [158,159]. Studies have also investigated the impact of acute death of oligodendroglia on neuron function and survival. Selective ablation of mature oligodendrocytes induced by diphtheria toxin produces axonal injury characterized by accumulation of non-phosphorylated neurofilaments and APP, without spread of myelin degradation Although some mice exhibited abnormalities in myelin composition, overall myelination was not affected, suggesting axonal injury is not due to demyelination [161]. Taken together, these observations from animal models suggest that the myelin-producing function of oligodendrocytes is not coupled to their role in axon preservation, and that oligodendrocytes themselves are critical for axonal function maintenance and survival in adult life.

During development oligodendrocytes import glucose and lactate to allow rapid myelination synthesize large amounts of lipids. When myelination is complete, oligodendrocytes-derived lactate and piruvate can be taken up by energy-deprived axons for mitochondrial ATP production supporting their energy needs [162]. Several experiments indicate monocarboxylic acid transporters (MCTs) are critical to maintain axonal integrity. Based on sequence homology, 16 MCTs members have been identified, of which only MCT1, 2 and 4 are found in the CNS [163]. As oligodendrocytes accumulate intracellular lactate, this substrate can flow through MCT1 into the periaxonal space, where neurons capture it through MCT2 and metabolize it to supplement energy requirements [162,164]. (Figure 2C). Notably, both genetic and pharmacologic down-regulation of MCT1, which is present almost exclusively in oligodendrocytes, results in axon degeneration and neuronal loss both in vivo and in vitro, without obvious oligodendrocyte damage [165]. Although the observations mentioned above provide strong evidence for a role of oligodendrocytes in directly supplying energy support to axons, other cells including astrocytes may also participate [166]. Astrocytes are essentially the only cells containing glycogen in the adult CNS, and glycogen metabolism followed by glyscolisis provides a source of lactate for other cells [167]. Studies show astrocytes transfer energy metabolites directly to oligodendrocytes, which in turn support neurons and axons metabolism as previously discussed (Figure 2C). Connections between astrcytes and myelinating cells occur via gap junctions formed by connexins (Cx). These gap junctions comprise Cx32 and Cx47 expressed on oligodendrocytes which form heteromeric channels with astrocytes through Cx30 and Cx43 respectively. Double mutant CX32- and Cx43-deficient mice exhibit profound CNS demyelination and axonal injury [168]. Likewise, CX47 and Cx30 double null mice, in which connections between astrocytes and oligodendrcoytes are altered, also developed myelin pathology and severe axonal degeneration [169]. Similarly, loss of Cx43 inhibits glucose delivery to progenitor oligodendrocytes cells and their proliferation, which can in turn influence oligodendrogenesis, and oligodendrocyte metabolic support [170]. Overall these findings provide new insights into the role of oligodendrocytes and astrocytes biology. Identification of bi-directional signaling pathways by which oligodendrocytes influence the axonal metabolism, is highly relevant to understanding MS progression.

7. Conclusions and Future Perspectives

Identification of effective therapies for progressive MS remains a priority and a challenge for the MS community. In order to develop new and effective treatment strategies it is necessary to better understand the pathological mechanisms driving disease. Unfortunately, absence of adequate animal models makes identification of potential therapeutic targets even more difficult. In this article we have recapitulated some of the main mechanisms involved in MS progression. Undoubtedly more research will lead to a better understanding of the processes of demyelination/remyelination, as well as of the importance of glial cells in neuronal homeostasis and neuronal degeneration. Clearly, identifying effective therapies for progressive MS would largely be contingent upon a comprehensive understanding of its pathogenesis, animal models incorporating these pathogenic characteristics, novel trial designs including more sensitive outcome measures, and new models of collaboration between physicians and basic science researchers.

Author Contributions: J.C. contributed to the conception and design of the manuscript, drafted the original, designed the figures, revised the draft and provided important intellectual contributions. M.M. contributed to drafting of the original manuscript, design of the figures, and providing important intellectual contributions.

M.C.Y. contributed to drafting the original manuscript, designing the figures, and providing important intellectual contributions.

Acknowledgments: We thank the collaboration of María Inés Gaitán, and Ismael Calandri for the preparation of the figures.

References

1. Thomson, A.J.; Baranzini, S.E.; Geurts, J.; Hemmer, B.; Ciccarelli, O. Multiple Sclerosis. *Lancet* **2018**, *391*, 1622–1636. [CrossRef]
2. Lassmann, H.; Brück, W.; Lucchinetti, C.F. The immunopathology of multiple sclerosis: An overview. *Brain Pathol.* **2007**, *17*, 210–218. [CrossRef] [PubMed]
3. Baecher-Allan, C.; Kaskow, B.J.; Weiner, H.L. Multiple sclerosis: Mechanisms and immunotherapy. *Neuron* **2018**, *97*, 742–768. [CrossRef] [PubMed]
4. Lublin, F.D.; Reingold, S.C. Defining the clinical course of multiple sclerosis: Results of an international survey. *Neurology* **1996**, *46*, 907–911. [CrossRef] [PubMed]
5. Skulina, C.; Schmidt, S.; Dornmair, K.; Babbe, H.; Roers, A.; Rajewsky, K.; Wekerle, H.; Hohlfeld, R.; Goebels, N. Multiple sclerosis: Brain-infiltrating $CD8^+$ T cells persist as clonal expansions in the cerebrospinal fluid and blood. *Proc. Natl. Acad. Sci. USA* **2004**, *101*, 2428–2433. [CrossRef] [PubMed]
6. Ghione, E.; Bergsland, N.; Ghione, E.; Bergsland, N.; Dwyer, M.G.; Hagemeier, J.; Jakimovski, D.; Paunkoski, I.; Ramasamy, D.P.; Silva, D.; et al. Brain Atrophy Is Associated with Disability Progression in Patients with MS followed in a Clinical Routine. *Am. J. Neuroradiol.* **2018**, *39*, 2237–2242. [CrossRef] [PubMed]
7. Trapp, B.D.; Peterson, J.; Ransohoff, R.M.; Rudick, R.; Mörk, S.; Bö, L. Axonal transection in lesions of Multiple Sclerosis. *N. Engl. J. Med.* **1998**, *338*, 278–285. [CrossRef] [PubMed]
8. Peterson, J.W.; Bö, L.; Mörk, S.; Chang, A.; Trapp, B.D. Transected neurites, apoptotic neurons, and reduced inflammation in cortical multiple sclerosis lesions. *Ann. Neurol.* **2001**, *50*, 389–400. [CrossRef]
9. Kutzelnigg, A.; Faber-Rod, J.C.; Bauer, J.; Lucchinetti, C.F.; Sorensen, P.S.; Laursen, H.; Stadelmann, C.; Brück, W.; Rauschka, H.; Schmidbauer, M.; et al. Widespread demyelination in the cerebellar cortex in multiple sclerosis. *Brain Pathol.* **2007**, *17*, 38–44. [CrossRef]
10. Geurts, J.J.; Bö, L.; Roosendaal, S.D.; Hazes, T.; Daniëls, R.; Barkhof, F.; Witter, M.P.; Huitinga, I.; van der Valk, P. Extensive hippocampal demyelination in multiple sclerosis. *J. Neuropathol. Exp. Neurol.* **2007**, *66*, 819–827. [CrossRef]
11. Vercellino, M.; Masera, S.; Lorenzatti, M.; Condello, C.; Merola, A.; Mattioda, A.; Tribolo, A.; Capello, E.; Mancardi, G.L.; Mutani, R.; et al. Demyelination, inflammation, and neurodegeneration in multiple sclerosis deep gray matter. *J. Neuropathol. Exp. Neurol.* **2009**, *68*, 489–502. [CrossRef] [PubMed]
12. Wegner, C.; Esiri, M.M.; Chance, S.A.; Palace, J.; Matthews, P.M. Neocortical neuronal, synaptic, and glial loss in multiple sclerosis. *Neurology* **2006**, *67*, 960–967. [CrossRef] [PubMed]
13. Kutzelnigg, A.; Lucchinetti, C.F.; Stadelmann, C.; Brück, W.; Rauschka, H.; Bergmann, M.; Schmidbauer, M.; Parisi, J.E.; Lassmann, H. Cortical demyelination and diffuse white matter injury in multiple sclerosis. *Brain* **2005**, *128*, 2705–2712. [CrossRef] [PubMed]
14. De Stefano, N.; Matthews, P.M. Evidence of early cortical atrophy in MS Relevance to white matter changes and disability. *Neurology* **2003**, *60*, 1157–1162. [CrossRef] [PubMed]
15. Montalban, X.; Gold, R.; Thompson, A.J.; Otero-Romero, S.; Amato, M.P.; Chandraratna, D.; Clanet, M.; Comi, G.; Derfuss, T.; Fazekas, F.; et al. ECTRIMS/EAN guideline on the pharmacological treatment of people with multiple sclerosis. *Eur. J. Neurol.* **2018**, *25*, 215–237. [CrossRef] [PubMed]
16. Rae-Grant, A.; Day, G.S.; Marrie, R.A.; Rabinstein, A.; Cree, B.A.C.; Gronseth, G.S.; Haboubi, M.; Halper, J.; Hosey, J.P.; Jones, D.E.; et al. Comprehensive systematic review summary: Disease-modifying therapies for adults with multiple sclerosis: Report of the Guideline Development, Dissemination, and Implementation Subcommittee of the American Academy of Neurology. *Neurology* **2018**, *90*, 789–800. [CrossRef] [PubMed]
17. Bø, L.; Vedeler, C.A.; Nyland, H.I.; Trapp, B.D.; Mørk, S.J. Subpial demyelination in the cerebral cortex of multiple sclerosis patients. *J. Neuropathol. Exp. Neurol.* **2003**, *62*, 723–732. [CrossRef] [PubMed]
18. Bø, L.; Geurts, J.J.G.; Nyland, H.I.; Trapp, B.D.; Mørk, S.J. Grey matter pathology in multiple sclerosis. *Acta Neurol. Scand.* **2006**, *113*, 48–50. [CrossRef]

19. Magliozzi, R.; Howell, O.; Vora, A.; Serafini, B.; Nicholas, R.; Puopolo, M.; Reynolds, R.; Aloisi, F. Meningeal B-cell follicles in secondary progressive multiple sclerosis associate with early onset of disease and severe cortical pathology. *Brain* **2007**, *130*, 1089–1104. [CrossRef]

20. Bevan, R.J.; Evans, R.; Griffiths, L.; Watkins, L.M.; Rees, M.I.; Magliozzi, R.; Allen, I.; McDonnell, G.; Kee, R.; Naughton, M.; et al. Meningeal inflammation and cortical demyelination in acute multiple sclerosis. *Ann. Neurol.* **2018**, *84*, 829–842. [CrossRef]

21. Eshaghi, A.; Prados, F.; Brownlee, W.J.; Altmann, D.R.; Tur, C.; Cardoso, M.J.; De Angelis, F.; van de Pavert, S.H.; Cawley, N.; De Stefano, N.; et al. Deep gray matter volume loss drives disability worsening in multiple sclerosis. *Ann. Neurol.* **2018**, *83*, 210–222. [CrossRef] [PubMed]

22. Lucchinetti, C.F.; Popescu, B.F.; Bunyan, R.F.; Moll, N.M.; Roemer, S.F.; Lassmann, H.; Brück, W.; Parisi, J.E.; Scheithauer, B.W.; Giannini, C.; et al. Inflammatory cortical demyelination in early multiple sclerosis. *N. Engl. J. Med.* **2011**, *365*, 2188–2197. [CrossRef] [PubMed]

23. Magliozzi, R.; Howell, O.W.; Reeves, C.; Roncaroli, F.; Nicholas, R.; Serafini, B.; Aloisi, F.; Reynolds, R. A gradient of neuronal loss and meningeal inflammation in multiple sclerosis. *Ann. Neurol.* **2010**, *68*, 477–493. [CrossRef] [PubMed]

24. Popescu, B.F.; Lucchinetti, C.F. Meningeal and cortical grey matter pathology in multiple sclerosis. *BMC Neurol.* **2012**, *12*, 11. [CrossRef] [PubMed]

25. Steenwijk, M.D.; Geurts, J.J.G.; Daams, M.; Tijms, B.M.; Wink, A.M.; Balk, L.J.; Tewarie, P.K.; Uitdehaag, B.M.; Barkhof, F.; Vrenken, H.; et al. Cortical atrophy patterns in multiple sclerosis are non-random and clinically relevant. *Brain* **2016**, *139*, 115–126. [CrossRef]

26. Granberg, T.; Fan, Q.; Treaba, C.A.; Ouellette, R.; Herranz, E.; Mangeat, G.; Louapre, C.; Cohen-Adad, J.; Klawiter, E.C.; Sloane, J.A.; et al. In vivo characterization of cortical and white matter neuroaxonal pathology in early multiple sclerosis. *Brain* **2017**, *140*, 2912–2926. [CrossRef] [PubMed]

27. Geurts, J.J.; Barkhof, F. Grey matter pathology in multiple sclerosis. *Lancet* **2008**, *7*, 841–851. [CrossRef]

28. Popescu, B.F.; Pirko, I.; Lucchinetti, C.F. Pathology of multiple sclerosis: Where do we stand? *Continuum* **2013**, *19*, 901–921. [CrossRef]

29. Lagumersindez-Denis, N.; Wrzos, C.; Mack, M.; Winkler, A.; van der Meer, F.; Reinert, M..; Hollasch, H.; Flach, A.; Brühl, H.; Cullen, E.; et al. Differential contribution of immune effector mechanisms to cortical demyelination in multiple scleosis. *Acta Neuropathol.* **2017**, *134*, 15–34. [CrossRef]

30. Chang, A.; Staugaitis, S.M.; Dutta, R.; Batt, C.E.; Easley, K.E.; Chomyk, A.M.; Yong, V.W.; Fox, R.J.; Kidd, G.J.; Trapp, B.D. Cortical remyelination: A new target for repair therapies in multiple sclerosis. *Ann. Neurol.* **2012**, *72*, 918–926. [CrossRef]

31. Bø, L.; Vedeler, C.A.; Nyland, H.; Trapp, B.D.; Mørk, S.J. Intracortical multiple sclerosis lesions are not associated with increased lymphocyte infiltration. *Mult. Scler.* **2003**, *9*, 323–331. [CrossRef] [PubMed]

32. Bö, L.; Geurts, J.J.; van der Valk, P.; Polman, C.; Barkhof, F. Lack of correlation between cortical demyelination and white matter pathologic changes in multiple sclerosis. *Arch. Neurol.* **2007**, *64*, 76–80. [CrossRef] [PubMed]

33. Fisniku, L.K.; Chard, D.T.; Jackson, J.S.; Anderson, V.M.; Altmann, D.R.; Miszkiel, K.A.; Thompson, A.J.; Miller, D.H. Gray matter atrophy is related to long-term disability in multiple sclerosis. *Ann. Neurol.* **2008**, *64*, 247–254. [CrossRef] [PubMed]

34. Fisher, E.; Lee, J.C.; Nakamura, K.; Rudick, R.A. Gray matter atrophy in multiple sclerosis: A longitudinal study. *Ann. Neurol.* **2008**, *64*, 255–265. [CrossRef] [PubMed]

35. Evangelou, N.; Konz, D.; Esiri, M.M.; Smith, S.; Palace, J.; Matthews, P.M. Size-selective neuronal changes in the anterior optic pathways suggest a differential susceptibility to injury in multiple sclerosis. *Brain* **2001**, *124*, 1813–1820. [CrossRef] [PubMed]

36. Azevedo, C.J.; Cen, S.Y.; Khadka, S.; Liu, S.; Kornak, J.; Shi, Y.; Zheng, L.; Hauser, S.L.; Pelletier, D. Thalamic atrophy in multiple sclerosis: A magnetic resonance imaging marker of neurodegeneration throughout disease. *Ann. Neurol.* **2018**, *83*, 223–234. [CrossRef] [PubMed]

37. Gaetano, L.; Häring, D.A.; Radue, E.W.; Mueller-Lenke, N.; Thakur, A.; Tomic, D.; Kappos, L.; Sprenger, T. Fingolimod effect on gray matter, thalamus, and white matter in patients with multiple sclerosis. *Neurology* **2018**, *90*, e1324–e1332. [CrossRef] [PubMed]

38. Fischer, M.T.; Wimmer, I.; Höftberger, R.; Gerlach, S.; Haider, L.; Zrzavy, T.; Hametner, S.; Mahad, D.; Binder, C.J.; Krumbholz, M.; et al. Disease-specific molecular events in cortical multiple sclerosis lesions. *Brain* **2013**, *136*, 1799–1815. [CrossRef]

39. Meuth, S.G.; Simon, O.J.; Grimm, A.; Melzer, N.; Herrmann, A.M.; Spitzer, P.; Landgraf, P.; Wiendl, H. CNS inflammation and neuronal degeneration is aggravated by impaired CD200–CD200R-mediated macrophage silencing. *J. Neuroimmunol.* **2008**, *194*, 62–69. [CrossRef]

40. Barnett, M.H.; Prineas, J.W. Relapsing and remitting multiple sclerosis: Pathology of the newly forming lesion. *Ann. Neurol.* **2004**, *55*, 458–468. [CrossRef]

41. Kassmann, C.M.; Lappe-Siefke, C.; Baes, M.; Brügger, B.; Mildner, A.; Werner, H.B.; Natt, O.; Michaelis, T.; Prinz, M.; Frahm, J.; Nave, K.A. Axonal loss and neuroinflammation caused by peroxisome-deficient oligodendrocytes. *Nat. Genet.* **2007**, *39*, 969. [CrossRef] [PubMed]

42. Hemmer, B.; Kerschensteiner, M.; Korn, T. Role of the innate and adaptive immune responses in the course of multiple sclerosis. *Lancet Neurol.* **2015**, *14*, 406–419. [CrossRef]

43. Magliozzi, R.; Howell, O.W.; Nicholas, R.; Cruciani, C.; Castellaro, M.; Romualdi, C.; Rossi, S.; Pitteri, M.; Benedetti, M.D.; Gajofatto, A.; et al. Inflammatory intrathecal profiles and cortical damage in multiple sclerosis. *Ann. Neurol.* **2018**, *83*, 739–755. [CrossRef] [PubMed]

44. Bar-Or, A.; Fawaz, L.; Fan, B.; Darlington, P.J.; Rieger, A.; Ghorayeb, C.; Calabresi, P.A.; Waubant, E.; Hauser, S.L.; Zhang, J.; et al. Abnormal B-cell cytokine responses a trigger of T-cell–mediated disease in MS? *Ann. Neurol.* **2010**, *67*, 452–461. [CrossRef] [PubMed]

45. Aloisi, F.; Pujol-Borrell, R. Lymphoid neogenesis in chronic inflammatory diseases. *Nat. Rev. Immunol.* **2006**, *6*, 205–217. [CrossRef] [PubMed]

46. Serafini, B.; Rosicarelli, B.; Magliozzi, R.; Stigliano, E.; Aloisi, F. Detection of ectopic B-cell follicles with germinal centers in the meninges of patients with secondary progressive multiple sclerosis. *Brain Pathol.* **2004**, *14*, 164–174. [CrossRef] [PubMed]

47. Pitzalis, C.; Jones, G.W.; Bombardieri, M.; Jones, S.A. Ectopic lymphoid-like structures in infection, cancer and autoimmunity. *Nat. Rev. Immunol.* **2014**, *14*, 447. [CrossRef] [PubMed]

48. Corsiero, E.; Nerviani, A.; Bombardieri, M.; Pitzalis, C. Ectopic lymphoid structures: Powerhouse of autoimmunity. *Front. Immunol.* **2016**, *7*, 430. [CrossRef] [PubMed]

49. Jones, G.W.; Jones, S.A. Ectopic lymphoid follicles: Inducible centers for generating antigen-specific immune responses within tissues. *Immunology* **2016**, *147*, 141–151. [CrossRef] [PubMed]

50. Lovato, L.; Willis, S.N.; Rodig, S.J.; Caron, T.; Almendinger, S.E.; Howell, O.W.; Reynolds, R.; O'Connor, K.C.; Hafler, D.A. Related B cell clones populate the meninges and parenchyma of patients with multiple sclerosis. *Brain* **2011**, *134*, 534–541. [CrossRef] [PubMed]

51. Howell, O.W.; Reeves, C.A.; Nicholas, R.; Carassiti, D.; Radotra, B.; Gentleman, S.M.; Serafini, B.; Aloisi, F.; Roncaroli, F.; Magliozzi, R.; et al. Meningeal inflammation is widespread and linked to cortical pathology in multiple sclerosis. *Brain* **2011**, *134*, 2755–2771. [CrossRef] [PubMed]

52. Corsiero, E.; Bombardieri, M.; Manzo, A.; Bugatti, S.; Uguccioni, M.; Pitzalis, C. Role of lymphoid chemokines in the development of functional ectopic lymphoid structures in rheumatic autoimmune diseases. *Immunol. Lett.* **2012**, *145*, 62–67. [CrossRef] [PubMed]

53. Vanguri, P.; Shin, M.L. Activation of complement by myelin: Identification of C1-binding proteins of human myelin from central nervous tissue. *J. Neurochem.* **1986**, *46*, 1535–1541. [CrossRef] [PubMed]

54. Huizinga, R.; Heijmans, N.; Schubert, P.; Gschmeissner, S.; 't Hart, B.A.; Herrmann, H.; Amor, S. Immunization with neurofilament light protein induces spastic paresis and axonal degeneration in Biozzi ABH mice. *J. Neuropathol. Exp. Neurol.* **2007**, *66*, 295–304. [CrossRef] [PubMed]

55. Mathey, E.K.; Derfuss, T.; Storch, M.K.; Williams, K.R.; Hales, K.; Woolley, D.R.; Al-Hayani, A.; Davies, S.N.; Rasband, M.N.; Olsson, T.; et al. Neurofascin as a novel target for autoantibody-mediated axonal injury. *J. Exp. Med.* **2007**, *204*, 2363–2372. [CrossRef] [PubMed]

56. Manzo, A.; Bombardieri, M.; Humby, F.; Pitzalis, C. Secondary and ectopic lymphoid tissue responses in rheumatoid arthritis: From inflammation to autoimmunity and tissue damage/remodeling. *Immunol. Rev.* **2010**, *233*, 267–285. [CrossRef] [PubMed]

57. Makshakov, G.; Magonov, E.; Totolyan, N.; Nazarov, V.; Lapin, S.; Mazing, A.; Verbitskaya, E.; Trofimova, T.; Krasnov, V.; Shumilina, M.; et al. Leptomeningeal contrast enhancement is associated with disability progression and grey matter atrophy in multiple sclerosis. *Neurol. Res. Int.* **2017**. [CrossRef] [PubMed]

58. Zivadinov, R.; Ramasamy, D.P.; Vaneckova, M.; Gandhi, S.; Chandra, A.; Hagemeier, J.; Bergsland, N.; Polak, P.; Benedict, R.H.; Hojnacki, D.; et al. Leptomeningeal contrast enhancement is associated with progression of cortical atrophy in MS: A retrospective, pilot, observational longitudinal study. *Mult. Scler.* **2016**, *23*, 1336–1345. [CrossRef] [PubMed]

59. Choi, S.R.; Howell, O.W.; Carassiti, D.; Magliozzi, R.; Gveric, D.; Muraro, P.A.; Nicholas, R.; Roncaroli, F.; Reynolds, R. Meningeal inflammation plays a role in the pathology of primary progressive multiple sclerosis. *Brain* **2012**, *135*, 2925–2937. [CrossRef] [PubMed]

60. Antel, J.; Antel, S.; Caramanos, Z.; Arnold, D.L.; Kuhlmann, T. Primary progressive multiple sclerosis: Part of the MS disease spectrum or separate disease entity? *Acta Neuropathol.* **2012**, *123*, 627–638. [CrossRef] [PubMed]

61. Ascherio, A.; Munger, K.L.; Lennette, E.T.; Spiegelman, D.; Hernán, M.A.; Olek, M.J.; Hankinson, S.E.; Hunter, D.J. Epstein-Barr virus antibodies and risk of multiple sclerosis: A prospective study. *JAMA* **2001**, *286*, 3083–3088. [CrossRef] [PubMed]

62. Warner, H.B.; Carp, R.I. Multiple Sclerosis and Epstein-Barr virus. *Lancet* **1981**, *2*, 1290. [CrossRef]

63. Serafini, B.; Rosicarelli, B.; Franciotta, D.; Magliozzi, R.; Reynolds, R.; Cinque, P.; Andreoni, L.; Trivedi., P.; Salvetti, M.; Faggioni, A.; et al. Dysregulated Epstein-Barr virus infection in the multiple sclerosis brain. *J. Exp. Med.* **2007**, *204*, 2899–2912. [CrossRef] [PubMed]

64. Küppers, R. B cells under influence: Transformation of B cells by Epstein–Barr virus. *Nat. Rev. Immunol.* **2003**, *3*, 801. [CrossRef] [PubMed]

65. Willis, S.N.; Stadelmann, C.; Rodig, S.J.; Caron, T.; Gattenloehner, S.; Mallozzi, S.S.; Roughan, J.E.; Almendinger, S.E.; Blewett, M.M.; Brück, W.; et al. Epstein–Barr virus infection is not a characteristic feature of multiple sclerosis brain. *Brain* **2009**, *132*, 3318–3328. [CrossRef] [PubMed]

66. Hislop, A.D.; Taylor, G.S.; Sauce, D.; Rickinson, A.B. Cellular responses to viral infection in humans: Lessons from Epstein-Barr virus. *Annu. Rev. Immunol.* **2007**, *25*, 587–617. [CrossRef] [PubMed]

67. Magliozzi, R.; Serafini, B.; Rosicarel, B.; Chiappetta, G.; Veroni, C.; Reynolds, R.; Aloisi, F. B-cell enrichment and Epstein-Barr virus infection in inflammatory cortical lesions in secondary progressive multiple sclerosis. *J. Neuropathol. Exp. Neurol.* **2013**, *72*, 29–41. [CrossRef] [PubMed]

68. Bitsch, A.; Schuchardt, J.; Bunkowski, S.; Kuhlmann, T.; Brück, W. Acute axonal injury in multiple sclerosis: Correlation with demyelination and inflammation. *Brain* **2000**, *123*, 1174–1183. [CrossRef] [PubMed]

69. Medana, I.M.; Gallimore, A.; Oxenius, A.; Martinic, M.M.; Wekerle, H.; Neumann, H. MHC class I-restricted killing of neurons by virus-specific CD8$^+$ T lymphocytes is effected through the Fas/FasL, but not the perforin pathway. *Eur. J. Immunol.* **2000**, *30*, 3623–3633. [CrossRef]

70. Meuth, S.G.; Herrmann, A.M.; Simon, O.J.; Siffrin, V.; Melzer, N.; Bittner, S.; Meuth, P.; Langer, H.F.; Hallermann, S.; Boldakowa, N.; et al. Cytotoxic CD8$^+$ T cell–neuron interactions: Perforin-dependent electrical silencing precedes but is not causally linked to neuronal cell death. *J. Neurosci.* **2009**, *29*, 15397–15409. [CrossRef] [PubMed]

71. Junker, A.; Ivanidze, J.; Malotka, J.; Eiglmeier, I.; Lassmann, H.; Wekerle, H.; Meinl, E.; Hohlfeld, R.; Dornmair, K. Multiple sclerosis: T-cell receptor expression in distinct brain regions. *Brain* **2007**, *130*, 2789–2799. [CrossRef] [PubMed]

72. Jacobsen, M.; Cepok, S.; Quak, E.; Happel, M.; Gaber, R.; Ziegler, A.; Schock, S.; Oertel, W.H.; Sommer, N.; Hemmer, B. Oligoclonal expansion of memory CD8$^+$ T cells in cerebrospinal fluid from multiple sclerosis patients. *Brain* **2002**, *125*, 538–550. [CrossRef] [PubMed]

73. Mars, L.T.; Saikali, P.; Liblau, R.S.; Arbour, N. Contribution of CD8 T lymphocytes to the immuno-pathogenesis of multiple sclerosis and its animal models. *Biochim. Biophys. Acta* **2011**, *1812*, 151–161. [CrossRef] [PubMed]

74. Kuhlmann, T.; Lingfeld, G.; Bitsch, A.; Schuchardt, J.; Brück, W. Acute axonal damage in multiple sclerosis is most extensive in early disease stages and decreases over time. *Brain* **2002**, *125*, 2202–2212. [CrossRef] [PubMed]

75. Ferguson, B.; Matyszak, M.K.; Esiri, M.M.; Perry, V.H. Axonal damage in acute multiple sclerosis lesions. *Brain* **1997**, *120*, 393–399. [CrossRef] [PubMed]

76. Höftberger, R.; Aboul-Enein, F.; Brueck, W.; Lucchinetti, C.; Rodriguez, M.; Schmidbauer, M.; Jellinger, K.; Lassmann, H. Expression of major histocompatibility complex class 1 molecules on the different cell types in multiple sclerosis lesions. *Brain Pathol.* **2004**, *14*, 43–50. [CrossRef] [PubMed]

77. Huse, M.; Quann, E.J.; Davis, M.M. Shouts, whispers and the kiss of death: Directional secretion in T cells. *Nat. Immunol.* **2008**, *9*, 1105. [CrossRef] [PubMed]

78. Mizuno, T.; Zhang, G.; Takeuchi, H.; Kawanokuchi, J.; Wang, J.; Sonobe, Y.; Jin, S.; Takada, N.; Komatsu, Y.; Suzumura, A. Interferon-γ directly induces neurotoxicity through a neuron specific, calcium-permeable complex of IFN-γ receptor and AMPA GluR1 receptor. *FASEB J.* **2008**, *22*, 1797–1806. [CrossRef] [PubMed]

79. Venters, H.D.; Dantzer, R.; Kelley, K.W. A new concept in neurodegeneration: TNFα is a silencer of survival signals. *Trend Neurosci.* **2000**, *23*, 175–180. [CrossRef]

80. Wang, T.; Allie, R.; Conant, K.; Haughey, N.; Turchan-Chelowo, J.; Hahn, K.; Rosen, A.; Steiner, J.; Keswani, S.; Jones, M.; et al. Granzyme B mediates neurotoxicity through a G-protein-coupled receptor. *FASEB J.* **2006**, *20*, 1209–1211. [CrossRef] [PubMed]

81. Giuliani, F.; Goodyer, C.G.; Antel, J.P.; Yong, V.W. Vulnerability of human neurons to T cell-mediated cytotoxicity. *J. Immunol.* **2003**, *171*, 368–379. [CrossRef] [PubMed]

82. Raveney, B.J.E.; Oki, O.; Hohjoh, H.; Nakamura, M.; Sato, W.; Murata, M.; Yamamura, T. Eomesodermin-expressing T-helper cells are essential for chronic neuroinflammation. *Nat. Commun.* **2015**, *6*, 8437. [CrossRef] [PubMed]

83. Broux, B.; Markovic-Plese, S.; Stinissen, P.; Hellings, N. Pathogenic features of CD4$^+$CD28$^-$ T cells in immune disorders. *Trends Mol. Med.* **2012**, *18*, 446–453. [CrossRef] [PubMed]

84. Kovalcsik, E.; Antunes, R.F.; Baruah, P.; Kaski, J.C.; Dumitriu, J.E. Proteasome-mediated reduction in proapoptotic molecule Bim renders CD4$^+$CD28^{null} T cell resistant to apoptosis in acute coronary syndrome. *Circulation* **2015**, *131*, 709–720. [CrossRef] [PubMed]

85. Thewissen, M.; Somers, V.; Hellings, N.; Fraussen, J.; Damoiseaux, J.; Stinissen, P. CD4$^+$CD28^{null} T cells in autoimmune disease: Pathogenic features and decreased susceptibility to immunoregualtion. *J. Immunol.* **2007**, *179*, 6514–6523. [CrossRef] [PubMed]

86. Markovic-Plese, S.; Cortese, I.; Wandinger, K.P.; McFarland, H.F.; Martin, R. CD4$^+$CD28$^-$ costimualtion-independent T cells in multiple sclerosis. *J. Clin. Investig.* **2001**, *108*, 1185–1194. [CrossRef] [PubMed]

87. Scholz, C.; Patton, K.T.; Anderson, D.E.; Freeman, G.J.; Hafler, D.A. Expansion of autoreactive T cells in multiple sclerosis is independent of exogenous B7 costimulation. *J. Immunol.* **1998**, *160*, 1532–1538. [PubMed]

88. Dumitriu, I.E.; Araguás, E.T.; Baboorian, C.; Kaski, J.C. CD4$^+$CD28^{null} T cells in coronary artery disease: When helpers become killers. *Cardiovasc. Res.* **2009**, *81*, 11–19. [CrossRef]

89. Peeters, L.M.; Vanheusden, M.; Somers, V.; Van Wijmeersch, B.; Stinissen, P.; Broux, B.; Hellings, N. Cytotoxic CD4$^+$ T cells drive multiple sclerosis progression. *Front. Immunol.* **2017**, *8*, 1160. [CrossRef]

90. Schmidt, D.; Goronzy, J.J.; Weyand, C.M. CD4$^+$ CD7$^-$ CD28$^-$ T cells are expanded in rheumatoid arthritis and are characterized by autoreactivity. *J. Clin. Investig.* **1996**, *97*, 2027–2037. [CrossRef]

91. Lassmann, H. Multiple sclerosis: Lessons from molecular neuropathology. *Exp. Neurol.* **2014**, *262*, 2–7. [CrossRef] [PubMed]

92. Kigerl, K.A.; de Rivero Vaccari, J.P.; Dietrich, W.D.; Popovich, P.G.; Keane, R.W. Pattern recognition recpetors and central nervous system repair. *Exp. Neurol.* **2014**, *258*, 5–16. [CrossRef] [PubMed]

93. De Groot, C.J.A.; Bergers, E.; Kamphorst, W.; Ravid, R.; Polman, C.H.; Barkhof, F.; van der Valk, P. Post-mortem MRI-guided sampling of multiple sclerosis brain lesions: Increased yield of active demyelinating and (p) reactive lesions. *Brain* **2001**, *124*, 1635–1645. [CrossRef] [PubMed]

94. Singh, S.; Metz, I.; Amor, S.; van der Valk, P.; Stadelmann, C.; Brück, W. Microglial nodules in early multiple sclerosis white matter are associated with degenerating axons. *Acta Neuropathol.* **2013**, *125*, 595–608. [CrossRef] [PubMed]

95. Correale, J. The role of microglial activation in disease progression. *Mult. Scler.* **2014**, *20*, 1288–1295. [CrossRef] [PubMed]

96. Campbell, G.R.; Ziabreva, I.; Ziabreva, I.; Reeve, A.K.; Krishnan, K.J.; Reynolds, R.; Howell, O.; Lassmann, H.; Turnbull, D.M.; Mahad, D.J. Mitochondrial DNA deletions and neurodegeneration in multiple sclerosis. *Ann. Neurol.* **2011**, *69*, 481–492. [CrossRef]

97. Nikić, I.; Merkler, D.; Sorbara, C.; Brinkoetter, M.; Kreutzfeldt, M.; Bareyre, F.M.; Brück, W.; Bishop, D.; Misgeld, T.; Kerschensteiner, M. A reversible form of axon damage in experimental autoimmune encephalomyelitis and multiple sclerosis. *Nat. Med.* **2011**, *17*, 495. [CrossRef]

98. Hametner, S.; Wimmer, I.; Haider, L.; Pfeifenbring, S.; Brück, W.; Lassmann, H. Iron and neurodegeneration in the multiple sclerosis brain. *Ann. Neurol.* **2013**, *74*, 848–861. [CrossRef]

99. Politis, M.; Su, P.; Piccini, P. Imaging of microglia in patients with neurodegenerative disorders. *Front. Pharmacol.* **2012**, *3*, 96. [CrossRef]

100. Cosenza-Nashat, M.; Zhao, M.L.; Suh, H.S.; Morgan, J.; Natividad., R.; Morgello, S.; Lee, S.C. Expression of the translocator protein of 18 kDa by microglia, macrophages and astrocytes based on immunohistochemical localization in abnormal human brain. *Neuropathol. Appl. Neurobiol.* **2009**, *35*, 306–328. [CrossRef]

101. Maeda, J.; Higuchi, M.; Inaji, M.; Ji, B.; Haneda, E.; Okauchi, T.; Zhang, M.R.; Suzuki, K.; Suhara, T. Phase-dependent roles of reactive microglia and astrocytes in nervous system injury as delineated by imaging of peripheral benzodiazepine receptor. *Brain Res.* **2007**, *1157*, 100–111. [CrossRef] [PubMed]

102. Banati, R.B.; Newcombe, J.; Gunn, R.N.; Cagnin, A.; Turkheimer, F.; Heppner, F.; Price, G.; Wegner, F.; Giovannoni, G.; Miller, D.H.; et al. The peripheral benzodiazepine binding site in the brain in multiple sclerosis: Quantitative in vivo imaging of microglia as a measure of disease activity. *Brain* **2000**, *123*, 2321–2337. [CrossRef] [PubMed]

103. Versijpt, J.; Debruyne, J.C.; Van Laere, K.J.; De Vos, F.; Keppens, J.; Strijckmans, K.; Achten, E.; Slegers, G.; Dierckx, R.A.; Korf, J.; et al. Microglial imaging with positron emission tomography and atrophy measurements with magnetic resonance imaging in multiple sclerosis: A correlative study. *Mult. Scler.* **2005**, *11*, 127–134. [CrossRef] [PubMed]

104. Politis, M.; Giannetti, P.; Su, P.; Turkheimer, F.; Keihaninejad, S.; Wu, K.; Waldman, A.; Malik, O.; Matthews, P.M.; Reynolds, R.; et al. Increased PK11195 PET binding in the cortex of patients with MS correlates with disability. *Neurology* **2012**, *79*, 523–530. [CrossRef] [PubMed]

105. Airas, L.; Nylund, M.; Rissanen, E. Evaluation of Microglial Activation in Multiple Sclerosis Patients Using Positron Emission Tomography. *Front. Neurol.* **2018**, *9*, 181. [CrossRef] [PubMed]

106. Sharma, R.; Fischer, M.T.; Bauer, J.; Felts, P.A.; Smith, K.J.; Misu, T.; Fujihara, K.; Bradl, M.; Lassmann, H. Inflammation induced by innate immunity in the central nervous system leads to primary astrocyte dysfunction followed by demyelination. *Acta Neuropathol.* **2010**, *120*, 223–236. [CrossRef] [PubMed]

107. Grinnell, A.D.; Chen, B.M.; Kashani, A.; Lin, J.; Suzuki, K.; Kidokoro, Y. The role of integrins in the modulation of neurotransmitter release from motor nerve terminals by stretch and hypertonicity. *J. Neurocytol.* **2003**, *32*, 489–503. [CrossRef] [PubMed]

108. Cuddapah, V.A.; Robel, S.; Watkins, S.; Sontheimer, H. A neurocentric perspective on glioma invasion. *Nat. Rev. Neurosci.* **2014**, *15*, 455. [CrossRef] [PubMed]

109. Goddard, D.R.; Berry, M.; Butt, A.M. In vivo actions of fibroblast growth factor-2 and insulin-like growth factor-I on oligodendrocyte development and myelination in the central nervous system. *J. Neurosci. Res.* **1999**, *57*, 74–85. [CrossRef]

110. Sherman, L.S.; Struve, J.N.; Rangwala, R.; Wallingford, N.M.; Tuohy, T.M.; Kuntz, C., 4th. Hyaluronate-based extracellular matrix: Keeping glia in their place. *Glia* **2002**, *38*, 93–102. [CrossRef]

111. Soilu-Hänninen, M.; Laaksonen, M.; Hänninen, A.; Erälinna, J.P.; Panelius, M. Downregulation of VLA-4 on T cells as a marker of long term treatment response to interferon beta-1a in MS. *J. Neuroimmunol.* **2005**, *167*, 175–182. [CrossRef] [PubMed]

112. Johnson-Green, P.C.; Dow, K.E.; Riopelle, R.J. Characterization of glycosaminoglycans produced by primary astrocytes in vitro. *Glia* **1991**, *4*, 314–321. [CrossRef]

113. Bradbury, E.J.; Moon, L.D.; Popat, R.J.; King, V.R.; Bennett, G.S.; Patel, P.N.; Fawcett, J.W.; McMahon, S.B. Chondroitinase ABC promotes functional recovery after spinal cord injury. *Nature* **2002**, *416*, 636. [CrossRef] [PubMed]

114. Yiu, G.; He, Z. Glial inhibition of CNS axon regeneration. *Nat. Rev. Neurosci.* **2006**, *7*, 617. [CrossRef] [PubMed]

115. Fujita, Y.; Takashima, R.; Endo, S.; Takai, T.; Yamashita, T. The p75 receptor mediates axon growth inhibition through an association with PIR-B. *Cell Death Dis.* **2011**, *2*, e198. [CrossRef] [PubMed]

116. Gimenez, M.A.T.; Sim, J.E.; Russell, J.H. TNFR1-dependent VCAM-1 expression by astrocytes exposes the CNS to destructive inflammation. *J. Neuroimmunol.* **2004**, *151*, 116–125. [CrossRef] [PubMed]

117. Sobel, R.A.; Mitchell, M.E.; Fondren, G. Intercellular adhesion molecule-1 (ICAM-1) in cellular immune reactions in the human central nervous system. *Am. J. Pathol.* **1990**, *136*, 1309.

118. Dong, Y.; Benveniste, E.N. Immune function of astrocytes. *Glia* **2001**, *36*, 180–190. [CrossRef]

119. DeWitt, D.A.; Perry, G.; Cohen, M.; Doller, C.; Silver, J. Astrocytes regulate microglial phagocytosis of senile plaque cores of Alzheimer's disease. *Exp. Neurol.* **1998**, *149*, 329–340. [CrossRef]

120. Mayo, L.; Trauger, S.A.; Blain, M.; Nadeau, M.; Patel, B.; Alvarez, J.I.; Mascanfroni, I.D.; Yeste, A.; Kivisäkk, P.; Kallas, K.; et al. Regulation of astrocyte activation by glycolipids drives chronic CNS inflammation. *Nat. Med.* **2014**, *20*, 1147. [CrossRef]

121. Pannu, R.; Won, J.S.; Khan, M.; Singh, A.K.; Singh, I. A novel role of lactosylceramide in the regulation of lipopolysaccharide/interferon-γ-mediated inducible nitric oxide synthase gene expression: Implications for neuroinflammatory diseases. *J. Neurosci.* **2004**, *24*, 5942–5954. [CrossRef] [PubMed]

122. Krumbholz, M.; Theil, D.; Cepok, S.; Hemmer, B.; Kivisäkk, P.; Ransohoff, R.M.; Hofbauer, M.; Farina, C.; Derfuss, T.; Hartle, C.; et al. Chemokines in multiple sclerosis: CXCL12 and CXCL13 up-regulation is differentially linked to CNS immune cell recruitment. *Brain* **2005**, *129*, 200–211. [CrossRef] [PubMed]

123. Chastain, E.M.; D'Anne, S.D.; Rodgers, J.M.; Miller, S.D. The role of antigen presenting cells in multiple sclerosis. *Biochim. Biophys. Acta* **2011**, *1812*, 265–274. [CrossRef] [PubMed]

124. Kort, J.J.; Kawamura, K.; Fugger, L.; Weissert, R.; Forsthuber, T.G. Efficient presentation of myelin oligodendrocyte glycoprotein peptides but not protein by astrocytes from HLA-DR2 and HLA-DR4 transgenic mice. *J. Neuroimmunol.* **2006**, *173*, 23–34. [CrossRef] [PubMed]

125. Bal-Price, A.; Brown, G.C. Inflammatory neurodegeneration mediated by nitric oxide from activated glia-inhibiting neuronal respiration, causing glutamate release and excitotoxicity. *J. Neurosci.* **2001**, *21*, 6480–6491. [CrossRef] [PubMed]

126. Hamby, M.E.; Hewett, J.A.; Hewett, S.J. TGF-β1 potentiates astrocytic nitric oxide production by expanding the population of astrocytes that express NOS-2. *Glia* **2006**, *54*, 566–577. [CrossRef] [PubMed]

127. Lee, S.J.; Benveniste, E.N. Adhesion molecule expression and regulation on cells of the central nervous system. *J. Neuroimmunol.* **1999**, *98*, 77–88. [CrossRef]

128. Stojanovic, I.R.; Kostic, M.; Ljubisavljevic, S. The role of glutamate and its receptors in multiple sclerosis. *J. Neural Transm.* **2014**, *121*, 945–955. [CrossRef]

129. Kumar, P.; Kalonia, H.; Kumar, A. Possible GABAergic mechanism in the neuroprotective effect of gabapentin and lamotrigine against 3-nitropropionic acid induced neurotoxicity. *Eur. J. Pharmacol.* **2012**, *674*, 265–274. [CrossRef]

130. Rossi, S.; Motta, C.; Studer, V.; Barbieri, F.; Buttari, F.; Bergami, A.; Sancesario, G.; Bernardini, S.; De Angelis, G.; Martino, G.; et al. Tumor necrosis factor is elevated in progressive multiple sclerosis and causes excitotoxic neurodegeneration. *Mult. Scler.* **2014**, *20*, 304–312. [CrossRef]

131. Matute, C. Excitotoxicity in glial cells. *Proc. Natl. Acad. Sci. USA* **1997**, *94*, 8830–8835. [CrossRef] [PubMed]

132. Nicholls, D.G. Mitochondrial dysfunction and glutamate excitotoxicity studied in primary neuronal cultures. *Curr. Mol. Med.* **2004**, *4*, 149–177. [CrossRef] [PubMed]

133. Correale, J.; Farez, M.F. The role of astrocytes in multiple sclerosis progression. *Front. Neurol.* **2015**, *6*, 180. [CrossRef] [PubMed]

134. Williams, A.; Piaton, G.; Lubetzki, C. Astrocytes—friends or foes in multiple sclerosis? *Glia* **2007**, *55*, 1300–1312. [CrossRef] [PubMed]

135. Frischer, J.M.; Bramow, S.; Dal-Bianco, A.; Lucchinetti, C.F.; Rauschka, H.; Schmidbauer, M.; Laursen, H.; Sorensen, P.S.; Lassmann, H. The relation between inflammation and neurodegeneration in multiple sclerosis brains. *Brain* **2009**, *132*, 1175–1182. [CrossRef] [PubMed]

136. Haider, L.; Fischer, M.T.; Frischer, J.M.; Bauer, J.; Höftberger, R.; Botond, G.; Esterbauer, H.; Binder, C.J.; Witztum, J.L.; Lassmann, H. Oxidative damage in multiple sclerosis lesions. *Brain* **2011**, *134*, 1914–1924. [CrossRef]

137. Mahad, D.J.; Ziabreva, I.; Campbell, G.; Lax, N.; White, K.; Hanson, P.S.; Lassmann, H.; Turnbull, D.M. Mitochondrial changes within axons in multiple Sclerosis. *Brain* **2009**, *132*, 1161–1174. [CrossRef]

138. Campbell, G.R.; Worrall, J.T.; Mahad, D.J. The central role of mitochondria in axonal degeneration in multiple sclerosis. *Mult. Scler.* **2014**, *20*, 1806–1813. [CrossRef]

139. Hirokawa, N.; Niwa, S.; Tanaka, Y. Molecular motors in neurons: Transport mechanisms and roles in brain function, development and disease. *Neuron* **2010**, *68*, 610–638. [CrossRef]

140. Campbell, G.; Mahad, D. Neurodegeneration in progressive multiple sclerosis. *Cold Spring Harb. Perspect. Med.* **2018**, *8*. [CrossRef]

141. Hares, K.; Kemp, K.; Rice, C.; Gray, E.; Scolding, N.; Wilkins, A. Reduced axonal motor protein expression in non-lesional grey matter in multiple sclerosis. *Mult. Scler.* **2014**, *20*, 812–821. [CrossRef] [PubMed]

142. Friese, M.A.; Schattling, B.; Fugger, L. Mechanisms of neurodegeneration and axonal dysfunction in multiple sclerosis. *Nat. Rev. Neurol.* **2014**, *10*, 225–238. [CrossRef] [PubMed]

143. Murphy, M.P. How mitochondria produce reactive oxygen species. *Biochem. J.* **2009**, *417*, 1–13. [CrossRef] [PubMed]

144. Craner, M.J.; Hains, B.C.; Lo, A.C.; Black, J.A.; Waxman, S.G. Co-localization of sodium channel Na$_v$1. 6 and the sodium-calcium exchanger at sites of axonal injury in the spinal cord in EAE. *Brain* **2004**, *127*, 294–303. [CrossRef] [PubMed]

145. Craner, M.J.; Newcombe, J.; Black, J.A.; Hartle, C.; Cuzner, M.L.; Waxman, S.G. Molecualr changes in neurons in multiple sclerosis: Altered axonal expression of Na$_v$1.2 and Na$_v$1.6 sodium channels and Na$^+$/Ca^{2+} exchanger. *Proc. Natl. Acad. Sci. USA* **2004**, *101*, 8168–8173. [CrossRef] [PubMed]

146. Rush, A.M.; Dib-Hajj, S.D.; Waxman, S.G. Electrophysiological properties of two axonal sodium channels, Na$_v$1. 2 and Na$_v$1. 6, expressed in mouse spinal sensory neurons. *J. Physiol.* **2005**, *564*, 803–815. [CrossRef] [PubMed]

147. Stys, P.K. General mechanisms of axonal damage and its prevention. *J. Neurol. Sci.* **2005**, *233*, 3–13. [CrossRef]

148. Kornek, B.; Storch, M.K.; Bauer, J.; Djamshidian, A.; Weissert, R.; Wallstroem, E.; Stefferl, A.; Zimprich, F.; Olsson, T.; Linington, C.; et al. Distribution of a calcium channel subunit in dystrophic axons in multiple sclerosis and experimental autoimmune encephalomyelitis. *Brain* **2001**, *124*, 1114–1124. [CrossRef]

149. Stirling, D.P.; Stys, P.K. Mechanisms of axonal injury: Intermodal nanocomplexes and calcium deregulation. *Trends Mol. Med.* **2010**, *16*, 160–170. [CrossRef]

150. Khalil, M.; Teunissen, C.E.; Otto, M.; Piehl, F.; Sormani, M.P.; Gattringer, T.; Barro, C.; Kappos, L.; Comabella, M.; Fazekas, F.; et al. Neurofilaments as biomarkers in neurological disorders. *Nat. Rev. Neurol.* **2018**, *14*, 577–589. [CrossRef]

151. Lycke, J.N.; Karlsson, J.E.; Andersen, O.; Rosengren, L.E. Neurofilament protein in cerebrospinal fluid: A potential marker of activity in multiple sclerosis. *J. Neurol. Neurosurg. Psychiatry* **1998**, *64*, 402–404. [CrossRef] [PubMed]

152. Rosengren, L.E.; Karlsson, J.E.; Karlsson, J.O.; Persson, L.I.; Wikkelsø, C. Patients with amyotrophic lateral sclerosis and other neurodegenerative diseases have increased levels of neurofilament protein in CSF. *J. Neurochem.* **1996**, *67*, 2013–2018. [CrossRef] [PubMed]

153. Novakova, L.; Axelsson, M.; Khademi, M.; Zetterberg, H.; Blennow, K.; Malmeström, C.; Piehl, F.; Olsson, T.; Lycke, J. Cerebrospinal fluid biomarkers of inflammation and degeneration as measures of fingolimod efficacy in multiple Sclerosis. *Mult. Scler.* **2017**, *23*, 62–71. [CrossRef] [PubMed]

154. Gunnarsson, M.; Malmeström, C.; Axelsson, M.; Sundström, P.; Dahle, C.; Vrethem, M.; Olsson, T.; Piehl, F.; Norgren, N.; Rosengren, L.; et al. Axonal damage in relapsing multiple Sclerosis is markedly reduced by natalizumab. *Ann. Neurol.* **2011**, *69*, 83–89. [CrossRef] [PubMed]

155. Disanto, G.; Barro, C.; Benkert, P.; Naegelin, Y.; Schädelin, S.; Giardiello, A.; Zecca, C.; Blennow, K.; Zetterberg, H.; Leppert, D.; et al. Serum neurofialments light: A biomarker of neuronal damage in multiple Sclerosis. *Ann. Neurol.* **2017**, *81*, 857–870. [CrossRef] [PubMed]

156. Barro, C.; Benkert, P.; Disanto, G.; Tsagkas, C.; Amann, M.; Naegelin, Y.; Leppert, D.; Gobbi, C.; Granziera, C.; Yaldizli, Ö.; et al. Serum neurfilament as a predictor of disease worsening and brain and spinal cord atrophy in multiple Sclerosis. *Brain* **2018**. [CrossRef] [PubMed]

157. Simons, M.; Nave, K.A. Oligodendrocytes: Myelination and axonal support. *Cold Spring Harb. Perspect. Biol.* **2015**, *8*, a020479. [CrossRef] [PubMed]

158. Griffiths, I.; Klugmann, M.; Anderson, T.; Yool, D.; Thomson, C.; Schwab, M.H.; Schneider, A.; Zimmermann, F.; McCulloch, M.; Nadon, N.; et al. Axonal swellings and degeneration in mice lacking the major proteolipid protein. *Science* **1998**, *280*, 1610–1613. [CrossRef] [PubMed]

159. Lappe-Siefke, C.; Goebbels, S.; Gravel, M.; Nicksch, E.; Lee, J.; Braun, P.E.; Griffiths, I.R.; Nave, K.A. Dysruption of Cnp1 uncouples oligodendroglial functions in axonal support and myelination. *Nat. Gen.* **2003**, *33*, 366. [CrossRef] [PubMed]

160. Edgar, J.M.; McLaughlin, M.; Werner, H.B.; McCulloch, M.C.; Barrie, J.A.; Brown, A.; Faichney, A.B.; Snaidero, N.; Nave, K.A.; Griffiths, I.R. Early ultrastructural defects of axons and axon-glia junctions in mice lacking expression of Cnp1. *Glia* **2009**, *57*, 1815–1824. [CrossRef] [PubMed]

161. Oluich, L.J.; Stratton, J.A.; Xing, Y.L.; Ng, S.W.; Cate, H.S.; Sah, P.; Windels, F.; Kilpatrick, T.J.; Merson, T.D. Targeted ablation of oligodendrocytes induces axonal pathology independent of overt demyelination. *J. Neurosci.* **2012**, *32*, 8317–8330. [CrossRef] [PubMed]

162. Fünfschilling, U.; Supplie, L.M.; Mahad, D.; Boretius, S.; Saab, A.S.; Edgar, J.; Brinkmann, B.G.; Kassmann, C.M.; Tzvetanova, I.D.; Möbius, W.; et al. Glycolytic oligodendrocytes maintain myelin and long-term axonal integrity. *Nature* **2012**, *485*, 517–521. [CrossRef] [PubMed]

163. Correale, J.; Ysrraelit, M.C.; Benarroch, E.E. Metabolic coupling of axons and glial cells: Implications for multiple sclerosis progression. *Neurology* **2018**, *90*, 737–744. [CrossRef] [PubMed]

164. Philips, T.; Rothstein, J.D. Oligodendroglia: Metabolic supporters of neurons. *J. Clin. Investig.* **2017**, *127*, 3271–3280. [CrossRef] [PubMed]

165. Lee, Y.; Morrsion, B.M.; Li, Y.; Lengacher, S.; Farah, M.H.; Hoffman, P.N.; Liu, Y.; Tsingalia, A.; Jin, L.; Zhang, P.W.; et al. Oligodendroglia metabolically support axons and contribute to neurodegeneration. *Nature* **2012**, *487*, 443–448. [CrossRef] [PubMed]

166. Bélanger, M.; Allaman, I.; Magistretti, P.J. Barin metabolism: Focus on astrcoyte-neuron metabolic cooperation. *Cell Metab.* **2011**, *14*, 724–738. [CrossRef] [PubMed]

167. Brown, A.M.; Baltan Tekkök, S.; Ramson, B.R. Energy transfer from astrcoytes to axons: The role of CNS glycogen. *Neurochem. Int.* **2004**, *45*, 529–536. [CrossRef] [PubMed]

168. Menichella, D.M.; Goodenough, D.A.; Sirkowski, E.; Scherer, S.S.; Paul, D.L. COnnexins are critical for normal myelination in the CNS. *J. Neurosci.* **2003**, *23*, 5963–5973. [CrossRef] [PubMed]

169. Tress, O.; Maglione, M.; May, D.; Pivneva, T.; Richter, N.; Seyfarth, J.; Binder, S.; Zlomuzica, A.; Seifert, G.; Theis, M.; et al. Panglial gap junctional communication is essential for maintenance of myelin in the CNS. *J. Neurosci.* **2012**, *32*, 7499–7518. [CrossRef] [PubMed]

170. Niu, J.; Li, T.; Yi, C.; Huang, N.; Koulakoff, A.; Weng, C.; Li, C.; Zhao, C.J.; Giaume, C.; Xiao, L. Connexin-based channels contribute to metabolic pathways in the oligodendroglial lineage. *J. Cell Sci.* **2016**, *129*, 1902–1914. [CrossRef] [PubMed]

5

Sample Size for Oxidative Stress and Inflammation When Treating Multiple Sclerosis with Interferon-β1a and Coenzyme Q10

Marcello Moccia [1],*, Antonio Capacchione [2], Roberta Lanzillo [1], Fortunata Carbone [3,4], Teresa Micillo [5], Giuseppe Matarese [4,6], Raffaele Palladino [7,8] and Vincenzo Brescia Morra [1]

[1] Multiple Sclerosis Clinical Care and Research Centre, Department of Neuroscience, Reproductive Science and Odontostomatology, Federico II University, 80131 Naples, Italy; robertalanzillo@libero.it (R.L.); vincenzo.bresciamorra2@unina.it (V.B.M.)
[2] Medical Affairs Department, Merck, 00176 Rome, Italy; antonio.capacchione@merckgroup.com
[3] Neuroimmunology Unit, IRCCS Fondazione Santa Lucia, 00142 Rome, Italy; fortunata.carbone@alice.it
[4] Laboratory of Immunology, Institute of Experimental Endocrinology and Oncology, National Research Council (IEOS-CNR), 80131 Naples, Italy; giuseppe.matarese@unina.it
[5] Department of Biology, Federico II University, 80131 Naples, Italy; teresa.micillo2@unina.it
[6] Treg Cell Lab, Department of Molecular Medicine and Medical Biotechnologies, Federico II University, 80131 Naples, Italy
[7] Department of Primary Care and Public Health, Imperial College, London W68RP, UK; palladino.raffaele@gmail.com
[8] Department of Public Health, Federico II University, 80131 Naples, Italy
* Correspondence: moccia.marcello@gmail.com;

Abstract: Studying multiple sclerosis (MS) and its treatments requires the use of biomarkers for underlying pathological mechanisms. We aim to estimate the required sample size for detecting variations of biomarkers of inflammation and oxidative stress. This is a post-hoc analysis on 60 relapsing-remitting MS patients treated with Interferon-β1a and Coenzyme Q10 for 3 months in an open-label crossover design over 6 months. At baseline and at the 3 and 6-month visits, we measured markers of scavenging activity, oxidative damage, and inflammation in the peripheral blood (180 measurements). Variations of laboratory measures (treatment effect) were estimated using mixed-effect linear regression models (including age, gender, disease duration, baseline expanded disability status scale (EDSS), and the duration of Interferon-β1a treatment as covariates; creatinine was also included for uric acid analyses), and were used for sample size calculations. Hypothesizing a clinical trial aiming to detect a 70% effect in 3 months (power = 80% alpha-error = 5%), the sample size per treatment arm would be 1 for interleukin (IL)-3 and IL-5, 4 for IL-7 and IL-2R, 6 for IL-13, 14 for IL-6, 22 for IL-8, 23 for IL-4, 25 for activation-normal T cell expressed and secreted (RANTES), 26 for tumor necrosis factor (TNF)-α, 27 for IL-1β, and 29 for uric acid. Peripheral biomarkers of oxidative stress and inflammation could be used in proof-of-concept studies to quickly screen the mechanisms of action of MS treatments.

Keywords: multiple sclerosis; inflammation; oxidative; biomarker; sample size

1. Introduction

Monitoring multiple sclerosis (MS) and developing new disease modifying treatments (DMTs) requires the use of biomarkers for underlying pathological mechanisms [1,2]. Thus, it is crucial to define a set of biomarkers that can be easily measured (e.g., in accessible body fluids), are quickly responsive to change, and reflect MS clinical features accurately [2,3].

Experimental evidence supports the important role of inflammation and oxidative stress in the pathogenesis of MS [4]. In the initial relapsing-remitting (RR) phase, oxidative stress is strictly associated with inflammatory activity, whereas the progressive phase is characterized by chronic inflammation and neurodegeneration, further amplifying the oxidative damage [4,5]. In our recent study [6], supplementation with Coenzyme Q10, a natural anti-oxidant, along with Interferon-β1a 44 mcg treatment, was associated with an improved oxidative balance, with a shift toward an anti-inflammatory milieu and with related clinical benefits. However, in this study we used a large number of peripheral biomarkers of oxidative stress and inflammation, which was time-and resource-consuming, and ultimately resulted in a significant statistical challenge due to multiple comparisons [6]. Thus, future studies would benefit from a subset of biomarkers that are sensitive to change in a short time and on a small sample.

In the present post-hoc analysis of our previous longitudinal study, we aim to estimate the sample size needed in RR-MS for different peripheral biomarkers of oxidative stress and inflammation.

2. Materials and Methods

2.1. Study Design and Population

This is a post-hoc analysis on a prospective cohort that was fully described elsewhere [6]. Briefly, in 2016–2017, we included 60 RRMS patients on clinical stability and on treatment with subcutaneous high-dose Interferon-β1a (Rebif®, 44 mcg, Merck, Rome, Italy), either alone or with Coenzyme Q10 (Skatto®, 100 mg/ml, Chiesi Farmaceutici SpA, Parma, Italy) for 3 months, with a cross-over design. In particular, group 1 ($n = 30$) was treated with Interferon-β1a and Coenzyme Q10 from baseline to a 3-month visit, and then with Interferon-β1a alone until a 6-month visit; meanwhile, group 2 ($n = 30$) was treated with Interferon-β1a alone from baseline to a 3-month visit, and then with Interferon-β1a and Coenzyme Q10 until a 6-month visit. This design used within-subjects comparison of treatments, and therefore minimized confounding variables by removing any natural biological variation that may have occurred in the measurement of the outcome measures [6,7].

2.2. Laboratory Analyses

Blood samples were collected at baseline and after 3 and 6 months (60 patients with 3 laboratory measurements, with 180 measurements overall) in fasting conditions in lithium heparin tubes, immediately centrifuged, stored at −80 °C, and then analyzed for:

(1) Markers of free radical scavenging activity: uric acid and bilirubin were measured by using the UA2 and the BILTS enzymatic methods (COBAS® c501 analyser, Roche Diagnostic, Mannheim, Germany);

(2) Markers of serum oxidative damage: 8-hydroxy-2-deoxyguanosine (8-OHdG, an end product of oxidative DNA damage) and protein carbonyls (an end product of oxidative protein damage) were measured by using the OxiSelect™ Oxidative DNA Damage ELISA kit, and the OxiSelect™ Protein Carbonyl ELISA Kit (both from Cell Biolabs, San Diego, CA, USA);

(3) Markers of inflammation: the Human Cytokine Magnetic 35-Plex Panel (Invitrogen by Thermo Fisher Scientific, Waltham, MA, USA) was used for the quantitative detection of epidermal growth factor (EGF), eotaxin, basic-fibroblast growth factor (FGF), granulocyte-colony stimulating factor (G-CSF), granulocyte-macrophage colony-stimulating factor (GM-CSF), hepatocyte growth factor (HGF), Interferon (IFN)-α, IFN-γ, interleukin (IL)-1α, IL-1β, IL-1RA, IL-2, IL-2R, IL-3, IL-4, IL-5, IL-6, IL-7, IL-8, IL-9, IL-10, IL-12, IL-13, IL-15, IL-17A, IL-17F, IL-22, IFN-γ-inducible protein (IP)-10, monocyte chemoattractant protein (MCP)-1, monokine induced by IFN-γ (MIG), macrophage inflammatory proteins (MIP)-1α, MIP-1β, regulated on activation-normal T cell expressed and secreted (RANTES), tumor necrosis factor (TNF)-α, and vascular endothelial growth factor (VEGF).

CellROX® Orange Reagent (Life Technologies, Carlsbad, CA, USA) was used for measuring intracellular reactive oxygen species (ROS) production in peripheral blood mononuclear cells (PBMCs) using a FACScanto II analyzer (Becton–Dickinson, San Diego, CA, USA) and Flow-Jo v10 software (Tree Star Inc., Ashland, OR, USA); intracellular ROS production (CellROX) was measured as percent positive cells (%) and mean fluorescence intensity (MFI).

2.3. Statistics

The sample size needed to detect a treatment effect on different markers of oxidative stress and inflammation was computed using the formula $n = \frac{2(Z_\alpha + Z_{1-\beta})^2 \sigma^2}{\Delta^2}$, where n is the required sample size per treatment arm in 1:1 controlled trials, Z_α and $Z_{1-\beta}$ are constants (set at 5% alpha-error and 80% power, respectively), σ is the standard deviation, and Δ the estimated effect size [8,9]. The treatment effect was defined as the actual observed effect in our previous study (i.e., variation in each laboratory measure between treated and untreated groups), estimated using mixed-effect linear regression models (including age, gender, disease duration, baseline expanded disability status scale (EDSS), and duration of Interferon-β1a treatment prior to study inclusion as covariates; creatinine was also included for uric acid analyses) [6,8,9]. The crossover model included random effects for patient ID, and fixed-effects for time (baseline, 3 and 6 months), and for the visit after Coenzyme Q10 exposure, overall accounting for possible carry-over effects. Adjusted beta-coefficients of 3-month variations were obtained for each laboratory measure. We assumed that the observed variation, as estimated by the adjusted beta-coefficients, was the highest achievable treatment effect (100%) over 3 months. From there, with a conservative approach, we hypothesized a number of effect sizes—e.g., 30%, 50%, 70%, and 90%—that were smaller than the observed effect. Standard deviations were calculated from the variation of each laboratory measure after 3 months. Then, we hypothesized a clinical trial where two different biomarkers were included as primary outcome measures for sample size estimates (alpha-error was set at 2.5%). Finally, we considered that the study was designed to include one or two interim analyses in addition to the final analysis (alpha-error was set at 2.94% and 2.21%, respectively, according to the Pocock method) [10,11].

Stata 15.0 (StataCorp LLC, College Station, TX, USA) was used for data processing and analysis.

3. Results

Sixty RRMS patients were included in the present study (age: 41.5 ± 9.7 years; female: $n = 42$ (70%); disease duration: 11.0 ± 1.7 years; baseline EDSS: 2.5 (1.0–5.0)). Four patients presented with a clinical relapse (6.6%) during the study period.

Hypothesizing a clinical trial aiming to detect 70% effect in 3 months (power = 80% alpha-error = 5%), the sample size per treatment arm would be 1 for IL-3 and IL-5, 4 for IL-7 and IL-2R, 6 for IL-13, 14 for IL-6, 22 for IL-8, 23 for IL-4, 25 for RANTES, 26 for TNF-α, 27 for IL-1β, and 29 for uric acid (Figure 1, Table 1). Other investigated markers presented with a sample size per treatment arm larger than 30 (Table 1).

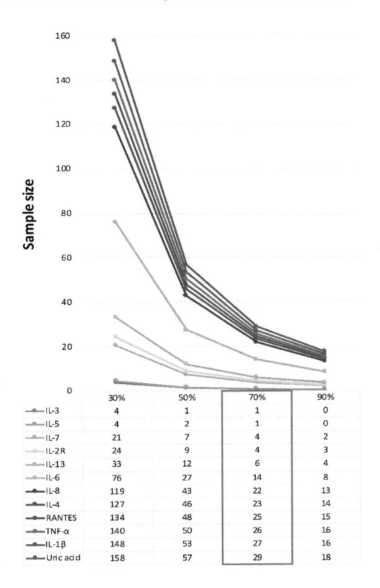

	30%	50%	70%	90%
IL-3	4	1	1	0
IL-5	4	2	1	0
IL-7	21	7	4	2
IL-2R	24	9	4	3
IL-13	33	12	6	4
IL-6	76	27	14	8
IL-8	119	43	22	13
IL-4	127	46	23	14
RANTES	134	48	25	15
TNF-α	140	50	26	16
IL-1β	148	53	27	16
Uric acid	158	57	29	18

Figure 1. Profile plot for sample size estimates for a treatment arm. Figure shows sample sizes for laboratory markers of oxidative stress and inflammation (<30 patients for a treatment arm with a 70% treatment effect). Sample size per treatment arm is reported hypothesizing a 30%, 50%, 70%, and 90% treatment effect compared with the observed effect. Power was set at 80% and alpha-error at 5%. Abbreviations: interleukin (IL), regulated on activation-normal T cell expressed and secreted (RANTES), and tumor necrosis factor (TNF).

Hypothesizing the combination of two different biomarkers as primary outcome measures (alpha-error = 2.5%), sample size estimates per treatment arm remained substantially favorable (3 for IL-3 and IL-5, 7 for IL-7, 8 for IL-2R, 9 for IL-13, 19 for IL-6, 28 for IL-8, 30 for IL-4, 32 for RANTES, 33 for TNF-α, 35 for IL-1β, and 37 for uric acid) (Table 1).

Sample size estimates for a study with one or two interim analyses (Pocock method, setting alpha-error = 2.94% and 2.21% respectively), in addition to the final analysis, are presented in Table 1; this design would reduce study participants' exposure to an inferior or useless treatment.

Table 1. Sample size estimates for a treatment arm for 3-month variations of peripheral biomarkers of oxidative stress and inflammation.

	Baseline	Adj. Coeff. (3-Month Variation)	SD (3-Month Variation)	Sample Size (70% Treatment Effect)		Interim Analyses (Pocock Method)	
				One Primary Outcome	Two Primary Outcomes	One Interim	Two Interim
				5% alpha	2.5% alpha	2.94% alpha	2.21% alpha
Markers of scavenging activity							
Uric acid (mg/dL)	4.670 ± 0.566	0.123 *	0.117	29	37	15	11
Bilirubin (mg/dL)	1.466 ± 0.268	0.066	0.190	265	323	134	98
Markers of oxidative damage							
CellROX cells (%)	76.405 ± 9.348	−9.925 *	11.25	41	52	21	15
CellROX cells (MFI)	2605.320 ± 828.707	−523.308 *	1124.538	148	181	75	55
Protein carbonyls (nmol/mg)	2.976 ± 1.402	−0.266	1.393	878	1066	444	326
8-OHdG (ng/mL)	6.379 ± 1.140	−0.630 *	0.708	40	51	20	15
Markers of inflammation							
EGF (pg/mL)	6.597 ± 12.877	−3.637	8.513	175	214	89	65
Eotaxin (pg/mL)	116.432 ± 46.800	−18.669 *	31.968	94	116	47	35
Basic-FGF (pg/mL)	53.218 ± 282.165	−2.736	4.863	101	124	51	38
G-CSF (pg/mL)	80.445 ± 48.370	−4.692	61.503	5498	6667	2783	2041
GM-CSF (pg/mL)	5.791 ± 4.953	−1.751 *	2.524	66	82	34	25
HGF (pg/mL)	64.959 ± 77.650	−26.397 *	33.925	53	66	27	20
IFN-α (pg/mL)	80.869 ± 469.445	1.780	11.498	1335	1618	676	496
IFN-γ (pg/mL)	2.311 ± 1.952	−1.526 *	1.937	52	64	26	19
IL-1α (pg/mL)	4.427 ± 6.477	−2.460 *	2.526	34	43	17	13
IL-1β (pg/mL)	1.694 ± 7.274	−1.188	1.096	27	35	14	10
IL-1RA (pg/mL)	33.085 ± 39.824	−10.464	18.329	98	121	50	36
IL-2 (pg/mL)	20.979 ± 107.943	5.099	14.090	244	298	124	91

Table 1. *Cont.*

	Baseline	Adj. Coeff. (3-Month Variation)	SD (3-Month Variation)	Sample Size (70% Treatment Effect)		Interim Analyses (Pocock Method)	
				One Primary Outcome	Two Primary Outcomes	One Interim	Two Interim
				5% alpha	2.5% alpha	2.94% alpha	2.21% alpha
IL-2R (pg/mL)	105.950 ± 61.462	−29.971 *	11.182	4	8	2	2
IL-3 (pg/mL)	202.849 ± 1283.170	28.661	4.276	1	3	0	0
IL-4 (pg/mL)	4.421 ± 11.691	3.883 *	3.317	23	30	12	9
IL-5 (pg/mL)	8.177 ± 33.861	−12.890	2.069	1	3	0	0
IL-6 (pg/mL)	62.945 ± 363.131	5.559	3.671	14	19	7	5
IL-7 (pg/mL)	12.871 ± 40.625	−16.428	5.639	4	7	2	1
IL-8 (pg/mL)	12.095 ± 7.422	−11.418	9.425	22	28	11	8
IL-9 (pg/mL)	2.248 ± 4.814	−3.749 *	4.212	40	51	20	15
IL-10 (pg/mL)	1079.590 ± 6456.040	1615.546	2417.951	72	89	36	27
IL-12 (pg/mL)	58.932 ± 110.51	2.498	14.365	1058	1284	536	393
IL-13 (pg/mL)	1.714 ± 3.341	3.732 *	1.628	6	9	3	2
IL-15 (pg/mL)	117.149 ± 673.398	21.693	21.658	32	40	16	12
IL-17A (pg/mL)	1.460 ± 2.265	−0.453	0.941	138	169	70	51
IL-17F (pg/mL)	35.954 ± 86.735	−68.854 *	72.039	35	44	18	13
IL-22 (pg/mL)	250.425 ± 642.791	−8.406	40.134	729	886	369	271
IP-10 (pg/mL)	26.279 ± 16.844	5.699	30.460	914	1110	463	339
MCP-1 (pg/mL)	232.083 ± 79.633	39.540	96.247	190	232	96	70
MIG (pg/mL)	32.386 ± 13.580	−5.409	13.555	201	245	102	75
MIP-1α (pg/mL)	7.830 ± 11.718	−5.327 *	5.338	32	41	16	12
MIP-1β (pg/mL)	182.476 ± 1024.490	17.125	17.060	32	40	16	12
RANTES (pg/mL)	1739.970 ± 1475.350	−2331.281 *	2041.081	25	32	12	9

Table 1. *Cont.*

	Baseline	Adj. Coeff. (3-Month Variation)	SD (3-Month Variation)	Sample Size (70% Treatment Effect)				
				One Primary Outcome	Two Primary Outcomes	Interim Analyses (Pocock Method)		
						One Interim	Two Interim	
				5% alpha	2.5% alpha	2.94% alpha	2.21% alpha	
TNF-α (pg/mL)	2.725 ± 4.310	−1.795 *	1.608	26	33	13	10	
VEGF (pg/mL)	0.619 ± 0.777	−0.398 *	0.519	54	68	28	20	

Table shows absolute values of biomarkers of oxidative stress and inflammation at the baseline visit. Adjusted beta-coefficients (adj. coeff.) of 3-month variation for each laboratory measure were obtained with mixed-effect linear regression models (including age, gender, disease duration, baseline EDSS, and duration of Interferon-β1a treatment prior to study inclusion as covariates; creatinine was also included for uric acid analyses) (* indicates $p < 0.05$). Standard deviation (SD) was calculated from the variation of each laboratory measure after 3 months. Sample size per treatment arm is reported, hypothesizing a 70% treatment effect, compared with the observed effect, over 3 months (power was set at 80%, alpha-error was set at 5%). Then, we also performed calculations hypothesizing additional scenarios: (i) two different biomarkers were included as combined primary outcome measures for sample size estimates (alpha-error was set at 2.5%); (ii) the study was designed to include one or two interim analyses in addition to the final analysis in order to obtain early evidence of inferior or useless treatment (alpha-error was set to be 0.0294 and 0.0221, respectively, according to the Pocock method). Abbreviations: intracellular ROS production (CellROX), mean fluorescence intensity (MFI), 8-hydroxy-2-deoxyguanosine (8-OHdG), epidermal growth factor (EGF), eotaxin, basic-fibroblast growth factor (FGF), granulocyte-colony stimulating factor (G-CSF), granulocyte-macrophage colony-stimulating factor (GM-CSF), hepatocyte growth factor (HGF), interferon (IFN)- α, IFN-γ, interleukin (IL)-1α, IL-1β, IL-1RA, IL-2, IL-2R, IL-3, IL-4, IL-5, IL-6, IL-7, IL-8, IL-9, IL-10, IL-12, IL-13, IL-15, IL-17A, IL-17E, IL-22, IFN-γ-inducible protein (IP)-10, monocyte chemoattractant protein (MCP)-1, monokine induced by IFN-γ (MIG), macrophage inflammatory proteins (MIP)-1α, MIP-1β, regulated on activation-normal T cell expressed and secreted (RANTES), tumor necrosis factor (TNF)-α, and vascular endothelial growth factor (VEGF).

4. Discussion

Peripheral biomarkers of inflammation, scavenging activity, and oxidative damage gave realistically achievable sample size estimates, and could be used in exploratory clinical trials and observational studies to screen new or already existing medications with putative effects on inflammation and oxidative stress over a 3-month period. Not least, interim analyses could detect an inferior or useless treatment even earlier, with subsequent study termination or treatment switch within adaptive designs [12].

Current sample size calculations were rather conservative. In particular, in the Results (Section 3) and in Figure 1, we specifically focused on a 70% treatment effect, which was smaller than what we actually observed (100% treatment effect) [6,9]. However, greater treatment effects could be hypothesized with different medications and doses, leading to even smaller sample size estimates. Also, the inclusion of multiple markers as primary outcome measures would remain feasible for sample size calculations. Of note, present estimates are based on the combination of subcutaneous high-dose Interferon-β1a (Rebif®, 44 mcg, Merck, Rome, Italy) and Coenzyme Q10. For a subgroup of patients (50%), the Interferon-β1a treatment was also administered prior to study inclusion. Drug naïve patients were equally distributed between Coenzyme Q10 treatment groups, and we also included the duration of the Interferon-β1a treatment as a covariate in the statistical models, but, of course, we cannot exclude the possibility that previous treatment has affected the study outcomes. However, if we assume Interferon-β1a could have exerted its effects before inclusion in the study, we would have observed smaller Coenzyme Q10-related effects, resulting in subsequently more conservative sample size estimates. Interferon-β1a is an approved treatment for MS, with a well-established long-term efficacy and safety profile [13]. On the contrary, Coenzyme Q10 has proven effect on biomarkers of oxidative stress and inflammation and on MS symptoms [14–16], but its disease-modifying effect remains to be established. As such, future studies should evaluate the reproducibility of our findings on more recent medications (e.g., cladribine).

Most promising inflammatory biomarkers are strongly related to MS pathogenesis, and in particular, to acute (e.g., IL-1β, IL-3) and chronic inflammation (e.g., IL-2R, IL-6, IL-7, IL-8, TNF-α) within the central nervous system [17–21], to suppression of the activity of microglia toward brain repair (i.e., RANTES), and to neuroprotective modulation of pathologically-active macrophages and microglia (e.g., IL-4, IL-13) [17,22]. Markers of oxidative stress also resulted in rather small sample sizes, with particular regard to markers of serum scavenging activity (uric acid), and of oxidative damage in inflammatory cells and DNA (CellROX, %, and 8-OHdG). Biomarkers of oxidative stress and inflammation are not only related to MS pathogenesis [17,23], but are also clinically relevant to MS, being associated with MS risk and progression [6,17,21,24–26], and also being used as therapeutic targets [17]. For instance, IL-6, IL-8, and RANTES have been associated with the risk of clinical relapses [27], radiological activity (e.g., lesions, atrophy) [28], treatment switch, and disability progression after up to 6 years [20]. Interestingly, clinical associations might be particularly sound in patients in apparent clinical stability [29]. As such, longitudinal measurements of oxidative stress and inflammation can provide pathologically and clinically relevant information in MS observational studies and clinical trials.

Of note, for some inflammatory biomarkers (e.g., IL-3 and IL-5) sample size estimates were unexpectedly low and should be interpreted with caution. If we assume we are studying a compound with a specific molecular target (e.g., anti-TNF-α or anti-CD20 antibodies), then only a very small sample is necessary to detect biological effect [30,31]. On the contrary, for compounds with multimodal mechanisms of action, a larger sample would be needed or, at least, profiles of inflammatory pathology should be considered [26].

Limitations of this study include possible confounding factors. In our previous study, we excluded patients with possible confounding factors (e.g., contraceptive and immunosuppressive medication), we used within-patients comparison of treatments (minimizing confounding effects by removing any natural biological variation), and we accounted for a number of covariates in our statistical models [6], but factors influencing oxidative stress and inflammation are multiple and virtually impossible to exclude completely. For instance, four patients presented with a clinical relapse (6.6%) that we did not account for considering that patients were equally distributed in the Coenzyme-Q10-treated and untreated groups. Specificity of peripheral biomarkers to MS-related pathology remains to be further investigated, and based on current knowledge, these markers cannot replace conventional biomarkers of disability (e.g., neuroimaging) [32]. We included 180 measurements at three timepoints from 60 patients to estimate coefficients of variation for sample estimates. As such, included sample could have been larger, but was based on sample size calculations from our previous study, and not least, was in line with previous studies with similar goals [6,8,33]. Also, measurements over short intervals may be prone to increased measurement errors leading to a greater variability and larger sample, but apparently, this was not the case in our cohort. A control group (untreated or treated with a medication different from Interferon-β1a) was unfortunately not available, with difficulties in drawing formal conclusions on the observed effects.

5. Conclusions

In conclusion, peripheral biomarkers of oxidative stress and inflammation could be used in exploratory, proof-of-concept studies aiming to evaluate the activity profile of new or already existing medications. Medications with putative anti-oxidant and anti-inflammatory effects could be tested in a short time (3 months) and on small samples (<30 per treatment arm) by using a limited subset of biomarkers, before being moved toward larger and more expensive clinical trials.

Author Contributions: M.M., A.C. and V.B.M. conceived and designed the experiments; R.L., F.C., T.M., G.M. and R.P. performed the experiments; M.M., R.L., R.P. and V.B.M. analyzed the data; A.C., F.C., T.M. and G.M. contributed reagents/materials/analysis tools; M.M., A.C., R.L., F.C., T.M., G.M., R.P. and V.B.M. wrote the paper.

References

1. Tur, C.; Moccia, M.; Barkhof, F.; Chataway, J.; Sastre-Garriga, J.; Thompson, A.J.; Ciccarelli, O. Assessing treatment outcomes in multiple sclerosis trials and in the clinical setting. *Nat. Rev. Neurol.* **2018**, *14*, 75–93. [CrossRef]

2. Thompson, A.J.; Baranzini, S.E.; Geurts, J.; Hemmer, B.; Ciccarelli, O. Multiple sclerosis. *Lancet* **2018**, *391*, 1622–1636. [CrossRef]

3. Zaratin, P.; Comi, G.; Coetzee, T.; Ramsey, K.; Smith, K.; Thompson, A.; Panzara, M. Progressive MS Alliance Industry Forum: Maximizing Collective Impact to Enable Drug Development. *Trends Pharmacol. Sci.* **2016**, *37*, 808–810. [CrossRef]

4. Haider, L.; Zrzavy, T.; Hametner, S.; Höftberger, R.; Bagnato, F.; Grabner, G.; Trattnig, S.; Pfeifenbring, S.; Brück, W.; Lassmann, H. The topograpy of demyelination and neurodegeneration in the multiple sclerosis brain. *Brain* **2016**, *139*, 807–815. [CrossRef]

5. Friese, M.A.; Schattling, B.; Fugger, L. Mechanisms of neurodegeneration and axonal dysfunction in multiple sclerosis. *Nat. Rev. Neurol.* **2014**, *10*, 225–238. [CrossRef]

6. Moccia, M.; Capacchione, A.; Lanzillo, R.; Carbone, F.; Micillo, T.; Perna, F.; De Rosa, A.; Carotenuto, A.; Albero, R.; Matarese, G.; et al. Coenzyme Q10 supplementation reduces peripheral oxidative stress and inflammation in Interferon-Beta1a treated multiple sclerosis. *Ther. Adv. Neurol. Disord.* **2019**, *12*, 1–12. [CrossRef]

7. Sedgwick, P. What is a crossover trial? *BMJ* **2014**, *348*, 9–10. [CrossRef]

8. Altmann, D.R.; Jasperse, B.; Barkhof, F.; Beckmann, K.; Filippi, M.; Kappos, L.D.; Molyneux, P.; Polman, C.H.; Pozzilli, C.; Thompson, A.J.; et al. Sample sizes for brain atrophy outcomes in trials for secondary progressive multiple sclerosis. *Neurology* **2009**, *72*, 595–601. [CrossRef]

9. Moccia, M.; Prados, F.; Filippi, M.; Rocca, M.A.; Valsasina, P.; Brownlee, W.J.; Zecca, C.; Gallo, A.; Rovira, A.; Gass, A.; et al. Longitudinal spinal cord atrophy in multiple sclerosis using the generalised boundary shift integral. *Ann. Neurol.* **2019**. [CrossRef]

10. Li, G.; Taljaard, M.; Van den Heuvel, E.R.; Levine, M.A.; Cook, D.J.; Wells, G.A.; Devereaux, P.J.; Thabane, L. An introduction to multiplicity issues in clinical trials: The what, why, when and how. *Int. J. Epidemiol.* **2017**, *46*, 746–755. [CrossRef]

11. Pocock, S. Group sequential methods in the design and analysis of clinical trials. *Biometrika* **1977**, *64*, 191–199. [CrossRef]

12. Fox, R.; Chataway, J. Advancing Trial Design in Progressive Multiple Sclerosis. *Mult. Scler.* **2017**, *23*, 1573–1578. [CrossRef]

13. Moccia, M.; Palladino, R.; Carotenuto, A.; Saccà, F.; Russo, C.V.; Lanzillo, R.; Brescia Morra, V. A 8-year retrospective cohort study comparing Interferon-β formulations for relapsing-remitting multiple sclerosis. *Mult. Scler. Relat. Disord.* **2018**, *19*, 50–54. [CrossRef]

14. Sanoobar, M.; Eghtesadi, S.; Azimi, A.; Khalili, M.; Khodadadi, B.; Jazayeri, S.; Gohari, M.R.; Aryaeian, N. Coenzyme Q10 supplementation ameliorates inflammatory markers in patients with multiple sclerosis: A double blind, placebo, controlled randomized clinical trial. *Nutr. Neurosci.* **2015**, *18*, 169–176. [CrossRef]

15. Sanoobar, M.; Eghtesadi, S.; Azimi, A.; Khalili, M.; Jazayeri, S.; Gohari, M.R. Coenzyme Q10 supplementation reduces oxidative stress and increases antioxidant enzyme activity in patients with coronary artery disease. *Int. J. Neurosci.* **2013**, *123*, 776–782. [CrossRef]

16. Sanoobar, M.; Dehghan, P.; Khalil, M.; Azimi, A.; Seifar, F. Coenzyme Q10 as a treatment for fatigue and depression in multiple sclerosis patients: A double blind randomized clinical trial. *Nutr. Neurosci.* **2016**, *19*, 138–143. [CrossRef]

17. Göbel, K.; Ruck, T.; Meuth, S.G. Cytokine signaling in multiple sclerosis: Lost in translation. *Mult. Scler. J.* **2018**, *24*, 432–439. [CrossRef]

18. Lee, P.W.; Xin, M.K.; Pei, W.; Yang, Y.; Lovett-Racke, A.E. IL-3 Is a Marker of Encephalitogenic T Cells, but Not Essential for CNS Autoimmunity. *Front. Immunol.* **2018**, *9*, 1–7. [CrossRef]

19. Lin, C.-C.; Edelson, B.T. New Insights into the Role of IL-1β in Experimental Autoimmune Encephalomyelitis and Multiple Sclerosis. *J. Immunol.* **2017**, *198*, 4553–4560. [CrossRef]

20. Bassi, M.S.; Iezzi, E.; Landi, D.; Monteleone, F.; Gilio, L.; Simonelli, I.; Musella, A.; Mandolesi, G.; De Vito, F.; Furlan, R.; et al. Delayed treatment of MS is associated with high CSF levels of IL-6 and IL-8 and worse future disease course. *J. Neurol.* **2018**, *265*, 2540–2547. [CrossRef]

21. Tavakolpour, S. Interleukin 7 receptor polymorphisms and the risk of multiple sclerosis: A meta-analysis. *Mult. Scler. Relat. Disord.* **2016**, *8*, 66–73. [CrossRef]

22. Guglielmetti, C.; Le Blon, D.; Santermans, E.; Salas-Perdomo, A.; Daans, J.; De Vocht, N.; Shah, D.; Hoornaert, C.; Praet, J.; Peerlings, J.; et al. Interleukin-13 immune gene therapy prevents CNS inflammation and demyelination via alternative activation of microglia and macrophages. *Glia* **2016**, *64*, 2181–2200. [CrossRef]

23. Hu, W.T.; Howell, J.C.; Ozturk, T.; Gangishetti, U.; Kollhoff, A.L.; Hatcher-Martin, J.M.; Anderson, A.M.; Tyor, W.R. CSF Cytokines in Aging, Multiple Sclerosis, and Dementia. *Front. Immunol.* **2019**, *10*, 480. [CrossRef]

24. Moccia, M.; Lanzillo, R.; Palladino, R.; Russo, C.; Carotenuto, A.; Massarelli, M.; Vacca, G.; Vacchiano, V.; Nardone, A.; Triassi, M.; et al. Uric acid: A potential biomarker of multiple sclerosis and of its disability. *Clin. Chem. Lab. Med.* **2015**, *53*, 753–759. [CrossRef]

25. Moccia, M.; Lanzillo, R.; Costabile, T.; Russo, C.; Carotenuto, A.; Sasso, G.; Postiglione, E.; De Luca Picione, C.; Vastola, M.; Maniscalco, G.T.; et al. Uric acid in relapsing-remitting multiple sclerosis: A 2-year longitudinal study. *J. Neurol.* **2015**, *262*, 961–967. [CrossRef]

26. Magliozzi, R.; Howell, O.; Nicholas, R.; Cruciani, C.; Castellaro, M.; Romualdi, C.; Rossi, S.; Pittieri, M.; Benedetti, M.; Gajofatto, A.; et al. Inflammatory intrathecal profiles and cortical damage in multiple sclerosis. *Ann. Neurol.* **2018**, *83*, 739–755. [CrossRef]

27. Lanzillo, R.; Carbone, F.; Quarantelli, M.; Bruzzese, D.; Carotenuto, A.; De Rosa, V.; Colamatteo, A.; Micillo, T.; De Luca Picione, C.; Saccà, F.; et al. Immunometabolic profiling of patients with multiple sclerosis identifies new biomarkers to predict disease activity during treatment with interferon Interferon beta-1a. *Clin. Immunol.* **2017**, *183*, 249–253. [CrossRef]

28. Ziliotto, N.; Bernardi, F.; Jakimovski, D.; Baroni, M.; Bergsland, N.; Ramasamy, D.P.; Weinstock-Guttman, B.; Zamboni, P.; Marchetti, G.; Zivadinov, R.; et al. Increased CCL18 plasma levels are associated with neurodegenerative MRI outcomes in multiple sclerosis patients. *Mult. Scler. Relat. Disord.* **2018**, *25*, 37–42. [CrossRef]

29. Ghezzi, L.; Cantoni, C.; Cignarella, F.; Bollman, B.; Cross, A.H.; Salter, A.; Galimberti, D.; Cella, M.; Piccio, L. T cells producing GM-CSF and IL-13 are enriched in the cerebrospinal fluid of relapsing MS patients. *Mult. Scler.* **2019**, 1352458519852092. [CrossRef]

30. Gibellini, L.; De Biasi, S.; Bianchini, E.; Bartolomeo, R.; Fabiano, A.; Manfredini, M.; Ferrari, F.; Albertini, G.; Trenti, T.; Nasi, M.; et al. Anti-TNF-α drugs differently affect the TNFα-sTNFR system and monocyte subsets in patients with psoriasis. *PLoS ONE* **2016**, *11*, 1–16. [CrossRef]

31. Ellrichmann, G.; Bolz, J.; Peschke, M.; Duscha, A.; Hellwig, K.; Lee, D.H.; Linker, R.A.; Gold, R.; Haghikia, A. Peripheral CD19 + B-cell counts and infusion intervals as a surrogate for long-term B-cell depleting therapy in multiple sclerosis and neuromyelitis optica/neuromyelitis optica spectrum disorders. *J. Neurol.* **2019**, *266*, 57–67. [CrossRef] [PubMed]

32. Moccia, M.; de Stefano, N.; Barkhof, F. Imaging outcomes measures for progressive multiple sclerosis trials. *Mult. Scler.* **2017**, *23*, 1614–1626. [CrossRef] [PubMed]

33. Cawley, N.; Tur, C.; Prados, F.; Plantone, D.; Kearney, H.; Abdel-Aziz, K.; Ourselin, S.; Wheeler-Kingshott, C.A.M.G.; Miller, D.H.; Thompson, A.J.; et al. Spinal cord atrophy as a primary outcome measure in phase II trials of progressive multiple sclerosis. *Mult. Scler.* **2018**, *24*, 932–941. [CrossRef] [PubMed]

6

Neuromyelitis Optica Spectrum Disorder and Anti-MOG Syndromes

Marco A. Lana-Peixoto * and Natália Talim

CIEM MS Research Center, Federal University of Minas Gerais Medical School, Belo Horizonte, MG 30130-090, Brazil; talim.fono@gmail.com

* Correspondence: marco.lanapeixoto@gmail.com;

Abstract: Neuromyelitis optica spectrum disorder (NMOSD) and anti-myelin oligodendrocyte glycoprotein (anti-MOG) syndromes are immune-mediated inflammatory conditions of the central nervous system that frequently involve the optic nerves and the spinal cord. Because of their similar clinical manifestations and habitual relapsing course they are frequently confounded with multiple sclerosis (MS). Early and accurate diagnosis of these distinct conditions is relevant as they have different treatments. Some agents used for MS treatment may be deleterious to NMOSD. NMOSD is frequently associated with antibodies which target aquaporin-4 (AQP4), the most abundant water channel in the CNS, located in the astrocytic processes at the blood-brain barrier (BBB). On the other hand, anti-MOG syndromes result from damage to myelin oligodendrocyte glycoprotein (MOG), expressed on surfaces of oligodendrocytes and myelin sheaths. Acute transverse myelitis with longitudinally extensive lesion on spinal MRI is the most frequent inaugural manifestation of NMOSD, usually followed by optic neuritis. Other core clinical characteristics include area postrema syndrome, brainstem, diencephalic and cerebral symptoms that may be associated with typical MRI abnormalities. Acute disseminated encephalomyelitis and bilateral or recurrent optic neuritis are the most frequent anti-MOG syndromes in children and adults, respectively. Attacks are usually treated with steroids, and relapses prevention with immunosuppressive drugs. Promising emerging therapies for NMOSD include monoclonal antibodies and tolerization.

Keywords: neuromyelitis optica spectrum disorders; anti-MOG syndrome; aquaporin 4-IgG; myelin oligodendrocyte glycoprotein; multiple sclerosis

1. Introduction

Neuromyelitis optica spectrum disorders (NMOSD) and anti-myelin oligodendrocyte glycoprotein (anti-MOG) syndromes are immune-mediated inflammatory conditions of the central nervous system (CNS) that frequently involve the optic nerves and the spinal cord. Because of their clinical manifestations and habitual relapsing course, they are frequently confounded with multiple sclerosis (MS). Early and accurate diagnosis of these distinct conditions is very relevant as they have different therapeutic approaches. Even a more important reason is the observation that some agents used in MS treatment may be deleterious to patients with NMOSD [1–3].

Although NMOSD and anti-MOG syndromes share a number of clinical manifestations, they are independent nosological entities with distinct pathophysiological mechanisms and histopathological features [4–7].

Whereas NMOSD is most frequently associated with antibodies which target aquaporin-4 (AQP4), the most abundant water channel in the CNS, particularly expressed in the astrocytic processes at the blood-brain barrier (BBB) [8], anti-MOG syndromes result from damage to myelin oligodendrocyte glycoprotein (MOG), a membrane protein expressed on oligodendrocyte cell surfaces and on the outermost surface of myelin sheaths. Because of this particular location, MOG is a good antigen candidate for autoimmune demyelination [6,7,9–11]. Moreover, three fourths of NMOSD patients test positive for AQP4 antibody, while serum MOG antibody is only detected in a minority of seronegative AQP4-IgG NMOSD patients [12–14].

The lack of coexistence of AQP4-IgG and MOG-IgG in the serum of a same patient further suggests that AQP4-IgG NMOSD and anti-MOG syndromes are distinct diseases [15]. On the other hand, failure to identify either AQP4-IgG or MOG-IgG in a proportion of patients with NMOSD phenotype supports the view that other autoantibodies or factors may also play a role in NMOSD pathogenesis. In line with that, N-methyl-D-aspartate receptor-IgG and CV2/CRMP5-IgG have been described in association with NMOSD phenotype [16–19].

2. Neuromyelitis Optica Spectrum Disorders

The term *neuromyelitis optica* was introduced by Eugène Devic and Fernand Gault in 1894, who first recognized the association of amaurosis and myelitis as a new clinical entity. Devic [20] reported the case of a 45-year-old French woman who was seen at the Hôtel-Dieu hospital of Lyon because of an intractable headache and depression in addition to general asthenia. One month later, she developed urinary retention, complete paraplegia and blindness, and died few weeks later. Autopsy disclosed severe demyelinating and necrotic lesions extending 4–5 cm length in the lower thoracic and lumbar spinal cord. There was demyelination of the optic nerves, but a gross examination of the brain was unrevealing. In this paper, Devic emphasized the similarity of the pathological process involving the spinal cord and the optic nerves, named the syndrome "neuro-myélite optique", or "neuroptico-myélite", and discussed its relationship with MS. Fernand Gault, a disciple of Devic's, reviewed in detail 17 cases of this condition in his doctoral thesis named "De la neuromyélite optique aiguë" [21]. The eponym "Devic's disease" was suggested by Acchiote [22]. However, the association of myelitis and blindness had already been reported by other authors in the early and mid 19th century. The *case of Marquis de Causan*—known as the first description of this association by the French anatomist and pathologist Antoine Portal in 1803–1804—was characterized by relapsing myelitis followed by amaurosis and signs of brainstem involvement [23]. Other previously reported cases included those by Giovanni Battista Pescetto in 1844 [24], Christopher Mercer Durrant in 1850 [25], Jacob Augustus Lockhart Clarke in 1862 [26], Thomas Clifford Albutt in 1870 [27], and Wilhelm Heinrich Erb in 1879–1880 [28]. Also, in the American continent, the association of optic neuritis and myelitis was identified by Seguin (1880) [29] prior to Devic and Gault's pioneering publication. None of these previous authors however, had used the term "neuromyelitis optica", or considered their cases as expression of a new nosological entity. It was only in 1943 that the disease was first identified in Latin America, when Aluizio Marques, in Rio de Janeiro, described two female patients who developed bilateral blindness and acute transverse myelitis [30].

2.1. Pathophysiology

The discovery of NMO-IgG and AQP4 as its targeted antigen unequivocally confirmed neuromyelitis optica as a disease distinct from MS and allowed its early laboratorial recognition [31,32]. The serum identification of AQP4-IgG expanded the clinical spectrum of the disease to include its limited forms (single or recurrent longitudinally extensive transverse myelitis [LETM], defined by MRI as a lesion extending for three or more vertebral segments, or recurrent isolated optic neuritis) [33], along with a wide variety of brainstem, diencephalic, and cerebral manifestations [34,35].

Aquaporin-4 monomers assemble to form tetramers which further aggregate in cell plasma membranes to form supramolecular arrays called orthogonal arrays of particles (OAP). There are two major forms of AQP-4: the full-length 323 amino acid M1 isoform, and the shorter 301 amino acid M23 isoform. Only the M23 isoform forms large OAPs [14]. It has been shown that M1 isoform does not form OAPs on its own, but can co-assemble with M23 in heterotetramers that limit OAP size [36,37].

Aquaporin-4 is widely expressed throughout the CNS. It is also highly expressed in the optic nerves and spinal cord, explaining their preferential involvement in the disease. Other CNS sites expressing AQP-4 include the supraoptic nucleus of the hypothalamus, the periventricular structures such as area postrema and the vascular organ of lamina terminalis, which lack BBB and contain osmo-sensitive neurons that regulate fluid homeostasis and release arginine-vasopressin, which facilitates this process. Aquaporin-4 is also expressed in non-neural tissues including skeletal muscle cells, lung airway cells, gastric parietal cells, renal collecting duct cells, inner ear, retinal Muller cells, lacrimal gland and salivary duct cells, and olfactory epithelial cells [38]. Human and experimental studies have shown that AQP4-IgG belongs mainly to IgG1 class, a potent activator of complement. The antibody enters the CNS, binds the antigen at astrocyte processes, induces complement-mediated inflammation, granulocyte infiltration, and astrocyte death [37,39]. Complement-mediated inflammation with secondary neutrophils and eosinophil infiltration plays a key role in the pathophysiology of NMOSD attacks [40].

Aquaporin-4 antibodies are more abundant in the peripheral blood than in the cerebrospinal fluid (CSF) [41]. In the periphery, they are produced by a number of B cell subpopulations which are vulnerable to interleukin-6 (IL-6), which enhances their survival and AQP4-IgG secretion [42]. Although AQP4-IgG can gain direct access to AQP4 on astrocytes located at circumventricular organs where the endothelia lack tight junction, the mechanisms of its penetration into other CNS sites that are protected byBBB are still unclear. Recent findings have shown that AQP4-IgG is not sufficient or even necessary to cause BBB disruption [43]. Sera from NMO patients contain non-reactive AQP4 antibodies, identified as recombinant antibodies (rAb) ON-12-2-46 and ON-07-5-31 which target glucose-regulated protein 78 (GRP78) on the cell surface of brain microvascular endothelial cells (BMEC). GRP78 is a stress protein of the heat shock 70 family expressed in all CNS cells [44]. However, only rAb ON 12-2-46 induces nuclear translocation of nuclear factor kB (NF-kB) p65, which is a marker of cell activation [43]. BMECs activation causes increased secretion of vascular endothelium growth factor (VEGF) and metaloproteinases (MMP)-2/9 which result in a down regulation of claudin 5 and disruption of the BBB. Leakage of the BBB allows entrance of AQP4-IgG to the CNS and its binding to AQP4 in the astrocytic endfeet. Evidences showing the causal role of AQP4-IgG in NMOSD include its nearly absolute specificity for the disease; its correlation with disease activity, higher number of relapses and more severe course as compared with seronegative patients; some distinct demographic and clinical features; increased concentration of AQP4-positive plasmablasts in NMOSD patients, mainly during disease relapses; and decreased serum AQP4-IgG concentration following successful treatments and during disease remission [45–47]. Histopathological features such as a marked loss of astrocytes and accumulation of IgG and IgM around blood vessels, the site of AQP4 expression; spare of myelin and axons in some lesions suggesting that astrocytes (which have a higher expression of AQP4) are the initial cell target in the disease, whereas in more recent lesions there may be preservation of glial fibrillary acidic protein (GFAP), a marker of astrocyte damage, suggesting that AQP4 is the primary target of the immune attack. The initial loss of AQP4 with astrocyte preservation might reflect the internalization of AQP4 of either M1-AQP4 or both isoforms before a complement becomes locally available to mediate a lytic inflammatory process. This would account for the rapid reversal of some MRI abnormalities in the area postrema and some parts of the cerebrum. The disease individual clinical phenotype and severity may be related to the ratio of AQP4-M1 to M23 in the optic nerves, brain, and spinal cord. While CNS regions with a higher proportion of M1 would rapidly internalize, avoiding a cascade of tissue damage, areas richer in AQP4-M23 isoform would be more liable to necrotic lesions and cavitation [44–46].

Additionally, following a decreased serum concentration of AQP4-IgG, the AQP4-M1 isoform is rapidly replaced in the astrocytic membrane. Experimental studies have showed that a passive transfer of AQP4-IgG from NMOSD patients to animals with disrupted BBB by previous experimental autoimmune encephalomyelitis (EAE), or through pretreatment with Freund's adjunct, develop CNS typical NMO histopathological lesions [37,48–51].

2.2. Epidemiology

Some caveats are needed before looking at published data on the epidemiology of NMOSD. First, studies on the frequency and distribution of the disease across the world are still scanty and most of them are based on small cohorts. Additionally, they employed non-standardized methodology and inconsistent inclusion of seronegative patients, and differ regarding used diagnostic criteria and assays for AQP4 antibodies detection. In spite of these limitations, a number of issues related to disease prevalence, ethnicity and geography have been clarified. Studies in different populations and geographic regions show that NMOSD is a rare disorder with worldwide distribution [52]. However, an exception to these studies is the seroprevalence study from Olmsted County, in the United States, and Martinique [53] which showed a 2.5-fold higher prevalence rate of the disease in Martinique (10 per 100,000) than in Olmsted County (3.9 per 100,000), all other studies [52] indicated a fairly uniform prevalence rate below 5 per 100,000 people in different regions and populations (Table 1). Likewise, incidence rates were also homogeneous in different countries, ranging from 0.2 per 1 million per year, in Mexico [54] to 4.0 in Denmark [55]. Although most studies point to incidence rate below 1 per 1 million, a peak incidence rate of 7.3 per 1 million was again found in Martinique [53].

Table 1. Incidence and prevalence of NMOSD across the world.

Authors, Year	Country	Number of Cases	Incidence (95% CI) (per Million per Year)	Prevalence (95% CI) (per 100,000)
Rivera et al., 2008 [54]	Mexico	34	0.20 (0.05–0.35)	1
Cabrera-Gómez et al., 2009 [56]	Cuba	58	0.44 (0.3–0.62)	0.43 (0.29–0.61)
Asgari et al., 2011 [55]	Denmark	42	4 (3.0–5.4)	4.41 (3.1–5.7)
Aboul Enein et al., 2011 [57]	Austria	71	0.54 (0.01–0.03)	0.71 (0.17–0.96)
Cossburn et al., 2012 [58]	UK	14	NA	1.96 (1.22–2.97)
Houzen et al., 2012 [59]	Japan	3	0.8 (0.3–1.6)	0.72 (0.31–1.42)
Jacob et al., 2013 [60]	UK	13	0.8 (0.3–1.6)	0.72 (0.31–1.42)
Etemadifar et al., 2014 [61]	Iran	95	NA	1.95 (1.62–2.23)
Pandit et al., 2014 [62]	India	11	NA	2.6
Kashipazha et al., 2015 [63]	Iran	51	NA	0.8 (0.54–1.06)
Flanagan et al., 2016 [53]	USA	6	0.7 (0.0–2.1)	3.9 (0.8–7.1)
	Martinique	39	7.3 (4.1–10.1)	10.0 (6.8–13.2)
van Pelt et al., 2016 [64]	Netherlands		1.2	NA
Houzen et al., 2017 [65]	Japan	14	NA	4.1 (2.2–6.9)
Hor et al., 2017 [66]	Malaysia	14	NA	1.99 (1.09–3.35)
Bukhari et al., 2017 [67]	ANZ	81	0.37 (0.36–0.38)	0.7 (0.66–0.74)
Sepulveda et al., 2017 [68]	Spain	74	0.63 (0.45–0.8)	0.89 (0.87–0.91)
Holroyd et al., 2018 [69]	United Arab Emirates	10	0.59	0.34

NMOSD: neuromyelitis optica spectrum disorders; NA: not available; ANZ: Australia and New Zealand.

Although NMOSD has been regarded to have a predilection for non-Caucasians, the similarity of prevalence and incidence rates in different geographic regions and distinct ethnicities may suggest that, as in opposition to MS, latitude and genetic factors may not play a key role in NMOSD pathogenesis [70]. This contradicts the ethnicity-specific higher prevalence for blacks in Olmsted County, which was similar to that found in the black population of Martinique [53]. The Australian-New Zealand study also observed higher prevalence rate in people with Asian ancestry than in Caucasians [67].

Ethnicity, however, influences age at onset and phenotype of AQP4 seropositive NMOSD. A recent study comparing the clinical manifestations and outcome of 603 NMOSD patients of three different races (Asians, Caucasians and Afro-Americans/Afro-Europeans) showed that non-white patients are younger at disease onset, and more frequently have brain attacks at onset or during the disease course, as well as more frequent abnormalities on brain MRI. Afro-American and Afro-European patients have more severe attacks at onset than Asians and Caucasians, but the outcome at the last follow-up was similar in the different racial groups [71]. This observed that the similarity of the outcome at the last follow-up for all racial groups is in opposition to previous reports of a more severe outcome of NMOSD in Afro-Caribbean than in Caucasian patients [56,72,73].

Usually, the initial clinical manifestations of NMOSD occur at an age of around 35-45 years (median age at onset is 39), but children and the elderly account for 18% of cases. Women comprise 70% to 90% of all cases, but there is no gender predilection in children [74]. The estimated proportion of familial cases (3%) is greater than expected based on the disease prevalence [75]. In some populations, human leukocyte antigen (HLA) has been reported to be associated with susceptibility to NMOSD, such as HLA-DPB1*0501 allele in Japanese and Chinese populations [76,77] and HLA-DPB1*03 in Caucasian, Afro-Caribbean, and Indian patients [78–81]. These genetic factors may account for the phenotypic variability among racial groups.

2.3. Clinical Manifestations

For a long time, the hallmark of NMOSD had been considered as the preferential involvement of the optic nerves and the spinal cord in absence of brain symptoms. However, following the discovery of NMO-IgG in 2004, a wide variety of brainstem, diencephalic and cerebral signs were described in seropositive patients [34]. In 2015 the International Panel for NMO Diagnosis (IPND) added area postrema, brainstem, diencephalic and cerebral manifestations to optic neuritis and LETM to the revised diagnostic criteria for NMOSD [35]. Table 2 shows the clinical manifestations of NMOSD. Clinical analysis of the largest international cohort of AQP4-seropositive NMOSD so far published [71] shows that the disease was relapsing in 85% of the cases. Myelitis was the initial manifestation in 48%, optic neuritis in 42%, area postrema syndrome in 10%, brainstem/diencephalic/cerebral symptoms in 14%, and simultaneous optic neuritis and myelitis in 4%. During the disease course, 84% of the patients presented myelitis, 63% optic neuritis, 15% APS, 17% brainstem syndrome, 3% diencephalic syndrome and 14% cerebral syndrome. In almost one half of the patients (45%) the inaugural attack was severe (defined as an Expanded Disability Status Scale (EDSS) score at ≥6.0 or visual acuity ≤0.1 in at least one eye at nadir).

Severe transverse myelitis in NMOSD most commonly causes symmetrical motor and sensory loss, mainly of the lower limbs, associated with sphincter disturbances. Hiccups and respiratory failure may result from an extension of cervical lesions to the medulla oblongata. Intractable nausea, vomiting and hiccups indicate involvement of the area postrema. The area postrema is the chemosensitive vomiting center located in the dorsal part of the medulla oblongata. It is highly vascularized, lacks blood brain barrier and has a high AQP-4 expression. Its fenestrated capillaries and loosely apposed astrocytic processes likely facilitate IgG access to the CNS [82]. This increased exposure to AQP4-IgG may explain the frequent occurrence of incoercible nausea/vomiting/hiccups in AQP4-IgG seropositive patients. Cervical lesions with rostral extension to the area postrema as seen on MRI, have been observed in other conditions, such as sarcoidosis, lymphoma, paraneoplastic myelitis, spondylosis and dural arteriovenous fistula. However, area postrema lesions on MRI occurring in association with incoercible nausea, vomiting or hiccups are specific for NMOSD [83].

Table 2. Clinical manifestations of NMOSD according to anatomic involvement *.

Site	Symtoms
Optic nerve/chiasm	Eye pain or headache
	Blurred vision
	Disturbance of color vision
	Amaurosis
	Optic disc edema
	Optic atrophy
	Scotomas and other visual field defects
	Limb weakness
	Lower limb spasticity
	Gait abnormalities
	Sensory disturbances
	Radicular pain
Spinal cord	Pruritus
	Painful tonic spasms
	Trunk and limb ataxia
	Sphincter disturbances
	Respiratory weakness
	Lhermitte phenomenon
	Motor and sensory disturbances
	Incoercible nausea, vomiting and hiccups
	Intractable cough
	Weight loss
	Anorexia
	Diplopia/ocular movement disorders
Brainstem	Facial dysesthesia and trigeminal neuralgia
	Dysgeusia
	Facial paralysis
	Hearing loss, tinnitus
	Vertigo
	Dysarthria/dysphagia
	Narcolepsy
	Hypophyseal abnormalities
	Antidiuretic hormone syndrome
Diencephalon	Pre-syncopal symptoms
	Disturbances of body temperature
	Anhydrosis/excessive sweating
	Hyperphagia
	Posterior reversible encephalopathy syndrome (PRES)
	Mental confusion
Cerebrum	Seizures
	Aphasia
	Apraxia
	Cognitive dysfunction
	Psychiatric symptoms

* Modified from Lana-Peixoto and Callegaro, 2012 [34]. NMOSD: neuromyelitis optica spectrum disorders.

Optic neuritis in NMOSD may differ from isolated idiopathic optic neuritis, and from optic neuritis occurring in MS. In NMOSD, optic neuritis is characterized by more severe visual loss at onset, bilateral involvement of the optic nerves or optic chiasm, relapsing course, poor response to IV corticosteroid pulses, poor recovery with permanent visual deficits, and association with normal brain MRI, or with unspecific lesions on brain MRI. Bitemporal hemianopsia points to the presence of chiasmal involvement, which is more common in AQP4-IgG NMOSD than in MS or anti-MOG syndromes.

Brainstem symptoms occur in about one third of the NMOSD patients and are the inaugural manifestation of the disease in about one half of these cases. The most commonly observed brainstem symptoms are vomiting (33%), hiccups (22%), oculomotor dysfunction (20%), and pruritus (12%), followed by hearing loss, facial palsy, vertigo, and trigeminal neuralgia (about 2% each) [84].

In a study of a multi-racial cohort, associated systemic autoimmune diseases were observed in 30% of the Caucasian, 9% of Asian, and 19% of the Afro-American/Afro-European AQP4-seropositive patients [71]. Serum autoantibodies associated with autoimmune conditions are frequently found in NMOSD patients, even in the absence of clinical manifestations. The most common autoimmune abnormalities associated with NMOSD include those related to thyroid disease, systemic lupus erythematosus, and Sjögren syndrome [46].

2.4. Laboratorial Characteristics

Patients with suspected NMOSD need a careful history and physical examination followed by a comprehensive laboratory work-up to rule out mimickers. Laboratory evaluation should include tests for infectious diseases, sarcoidosis, lymphomas and other tumors, paraneoplastic disorders, metabolic and nutritional disorders as well as a number of other autoimmune conditions. Testing for serum AQP4-IgG and MOG-IgG has diagnostic relevance for all patients with suspected NMOSD. Previously employed techniques for serum detection of AQP4-IgG such as indirect immunofluorescence and enzyme-linked immunosorbent assay (ELISA) proved to have lower sensitivity and specificity than cell-based assays (CBA) (mean sensitivity of indirect immunofluorescence and ELISA were 63% and 64%, respectively). Moreover, ELISA may yield 0.5%–1.2% of false-positive results [85–87]. There is a marked variation in assay sensitivity, which ranges from 48.7% to 76.7%, with the highest sensitivity obtained with CBA [88]. The specificity of the different assays ranged from 86.9% to 100% with the commercial fixed CBA having higher specificity than the live CBA. False negative results are higher during remissions, after plasma exchange, or in use of immunosuppressive drugs [88].

Recommendations for testing for serum AQP4-IgG include: (1) patients with acute transverse myelitis associated with a LETM lesion on spinal MRI, or with myelitis associated with normal brain MRI or without evidences of MS or other causes; (2) patients with optic neuritis with atypical features, such as the occurrence of relapses, bilateral simultaneous involvement of the optic nerves or chiasmal involvement, poor recovery, or optic neuritis associated with a long lesion of the optic nerve; (3) patients with area postrema syndrome; (4) patients with diencephalic symptoms and MRI abnormalities of unknown etiology; and (5) patients with encephalopathy of unknown nature. Testing for AQP4-IgG is not recommended in patients with typical clinical and imaging evidences of MS [14,88].

Cerebrospinal fluid (CSF) analysis usually discloses distinct features from those found in MS. While oligoclonal bands (OCB) restricted to the CSF occur in more than 90% of the MS population [89], they were found in only 18% of a large NMOSD cohort [90]. Interestingly, OCB restricted to the CSF are less frequently observed in Asian than in Caucasian or African-American/African European NMOSD patients [71]. During acute relapses a variable pleocytosis with presence of neutrophils and eosinophils may be observed [46].

2.5. Diagnostic Criteria

Current diagnostic criteria for NMOSD were developed by the IPND in 2015 [35]. The panel took the following decisions: (1) unify NMO and NMOSD under the single term "NMOSD"; (2) define (i) optic neuritis; (ii) acute myelitis; (iii) area postrema syndrome or episode of otherwise unexplained hiccups or nausea and vomiting; (iv) acute brainstem syndrome; (v) symptomatic narcolepsy or acute diencephalic clinical syndrome with NMOSD-typical diencephalic MRI lesions; and (vi) symptomatic cerebral syndrome with NMOSD-typical brain lesions as the six "core clinical characteristics" of NMOSD, according to involvement of anatomic sites; (3) establish diagnostic criteria for both NMOSD with AQP4-IgG and NMOSD without AQP4-IgG (negative serology or not performed test) (Table 3); (4) require additional supportive MRI characteristics to diagnostic criteria for NMOSD without AQP4-IgG or with unknown AQP4-IgG in order to enhancing specificity; (5) recommend the use of CBA for AQP4-IgG detection due to their higher sensitivity and specificity; (6) list some clinical features as well as laboratory and imaging findings that may point to alternative diagnoses, and therefore must be seen as "red flags".

Table 3. International consensus diagnostic criteria for NMOSD *.

---

1. Diagnostic criteria for NMOSD with AQP4-IgG
      1. At least one core clinical characteristic
      2. Exclusion of alternative diagnoses
2. Diagnostic criteria for NMOSD without AQP4-IgG or NMOSD with unknown AQP4-IgG status
      1. At least two core clinical characteristics meeting all of the following requirements:
        a. At least one core clinical characteristic must be optic neuritis, acute myelitis with LETM, or area postrema syndrome
        b. Dissemination in space (two or more different core clinical characteristics)
        c. Core clinical syndromes must be associated with respective MRI findings:
            i. Optic neuritis:
                1. Brain MRI is normal or with nonspecific lesions; OR
                2. Optic nerve lesion extending over $\frac{1}{2}$ of the optic nerve length; or chiasmal lesion
            ii. Acute myelitis: MRI with lesion or spinal atrophy extending over ≥3 contiguous segments
            iii. Area postrema syndrome: MRI with dorsal medulla/area postrema lesions
            iv. Acute brainstem syndrome: MRI with periependymal brainstem lesions
            v. Narcolepsy or acute diencephalic clinical syndrome: MRI with NMOSD-typical diencephalic lesions
      2. Exclusion of alternative diagnoses

---

* Modified from Wingerchuk et al., 2015 [35]. NMOSD: neuromyelitis optica spectrum disorders; AQP4: aquaporin-4; IgG: immunoglobulin G; LETM: longitudinally extensive transverse myelitis lesions.

Table 3 shows the international consensus diagnostic criteria for NMOSD with AQP4-IgG, and the diagnostic criteria for NMOSD without AQP4-IgG or with AQP4-IgG unknown status. For AQP4-IgG seropositive individuals, at least one of six "core clinical characteristics" must be present. For individuals without AQP4-IgG or with unknown AQP4-IgG status, diagnosis of NMOSD requires at least two of the six core clinical characteristics. One of the six core clinical characteristics must be optic neuritis, transverse myelitis or area postrema syndrome, and all of them need additional supportive MRI characteristics.

Clinical signs, CSF, MRI and optic coherence tomography (OCT) findings usually distinguish NMOSD from MS. Most frequently, atypical features for NMOSD ("red flags") point to the diagnosis of MS (Table 4). However, a number of other conditions may mimic NMOSD by involvement of the optic nerves and/or the spinal cord (Table 5) [91].

Table 4. Distinctive characteristics between MS and NMOSD.

Distinctive characteristics of MS
Progressive course
Partial transverse myelitis
Brain MRI features
        Perpendicular periventricular lesions (Dawson fingers)
        Periventricular lesions in the inferior temporal lobe
        Juxtacortical lesions involving subcortical U-fibers
        Cortical lesions
        More severe brain atrophy
Spinal cord MRI features
        Lesions <3 complete vertebral segments
        Lesions located predominantly in the peripheral cord
        Diffuse, indistinct signal change on T2-weighted sequences
Cerebrospinal fluid analysis
        Presence of oligoclonal bands
Optic coherence tomography features
        Predominant atrophy of temporal RNFL
Distinctive characteristics of NMOSD
Complete transverse myelitis
Brain MRI features
        Multiple patchy enhancement with blurred margin in adjacent regions
        (cloud-like enhancement)
        Large and edematous callosal lesions
        Large and confluent white matter lesions (as in PRES)
        Predominantly posterior brainstem lesions (around the fourth ventricle
        lesions and periaqueductal lesions)
        Hypothalamic lesions
        Extensive optic nerve lesions and chiasmal lesions
Spinal cord MRI features
        Longitudinally extensive transverse myelitis lesions (≥3 contiguous
        segments)
        Longitudinally extensive spinal cord atrophy (≥3 contiguous segments)
        Centrally-located or holomedullary spinal cord lesions
Cerebrospinal fluid analysis
        Moderate or marked pleocytosis
        Presence of neutrophils and eosinophils
Optic coherence tomography features
        Predominant atrophy of superior and inferior RNFL

MS: multiple sclerosis; NMOSD: neuromyelitis optica spectrum disorders; PRES: posterior reversible encephalopathy syndrome; RNFL: retinal nerve fiber layer.

Table 5. Differential diagnosis of NMOSD.

Multiple Sclerosis
Acute disseminated encephalomyelitis
MOG-related disorders
Sarcoidosis
Lymphoma
Paraneoplastic disease
Central nervous system infections
Syphilis
Tuberculosis
Human T-lymphotropic virus-I (HTLV-I) infection
Herpes virus infection
Dengue-virus infection
Lyme disease
Schistosomiasis
Sjogren syndrome
Systemic lupus erythematosus
Neuro-Behçet's disease
Spinal dural arteriovenous fistula

NMOSD: neuromyelitis optica spectrum disorders.

2.6. Magnetic Resonance Imaging

Magnetic resonance imaging of the brain and spinal cord is an essential tool for the diagnosis and management of demyelinating diseases of the CNS. The correct differentiation of NMOSD and anti-MOG syndromes from MS is important to provide patients with the most appropriate treatment.

Longitudinally extensive transverse myelitis, is the most specific imaging feature of NMOSD (Figure 1a). The length of the lesion has been considered the most distinguishing feature from MS, although long lesions may occur in MS and short lesions in NMOSD. Frequently, LETM lesions exhibit non-homogeneous contrast-enhancing that may persists for months following acute attacks. An extensive centrally-located hypointense signal in T1-sequence denotes cavitation secondary to tissue necrosis (Figure 1b). Cervical lesions may extend rostrally to the medulla oblongata (Figure 1c). Longitudinally extensive cord atrophy results from severe or recurring myelitis (Figure 1d). Short lesions, characterized by extension < three vertebral segments have been reported, predominantly at disease onset in 14% of the patients [92].

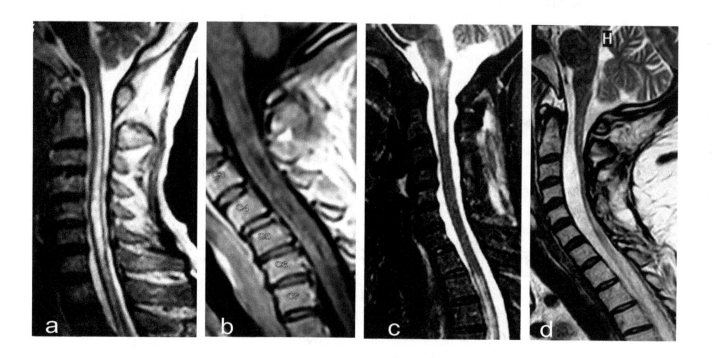

Figure 1. Examples of longitudinally extensive spinal cord lesions detected by MRI in AQP4- seropositive NMOSD patients. (**a**). T2-weighted central longitudinally extensive cervical lesion. (**b**). T1-weighted lesion with gadolinium showing multiple hypointensities (cavitations) throughout the cervical cord. (**c**). T2-weighted cervical lesion extending to brainstem. Another lesion is seen in the upper thoracic levels. (**d**). Longitudinally extensive spinal cord atrophy of the cervical cord.

Optic nerve abnormalities differ between, NMOSD and MS. Thickened, contrast-enhancing and long (≥ one-half the length of the optic nerve) lesions, as well as preference for involvement of the posterior segment of the nerve or chiasm are all in favor of NMOSD (Figure 2).

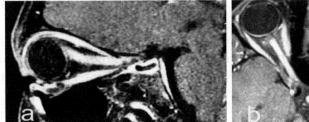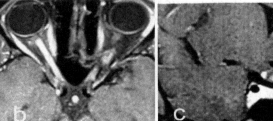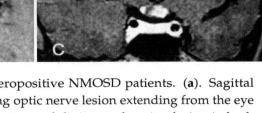

Figure 2. Optic nerve abnormalities on MRI in AQP4-seropositive NMOSD patients. (**a**). Sagittal T1-weighted MRI shows edematous gadolinium-enhancing optic nerve lesion extending from the eye to the intracranial segment. (**b**). Axial T1-weighted extensive gadolinium-enhancing lesion in both optic nerves. (**c**). Coronal T1-weighted MRI shows edematous gadolinium enhancing lesion in the optic chiasm.

Most NMOSD patients have abnormalities on brain MRI [93]. More commonly, brain MRI lesions are unspecific, but they fulfill Barkoff's criteria for MS in up to 42% of patients [93,94]. In a minority of cases, NMOSD typical brain lesions can be identified mainly in AQP4 enriched regions, such as around the lateral, third and fourth ventricles [93]. Brain lesions that favor NMOSD more than MS include peri-ependymal lesions surrounding the ventricles and aqueduct, hemispheric tumefactive lesions, extensive lesions involving corticospinal tracts, and "cloud-like" enhancing lesions [95]. One recent study [96] showed that criteria comprising (1) at least one lesion adjacent to the body of the lateral ventricle and in the inferior temporal lobe; or (2) the presence of an S-shaped U-fiber lesion; or (3) a Dawson's finger type lesion were fulfilled by 90.9% RRMS, 12.9% AQP4-IgG NMOSD, and 4.8% MOG-IgG NMOSD patients.

Adults and children with MOG antibody disease frequently had fluffy brainstem lesions, often located in pons and/or adjacent to fourth ventricle. Children across all conditions showed more frequent bilateral, large, brainstem and deep grey matter lesions. MOG antibody disease spontaneously separated from multiple sclerosis, but overlapped with AQP4 antibody disease. Multiple sclerosis was discriminated from MOG antibody disease and from AQP4 antibody disease with high predictive values, while MOG antibody disease could not be accurately discriminated from AQP4 antibody disease. The best classifiers between MOG antibody disease and multiple sclerosis were similar in adults and children, and included ovoid lesions adjacent to the body of lateral ventricles, Dawson's fingers T1 hypointense lesions (multiple sclerosis), fluffy lesions and three lesions or less (MOG antibody). In the validation cohort patients with antibody-mediated conditions were differentiated from multiple sclerosis with high accuracy [96].

2.7. Treatment

In spite of their clinical similarities, NMOSD and MS have different treatment. It has been shown that most MS disease modifying drugs, including beta-interferons, glatiramer acetate, natalizumab, alemtuzumab, fingolimod and dimethyl-fumarate are not only inefficacious in NMOSD, but may cause disease exacerbation [97].

In NMOSD the outcome of attacks is usually poor. Recent analysis of 871 attacks revealed that complete remission occurred in only 21% of them and 6% of them had no improvement [98]. The sequence of treatments is of fundamental importance to improve the outcome. Medical therapy, therefore, aims both to enfeeble an ongoing inflammatory attack, and avoid future relapses.

2.7.1. Therapy of Acute Relapses

Relapses are usually treated with intravenous pulses of methylprednisolone (one gram/day for five days). In severe NMOSD attacks, or when corticosteroids fail to stabilize progression of symptoms plasma exchange (PLEX) must be added [99]. Apheresis eliminates the pathogenic antibodies, from circulation and has higher therapeutic efficacy than IV corticosteroids. Its early use as first-line therapy following attack is a predictor of better remission.

Post-infusion oral prednisone is usually recommended, mainly when an immunosuppressive agent with delayed onset of action is prescribed as prophylaxis of new events [100]. Azathioprine, mycophenolate mofetil, and rituximab are the most commonly used immunosuppressive treatments for prevention of new attacks of the disease.

2.7.2. Therapy for Relapses Prevention

Table 6 shows the various drugs used for prevention of relapses in NMOSD. Prednisone, azathioprine, mycophenolate mofetil and rituximab are the first-line drugs. The choice of the initial treatment depends on availability, costs, co-morbidities, and disease course. Prednisone is inexpensive and has a rapid-onset therapeutic action, but adverse effects frequently restrain its continuation for a long time.

Table 6. Drugs used in relapse prevention in neuromyelitis optica spectrum disorders.

Drugs	Route	Regimen	Comments
Prednisone	Oral	≥30 mg/d	Keep until until azathioprine or mycophenolate fully effective, then taper over six months
Azathioprine	Oral	2-3 mg/kg/d in 2 doses	First line treatment; latency four to six months; target dose guided by ALC and MCV; monitor liver function
Mycophenolate mofetil	Oral	1500–3000 mg/d in 2 doses	Target dose guided by ALC and blood concentration (1–2 μg/mL)
Rituximab	IV	1000 mg given twice, 14 d apart.Repeat every 6 mo or based on reemergence of CD19 B cells	First-line therapy; CD19 B cells as a marker
Methotrexate	Oral	15–25.0 mg weekly	Supplement with folic acid 1 mg/d, monitor liver function
Ciclosporin A	Oral	2–5 mg/kg/day in 2 doses	Nephrotoxic, target dose guided by blood concentration (70–100 ng/mL)
Tacrolimus	Oral	1–6 mg/day in 2 doses	Nephrotoxic, target dose guided by blood concentration (5–10 ng/mL)
Mitoxantrone	IV	12 mg/m2 every 1–3 months	Cardiac monitoring (LVEF), target dose guided by leukocyte count; total cumulative dose 100 mg/m2
Tocilizumab	IV	8 mg/kg every 4 weeks	8 mg/kg every four weeks; monitoring for infections; CRP no reliable biomarker for infection

ALC = absolute lymphocyte count; MCV = mean corpuscular volume; IV = intravenously; LVEF = left ventricular ejection fraction; CRP = C-reactive protein.

Azathioprine is probably the most commonly used drug in the preventive treatment of attacks in NMOSD. Initially, it should be combined with prednisone for three to six months until its maximal therapeutic effect can be reached. The lymphocyte count should decrease to 600–1000/cubic millimeter and the mean erythrocyte volume should increase five points from baseline. Thiopurine methyltransferase enzyme activity testing, when available is recommended before the administration of the drug to avoid higher risk of adverse effects. Monitoring of blood cell count and liver function tests on a regular basis is mandatory.

Mycophenolate mofetil is recommended as an alternative treatment in patients who develop intolerance or poor response to azathioprine.

Rituximab is a chimeric monoclonal anti-CD20 antibody that produces rapid depletion of circulating CD20 B cells. A number of studies have showed its efficacy and tolerance in the treatment of NMOSD, but some aspects of treatment strategy and long-term safety still remain to be clarified [101].

Monoclonal antibodies will probably play a most important role in treatment of NMOSD in the coming years. Eculizumab and tocilizumab have already shown their efficacy in small groups of patients [102].

Eculizumab is a humanized monoclonal antibody that inhibits the complement protein C5 and blocks terminal complement activation [103]. The complement cascade is a fundamental part in the inflammation process in NMOSD lesions. In spite of eculizumab efficacy in preventing relapses the increased risk of patients developing meningococcal meningitis raises important safety concerns [104].

Tocilizumab is a monoclonal antibody that targets Interleukin-6 (IL-6) receptor and decrease survival of the antibody-producing plasmablasts. Inebelizumab is a humanized anti-CD19 monoclonal antibody that targets B cell lineage. Although there is still no open-label study supporting its use, it is probably more efficacious than rituximab, which targets the more mature CD20. Inebelizumab removes plasmablasts that express CD19, decreasing the production of AQP4-IgG [102].

Satralizumab is an anti-IL-6 receptor monoclonal antibody. A recent communication on results of a phase III study showed that Satralizumab is a promising therapeutic agent by reducing the risk of relapses by 62% in NMOSD patients [105].

Tolerization is a recent therapeutic approach that uses innovative techniques to restore immune tolerance to host antigens and suppress autoimmune diseases [106]. Tolerization techniques include inverse DNA vaccination, T-cell vaccination, peptide-coupling strategies, tolerogenic dendritic cell vaccination, as well as T-cell receptor engineering-, and chimeric antigen receptor-based therapeutics. As AQP-4 is a specific target to NMO-IgG, there is reason for optimism that this new approach might offer marked beneficial to NMOSD patients, avoiding the wide variety of adverse effects of chronic immunosuppressive agents.

3. Anti-Myelin Oligodendrocyte Glycoprotein Syndromes

Myelin oligodendrocyte glycoprotein is a component of myelin expressed exclusively in myelin produced by oligodendrocytes in the CNS, making up less than 0.05% of total myelin proteins. It presents a length of 245 amino acids with a molecular weight of approximately 26–28 kDa [107–109].

The introduction of experimental autoimmune encephalomyelitis (EAE) as an animal model of demyelination raised the interest in the search of anti-MOG antibodies in MS patients. Some investigators reported a prevalence as high as 41% of anti-MOG antibodies serum positivity in MS patients [110]. Others, however, found similar rates of positive MOG-IgG serostatus inpatients with MS, other neurological disorders and healthy controls [111–117]. Recently, the introduction of CBA in substitution to enzyme-linked immunosorbent assays and immunoprecipitation techniques for the detection of MOG-IgG, methods which were not reliable, led to a major change in the understanding of the relationship between MOG-IgG and CNS disorders in humans. Using CBA, a technique that preserve the conformational structure of full-length human MOG, antibodies targeting MOG have been identified in both children and adults with a variety of phenotypes such as ADEM, optic neuritis, transverse myelitis, NMOSD, and brainstem encephalitis [118–122]. Conversely, MOG-IgG has rarely been found in patients with MS phenotype [123,124].

3.1. Pathophysiology

While the role of AQP4-IgG in the pathophysiology of NMOSD has been established by a large number of clinical and experimental evidences the innermost mechanisms underlying the variety of human demyelinating phenotypes in association with anti-MOG antibodies remain to be better clarified.

Anti-MOG antibodies are produced peripherally and usually reach the CNS following a breakdown of the BBB secondary to infections. A history of preceding infectious prodrome is reported in almost 50% of the patients [124]. The absence of restrict oligoclonal bands in the CSF of patients with anti-MOG syndromes supports the notion of its peripheral origin. Circulating lymphocytes may also migrate to CNS with subsequent clonal expansion [125].

Both in vivo and in vitro studies have suggested the presence of complement in mediating demyelination [126,127]. The observation of complement-mediated cytotoxicity from in vitro studies, and the development of a NMOSD-like disorder in animal models are strong evidences in favor of MOG-IgG pathogenicity [18,128,129].

However, in some instances there are reversible alterations to myelin without complement activation or inflammatory cell infiltration [130]. This is in consonance with the better recovery of some patients with anti-MOG syndromes as compared with NMOSD [119,131].

There are few pathological studies on anti-MOG syndromes [7,10]. A brain biopsy from a patient with MOG-antibody-associated encephalomyelitis revealed typical MS-type II histopathological features characterized by deposition of IgG and activated complement at sites of ongoing demyelination. There were well demarcated areas of loss of myelin with relative preservation of axons and astrocytes, numerous lipid-laden macrophages containing myelin debris, and inflammatory infiltrates with predominately perivascular T cells and some perivascular B-cells [7]. However, search for MOG-IgG and a number of other autoantibodies in a series of patients with Type-II MS failed to show any direct relation between type II-MS and MOG-IgG [6]. In contrast with seropositive AQP4-IgG NMOSD, co-existing serum autoantibodies are rare in anti-MOG syndromes. Associated autoimmune disorders are found in over one third of patients with AQP4-IgG seropositive NMOSD, but in only 9% of the anti-MOG syndromes.

3.2. Epidemiology

Major published series show that anti-MOG syndromes have an earlier age at onset, a lower female to male ratio, and a different racial predisposition as compared with seropositive AQP4-IgG NMOSD [96,119,124,132]. In a recent analysis of 50 cases [6], the age at onset ranged from 6 to 70 years (median 31 years) and 64% were females. Caucasians comprised 73% of the 59 patients in Australia/New Zealand series [124].

3.3. Clinical Manifestations

Almost all patients with anti-MOG syndromes present a relapsing course. The proportion of patients with a monophasic disease declines with extension of the follow-up. Relapses occurred in 93% of patients with disease duration ≥8 years [6]. In a study of 276 relapses in 50 patients, optic neuritis occurred in 88%, acute myelitis in 56%, brainstem attacks in 24%, supratentorial encephalitis in 14%, and cerebellitis in 4% of the patients. Bilateral simultaneous optic neuritis occurred in 51% and simultaneous optic neuritis and myelitis in 18 % of the patients [6].

Anti-MOG syndromes have distinct clinical features in children and adults. In children MOG-IgG most frequently expresses clinically as ADEM phenotype, whereas optic neuritis, usually with bilateral involvement, predominates in adults. In a study of 59 patients with relapsing anti-MOG syndromes (33 children and 26 adults) [124] the inaugural symptoms in the pediatric group were ADEM (36%), bilateral optic neuritis (24%), unilateral optic neuritis (15%). In adults, optic neuritis was the presenting symptom in 73% (bilateral optic neuritis 42%; unilateral optic neuritis 31%). Simultaneous involvement of the optic nerves and spinal cord (NMOSD phenotype was the presenting symptom in two children (6%) and five adults (19%). ADEM did not occur in the adult group. Transverse myelitis was less common. Conversely, myelitis occurred at disease presentation in 34% of the patients in another series [6], whereas optic neuritis in 74%, brainstem encephalitis in 8%, cerebral symptoms in 6% and cerebellar symptoms in 2%. At presentation, most patients exhibit either isolated optic neuritis (64%), isolated myelitis (18%), or combined optic neuritis and myelitis (10%). [6]. Optic neuritis is usually severe. Visual acuity ≥20/200 is observed in almost 70% of patients and optic nerve head swelling in the vast majority of the cases [124,132].

Interestingly, 25% to 32% of the patients in both series fulfilled the 2015 International consensus criteria for NMOSD, whereas 15% to 33% of them fulfilled revised McDonald criteria for MS [124,132].

3.4. Anti-MOG Testing

The recently introduced CBA techniques to detect specific autoantibodies that recognize conformational epitopes of membrane proteins, are the currently recommended method for the detection of AQP4-IgG and MOG-IgG. Indications for testing are based on the presence of specific clinical and paraclinical abnormalities that are considered typical for these disorders and atypical for MS. As some patients with MOG-related disorders may test negative for MOG-IgG during disease remission and treatment with immunosuppressive agents, it is recommended that the search for the antibody should be performed during acute relapses.

Many factors influence the sensitivity and specificity for anti-MOG antibody detection and the discrepancies found in early studies are now considered as a result of the use of inappropriate methodology for antibody detection, such as ELISA and immunoblot techniques. Using CBA antibodies targeting MOG have been recently identified in both children and adults with demyelination disorders including acute disseminated encephalomyelitis (ADEM), optic neuritis (ON), transverse myelitis (TM), and AQP4-seronegative NMOSD [124].

3.5. Cerebrospinal Fluid Analysis

Pleocytosis is found in over one half of patients with anti-MOG syndromes. White cell counts ≥100 cell/μL have been reported in 28% of cases [132]. Neutrophils may be present in variable proportion. Intrathecal IgG synthesis as measured by the presence of restricted oligoclonal bands in CSF was found in 11% to 13% of patients [124,132].

3.6. MRI Features

Optic neuritis in anti-MOG syndrome exhibits some peculiar features that may distinguish it from optic neuritis in AQP4-IgG NMOSD and MS. Bilateral optic nerve lesions occur more commonly in MOG (and AQP4-IgG) optic neuritis than in MS optic neuritis (Figure 3a). Usually, lesions are longitudinally extensive and tend to locate in the retrobulbar and orbital segments of the optic nerve. Chiasmal involvement is very rare. Perioptic contrast enhancement which may extend to surrounding orbital tissues (Figure 3b) is observed in over one third of patients [132].

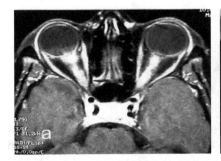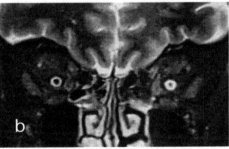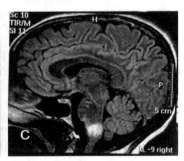

Figure 3. Examples of MRI abnormalities in anti-MOG syndrome. (**a**). Axial T1-weighted MRI reveals longitudinal extensive gadolinium enhancement of both optic nerves. (**b**). Coronal T2-weighted MRI shows hyperintense thickening of perioptic nerve sheath. (**c**). Sagittal T2/FLAIR-weighted image shows large fluffy lesion in the medulla.

Spinal MRI shows in patients with acute myelitis at disease onset LETM lesions in two thirds lesions occur and short lesions (<3 vertebral segments) in one third of patients. Swelling and contrast enhancement of the lesions are frequently observed [131].

Brain MRI is normal in a large majority of anti-MOG NMOSD patients. However, when brain MRI is abnormal, some lesion characteristics may discriminate between anti-MOG NMOSD and MS with high predictive values [96]. Imaging features that are useful to differ between the two conditions are the presence of three lesions or less, and of fluffy brainstem lesions in the pons/or adjacent to fourth ventricle (anti-MOG syndrome) (Figure 3c); and of ovoid lesions adjacent to the body of lateral ventricles, or Dawson's fingers T1 hypointense lesions (MS). On the other hand, brain MRI does not discriminate anti-MOG-NMOSD from AQP4-IgG NMOSD [96].

3.7. Diagnosis

Recently, an international panel of experts [133] formulated the diagnostic criteria for MOG-related disorders in adults. Accordingly, MOG-related disorders should be diagnosed in patients who meet all of the following criteria:

1. Monophasic or relapsing acute ON, myelitis, brainstem encephalitis, or any combination of these symptoms
2. MRI or electrophysiological (visual evoked potentials in patients with isolated ON) findings compatible with CNS demyelination
3. Seropositivity for MOG-IgG as detected by means of a cell-based assay employing full length human MOG as target antigen.

Clinical, laboratory and imaging features that favor the diagnosis of conditions other than MOG-related disorders ("red-flags") include:

a. Chronic progressive course (progressive MS, sarcoidosis and tumors) or acute onset (ischemia);
b. Clinical and paraclinical findings suggesting other conditions such as:

    i. Tuberculosis, borreliosis, syphilis, Behçet's disease, subacute combined degeneration of the spinal cord, Leber's hereditary optic neuropathy, lymphoma, and paraneoplastic disorders;
    ii. Peripheral demyelination

c. Brain MRI abnormalities such as:

    i. Lesion adjacent to lateral ventricle associated with inferior temporal lobe lesion, or Dawson's finger-type lesion;
    ii. Increasing number of lesions between relapses.

d. Serum MOG-IgG at low titers.

It is recommended that patients who test positive for MOG-IgG but in whom a "red flag" is suspected undergo retesting, preferably employing a different CBA [133].

3.8. Treatment

Patients with anti-MOG syndrome are usually responsive to steroids, but frequently relapse after prednisone withdrawal or with a rapid taper [134]. More severe attacks or those with suboptimal response to steroid may be treated with plasma exchange or IV immunoglobulin. As relapsing disease is the rule with extended follow-up long-term immunosuppression should follow first-line treatment [132]. Azathioprine, mycophenolate mofetil and rituximab have all been used but studies on their comparative efficacy are still lacking. Multicenter studies are needed to provide physicians with more robust data on the most appropriate way to treat this rare condition.

3.9. Conclusions

The understanding of NMOSD has enormously advanced in the last few years. Pathophysiological and clinical studies have cleared up a number of uncertainties and deeply changed the concept of the disease. Previously considered as a variant of MS, characterized by monophasic course and exclusive involvement of the optic nerves and spinal cord, NMOSD is now recognized as an independent disorder, most frequently with relapsing course and a variety of clinical manifestations. The 2015 diagnostic criteria [35] allows for the identification of NMOSD in both patients with AQP4-IgG seropositivity and without the antibody, or who were not tested. High doses of IV steroids and PLEX are the main therapeutic measures during relapses, whereas immunosupressive drugs and rituximab are most useful to prevent new attacks. Monoclonal antibodies and tolerization are emerging and promising therapeutic approaches. Recently, MOG-IgG was identified in patients with relapsing optic neurits, acute myelitis, NMOSD phenotypes, and brainstem encephalitis, in addition to ADEM. Although these patients are treated with IV corticosteroids and immunosupressive agents, data are too scanty to evaluate the real efficacy of these drugs.

As NMOSD and anti-MOG syndromes are rare conditions, international collaborative efforts are necessary to determine their distribution in different regions and populations, their intimate pathophysiological mechanisms and the most efficacious therapeutic approach, in order to improving patients care.

References

1.   Kleiter, I.; Hellwig, K.; Berthele, A.; Kumpfel, T.; Linker, R.A.; Hartung, H.P.; Paul, F.; Aktas, O. Failure of natalizumab to prevent relapses in neuromyelitis optica. *Arch. Neurol.* **2012**, *69*, 239–245. [CrossRef] [PubMed]
2.   Min, J.H.; Kim, B.J.; Lee, K.H. Development of extensive brain lesions following fingolimod (fty720) treatment in a patient with neuromyelitis optica spectrum disorder. *Mult. Scler.* **2012**, *18*, 113–115. [CrossRef] [PubMed]
3.   Trebst, C.; Jarius, S.; Berthele, A.; Paul, F.; Schippling, S.; Wildemann, B.; Borisow, N.; Kleiter, I.; Aktas, O.; Kumpfel, T. Update on the diagnosis and treatment of neuromyelitis optica: Recommendations of the neuromyelitis optica study group (nemos). *J. Neurol.* **2014**, *261*, 1–16. [CrossRef] [PubMed]
4.   van Pelt, E.D.; Wong, Y.Y.; Ketelslegers, I.A.; Hamann, D.; Hintzen, R.Q. Neuromyelitis optica spectrum disorders: Comparison of clinical and magnetic resonance imaging characteristics of aqp4-igg versus mog-igg seropositive cases in the netherlands. *Eur. J. Neurol.* **2016**, *23*, 580–587. [CrossRef] [PubMed]
5.   Narayan, R.; Simpson, A.; Fritsche, K.; Salama, S.; Pardo, S.; Mealy, M.; Paul, F.; Levy, M. Mog antibody disease: A review of mog antibody seropositive neuromyelitis optica spectrum disorder. *Mult. Scler. Relat. Disord.* **2018**, *25*, 66–72. [CrossRef] [PubMed]
6.   Jarius, S.; Metz, I.; Konig, F.B.; Ruprecht, K.; Reindl, M.; Paul, F.; Bruck, W.; Wildemann, B. Screening for mog-igg and 27 other anti-glial and anti-neuronal autoantibodies in 'pattern ii multiple sclerosis' and brain biopsy findings in a mog-igg-positive case. *Mult. Scler.* **2016**, *22*, 1541–1549. [CrossRef] [PubMed]
7.   Spadaro, M.; Gerdes, L.A.; Mayer, M.C.; Ertl-Wagner, B.; Laurent, S.; Krumbholz, M.; Breithaupt, C.; Hogen, T.; Straube, A.; Giese, A.; et al. Histopathology and clinical course of mog-antibody-associated encephalomyelitis. *Ann. Clin. Transl. Neurol.* **2015**, *2*, 295–301. [CrossRef] [PubMed]
8.   Misu, T.; Hoftberger, R.; Fujihara, K.; Wimmer, I.; Takai, Y.; Nishiyama, S.; Nakashima, I.; Konno, H.; Bradl, M.; Garzuly, F.; et al. Presence of six different lesion types suggests diverse mechanisms of tissue injury in neuromyelitis optica. *Acta Neuropathol.* **2013**, *125*, 815–827. [CrossRef] [PubMed]
9.   Reindl, M.; Rostasy, K. Mog antibody-associated diseases. *Neurol. Neuroimmunol. Neuroinflamm.* **2015**, *2*, e60. [CrossRef]
10.   Di Pauli, F.; Hoftberger, R.; Reindl, M.; Beer, R.; Rhomberg, P.; Schanda, K.; Sato, D.; Fujihara, K.; Lassmann, H.; Schmutzhard, E.; et al. Fulminant demyelinating encephalomyelitis: Insights from antibody studies and neuropathology. *Neurol. Neuroimmunol. Neuroinflamm.* **2015**, *2*, e175. [CrossRef]
11.   Ramanathan, S.; Dale, R.C.; Brilot, F. Anti-mog antibody: The history, clinical phenotype, and pathogenicity of a serum biomarker for demyelination. *Autoimmun. Rev.* **2016**, *15*, 307–324. [CrossRef] [PubMed]
12.   Jarius, S.; Probst, C.; Borowski, K.; Franciotta, D.; Wildemann, B.; Stoecker, W.; Wandinger, K.P. Standardized method for the detection of antibodies to aquaporin-4 based on a highly sensitive immunofluorescence assay employing recombinant target antigen. *J. Neurol. Sci.* **2010**, *291*, 52–56. [CrossRef] [PubMed]
13.   Waters, P.J.; McKeon, A.; Leite, M.I.; Rajasekharan, S.; Lennon, V.A.; Villalobos, A.; Palace, J.; Mandrekar, J.N.; Vincent, A.; Bar-Or, A.; et al. Serologic diagnosis of nmo: A multicenter comparison of aquaporin-4-igg assays. *Neurology* **2012**, *78*, 665–671; discussion 669. [CrossRef] [PubMed]

14. Waters, P.J.; Pittock, S.J.; Bennett, J.L.; Jarius, S.; Weinshenker, B.G.; Wingerchuk, D.M. Evaluation of aquaporin-4 antibody assays. *Clin. Exp. Neuroimmunol.* **2014**, *5*, 290–303. [CrossRef] [PubMed]

15. Jarius, S.; Ruprecht, K.; Kleiter, I.; Borisow, N.; Asgari, N.; Pitarokoili, K.; Pache, F.; Stich, O.; Beume, L.A.; Hummert, M.W.; et al. Mog-igg in nmo and related disorders: A multicenter study of 50 patients. Part 1: Frequency, syndrome specificity, influence of disease activity, long-term course, association with aqp4-igg, and origin. *J. Neuroinflamm.* **2016**, *13*, 279. [CrossRef] [PubMed]

16. Ishikawa, N.; Tajima, G.; Hyodo, S.; Takahashi, Y.; Kobayashi, M. Detection of autoantibodies against nmda-type glutamate receptor in a patient with recurrent optic neuritis and transient cerebral lesions. *Neuropediatrics* **2007**, *38*, 257–260. [CrossRef] [PubMed]

17. Kruer, M.C.; Koch, T.K.; Bourdette, D.N.; Chabas, D.; Waubant, E.; Mueller, S.; Moscarello, M.A.; Dalmau, J.; Woltjer, R.L.; Adamus, G. Nmda receptor encephalitis mimicking seronegative neuromyelitis optica. *Neurology* **2010**, *74*, 1473–1475. [CrossRef] [PubMed]

18. Mader, S.; Gredler, V.; Schanda, K.; Rostasy, K.; Dujmovic, I.; Pfaller, K.; Lutterotti, A.; Jarius, S.; Di Pauli, F.; Kuenz, B.; et al. Complement activating antibodies to myelin oligodendrocyte glycoprotein in neuromyelitis optica and related disorders. *J. Neuroinflamm.* **2011**, *8*, 184. [CrossRef] [PubMed]

19. Jarius, S.; Wandinger, K.P.; Borowski, K.; Stoecker, W.; Wildemann, B. Antibodies to cv2/crmp5 in neuromyelitis optica-like disease: Case report and review of the literature. *Clin. Neurol. Neurosurg.* **2012**, *114*, 331–335. [CrossRef] [PubMed]

20. Devic, E. Myelite subaigue compliquee de nevrite optique. *Bull. Med.* **1894**, *8*, 1033.

21. Gault, F. De la neuromyélite optique aiguë. Ph.D. Thesis, Alexandre Rey, imprimeur de la faculté de médecine, Faculté de Medicine et de Pharmacie de Lyon, Lyon, France, 1894.

22. Acchiote, P. Sur un cas de neuromyélite subaiguë ou maladie de devic. *Rev. Neurol.* **1907**, *20*, 775–777.

23. Jarius, S.; Wildemann, B. The case of the marquis de causan (1804): An early account of visual loss associated with spinal cord inflammation. *J. Neurol.* **2012**, *259*, 1354–1357. [CrossRef] [PubMed]

24. Jarius, S.; Wildemann, B. 'Noteomielite' accompanied by acute amaurosis (1844). An early case of neuromyelitis optica. *J. Neurol. Sci.* **2012**, *313*, 182–184. [CrossRef] [PubMed]

25. Jarius, S.; Wildemann, B. An early british case of neuromyelitis optica (1850). *BMJ Clin. Res. Ed.* **2012**, *345*, e6430. [CrossRef] [PubMed]

26. Jarius, S.; Wildemann, B. An early case of neuromyelitis optica: On a forgotten report by jacob lockhart clarke, frs. *Mult. Scler.* **2011**, *17*, 1384–1386. [CrossRef] [PubMed]

27. Allbutt, T.C. On the ophthalmoscopic signs of spinal disease. *Lancet* **1870**, *95*, 76–78. [CrossRef]

28. Erb, W. Ueber das zusammenvorkommen von neuritis optica und myelitis subacuta. *Eur. Arch. Psychiatry Clin. Neurosci.* **1880**, *10*, 146–157. [CrossRef]

29. Seguin, E.C. Art. I.—On the coincidence of optic neuritis and subacute transverse myelitis. *J. Nerv. Ment. Dis.* **1880**, *7*, 177–188. [CrossRef]

30. Marques, A. Da neuromielite ótica: Contribuição clínica e etiológica. *Hospital* **1943**, *24*, 49–63.

31. Lennon, V.A.; Wingerchuk, D.M.; Kryzer, T.J.; Pittock, S.J.; Lucchinetti, C.F.; Fujihara, K.; Nakashima, I.; Weinshenker, B.G. A serum autoantibody marker of neuromyelitis optica: Distinction from multiple sclerosis. *Lancet* **2004**, *364*, 2106–2112. [CrossRef]

32. Lennon, V.A.; Kryzer, T.J.; Pittock, S.J.; Verkman, A.S.; Hinson, S.R. Igg marker of optic-spinal multiple sclerosis binds to the aquaporin-4 water channel. *J. Exp. Med.* **2005**, *202*, 473–477. [CrossRef] [PubMed]

33. Wingerchuk, D.M.; Lennon, V.A.; Lucchinetti, C.F.; Pittock, S.J.; Weinshenker, B.G. The spectrum of neuromyelitis optica. *Lancet Neurol.* **2007**, *6*, 805–815. [CrossRef]

34. Lana-Peixoto, M.A.; Callegaro, D. The expanded spectrum of neuromyelitis optica: Evidences for a new definition. *Arq. Neuro-Psiquiatr.* **2012**, *70*, 807–813. [CrossRef]

35. Wingerchuk, D.M.; Banwell, B.; Bennett, J.L.; Cabre, P.; Carroll, W.; Chitnis, T.; de Seze, J.; Fujihara, K.; Greenberg, B.; Jacob, A.; et al. International consensus diagnostic criteria for neuromyelitis optica spectrum disorders. *Neurology* **2015**, *85*, 177–189. [CrossRef] [PubMed]

36. Jin, B.J.; Rossi, A.; Verkman, A.S. Model of aquaporin-4 supramolecular assembly in orthogonal arrays based on heterotetrameric association of m1-m23 isoforms. *Biophys. J.* **2011**, *100*, 2936–2945. [CrossRef] [PubMed]

37. Papadopoulos, M.C.; Verkman, A.S. Aquaporin 4 and neuromyelitis optica. *Lancet Neurol.* **2012**, *11*, 535–544. [CrossRef]

38. Verkman, A.S.; Anderson, M.O.; Papadopoulos, M.C. Aquaporins: Important but elusive drug targets. *Nat. Rev. Drug Discov.* **2014**, *13*, 259–277. [CrossRef]

39. Saadoun, S.; Waters, P.; Bell, B.A.; Vincent, A.; Verkman, A.S.; Papadopoulos, M.C. Intra-cerebral injection of neuromyelitis optica immunoglobulin g and human complement produces neuromyelitis optica lesions in mice. *Brain J. Neurol.* **2010**, *133*, 349–361. [CrossRef]

40. Lucchinetti, C.F.; Mandler, R.N.; McGavern, D.; Bruck, W.; Gleich, G.; Ransohoff, R.M.; Trebst, C.; Weinshenker, B.; Wingerchuk, D.; Parisi, J.E.; et al. A role for humoral mechanisms in the pathogenesis of devic's neuromyelitis optica. *Brain J. Neurol.* **2002**, *125*, 1450–1461. [CrossRef]

41. Jarius, S.; Franciotta, D.; Paul, F.; Ruprecht, K.; Bergamaschi, R.; Rommer, P.S.; Reuss, R.; Probst, C.; Kristoferitsch, W.; Wandinger, K.P.; et al. Cerebrospinal fluid antibodies to aquaporin-4 in neuromyelitis optica and related disorders: Frequency, origin, and diagnostic relevance. *J. Neuroinflamm.* **2010**, *7*, 52. [CrossRef]

42. Chihara, N.; Aranami, T.; Sato, W.; Miyazaki, Y.; Miyake, S.; Okamoto, T.; Ogawa, M.; Toda, T.; Yamamura, T. Interleukin 6 signaling promotes anti-aquaporin 4 autoantibody production from plasmablasts in neuromyelitis optica. *Proc. Natl. Acad. Sci. USA* **2011**, *108*, 3701–3706. [CrossRef] [PubMed]

43. Shimizu, F.; Schaller, K.L.; Owens, G.P.; Cotleur, A.C.; Kellner, D.; Takeshita, Y.; Obermeier, B.; Kryzer, T.J.; Sano, Y.; Kanda, T.; et al. Glucose-regulated protein 78 autoantibody associates with blood-brain barrier disruption in neuromyelitis optica. *Sci. Transl. Med.* **2017**, *9*, eaai9111. [CrossRef] [PubMed]

44. Shimizu, F.; Nishihara, H.; Kanda, T. Blood-brain barrier dysfunction in immuno-mediated neurological diseases. *Immunol. Med.* **2018**, *41*, 120–128. [CrossRef] [PubMed]

45. Jarius, S.; Wildemann, B.; Paul, F. Neuromyelitis optica: Clinical features, immunopathogenesis and treatment. *Clin. Exp. Immunol.* **2014**, *176*, 149–164. [CrossRef] [PubMed]

46. Weinshenker, B.G.; Wingerchuk, D.M. Neuromyelitis spectrum disorders. *Mayo Clin. Proc.* **2017**, *92*, 663–679. [CrossRef] [PubMed]

47. Hinson, S.R.; Pittock, S.J.; Lucchinetti, C.F.; Roemer, S.F.; Fryer, J.P.; Kryzer, T.J.; Lennon, V.A. Pathogenic potential of igg binding to water channel extracellular domain in neuromyelitis optica. *Neurology* **2007**, *69*, 2221–2231. [CrossRef]

48. Bennett, J.L.; Lam, C.; Kalluri, S.R.; Saikali, P.; Bautista, K.; Dupree, C.; Glogowska, M.; Case, D.; Antel, J.P.; Owens, G.P.; et al. Intrathecal pathogenic anti-aquaporin-4 antibodies in early neuromyelitis optica. *Ann. Neurol.* **2009**, *66*, 617–629. [CrossRef]

49. Bradl, M.; Misu, T.; Takahashi, T.; Watanabe, M.; Mader, S.; Reindl, M.; Adzemovic, M.; Bauer, J.; Berger, T.; Fujihara, K.; et al. Neuromyelitis optica: Pathogenicity of patient immunoglobulin in vivo. *Ann. Neurol.* **2009**, *66*, 630–643. [CrossRef]

50. Kinoshita, M.; Nakatsuji, Y.; Kimura, T.; Moriya, M.; Takata, K.; Okuno, T.; Kumanogoh, A.; Kajiyama, K.; Yoshikawa, H.; Sakoda, S. Neuromyelitis optica: Passive transfer to rats by human immunoglobulin. *Biochem. Biophys. Res. Commun.* **2009**, *386*, 623–627. [CrossRef]

51. Kinoshita, M.; Nakatsuji, Y.; Kimura, T.; Moriya, M.; Takata, K.; Okuno, T.; Kumanogoh, A.; Kajiyama, K.; Yoshikawa, H.; Sakoda, S. Anti-aquaporin-4 antibody induces astrocytic cytotoxicity in the absence of cns antigen-specific t cells. *Biochem. Biophys. Res. Commun.* **2010**, *394*, 205–210. [CrossRef]

52. Etemadifar, M.; Nasr, Z.; Khalili, B.; Taherioun, M.; Vosoughi, R. Epidemiology of neuromyelitis optica in the world: A systematic review and meta-analysis. *Mult. Scler. Int.* **2015**, *2015*, 174720. [CrossRef] [PubMed]

53. Flanagan, E.P.; Cabre, P.; Weinshenker, B.G.; Sauver, J.S.; Jacobson, D.J.; Majed, M.; Lennon, V.A.; Lucchinetti, C.F.; McKeon, A.; Matiello, M.; et al. Epidemiology of aquaporin-4 autoimmunity and neuromyelitis optica spectrum. *Ann. Neurol.* **2016**, *79*, 775–783. [CrossRef] [PubMed]

54. Rivera, J.F.; Kurtzke, J.F.; Booth, V.A.; Corona, T. Characteristics of devic's disease (neuromyelitis optica) in mexico. *J. Neurol.* **2008**, *255*, 710–715. [CrossRef] [PubMed]

55. Asgari, N.; Lillevang, S.T.; Skejoe, H.P.; Falah, M.; Stenager, E.; Kyvik, K.O. A population-based study of neuromyelitis optica in caucasians. *Neurology* **2011**, *76*, 1589–1595. [CrossRef] [PubMed]

56. Cabrera-Gomez, J.A.; Kurtzke, J.F.; Gonzalez-Quevedo, A.; Lara-Rodriguez, R. An epidemiological study of neuromyelitis optica in cuba. *J. Neurol.* **2009**, *256*, 35–44. [CrossRef] [PubMed]

57. Aboul-Enein, F.; Seifert-Held, T.; Mader, S.; Kuenz, B.; Lutterotti, A.; Rauschka, H.; Rommer, P.; Leutmezer, F.; Vass, K.; Flamm-Horak, A.; et al. Neuromyelitis optica in austria in 2011: To bridge the gap between neuroepidemiological research and practice in a study population of 8.4 million people. *PLoS ONE* **2013**, *8*, e79649. [CrossRef] [PubMed]

58. Cossburn, M.; Tackley, G.; Baker, K.; Ingram, G.; Burtonwood, M.; Malik, G.; Pickersgill, T.; te Water Naude, J.; Robertson, N. The prevalence of neuromyelitis optica in south east wales. *Eur. J. Neurol.* **2012**, *19*, 655–659. [CrossRef] [PubMed]

59. Houzen, H.; Niino, M.; Hirotani, M.; Fukazawa, T.; Kikuchi, S.; Tanaka, K.; Sasaki, H. Increased prevalence, incidence, and female predominance of multiple sclerosis in northern japan. *J. Neurol. Sci.* **2012**, *323*, 117–122. [CrossRef] [PubMed]

60. Jacob, A.; Panicker, J.; Lythgoe, D.; Elsone, L.; Mutch, K.; Wilson, M.; Das, K.; Boggild, M. The epidemiology of neuromyelitis optica amongst adults in the merseyside county of united kingdom. *J. Neurol.* **2013**, *260*, 2134–2137. [CrossRef] [PubMed]

61. Etemadifar, M.; Dashti, M.; Vosoughi, R.; Abtahi, S.H.; Ramagopalan, S.V.; Nasr, Z. An epidemiological study of neuromyelitis optica in isfahan. *Mult. Scler.* **2014**, *20*, 1920–1922. [CrossRef] [PubMed]

62. Pandit, L.; Kundapur, R. Prevalence and patterns of demyelinating central nervous system disorders in urban mangalore, south india. *Mult. Scler.* **2014**, *20*, 1651–1653. [CrossRef] [PubMed]

63. Kashipazha, D.; Mohammadianinejad, S.E.; Majdinasab, N.; Azizi, M.; Jafari, M. A descriptive study of prevalence, clinical features and other findings of neuromyelitis optica and neuromyelitis optica spectrum disorder in khuzestan province, iran. *Iran. J. Neurol.* **2015**, *14*, 204–210. [PubMed]

64. Danielle van Pelt, E.; Wong, Y.Y.M.; Ketelslegers, I.A.; Siepman, D.A.; Hamann, D.; Hintzen, R.Q. Incidence of aqp4-igg seropositive neuromyelitis optica spectrum disorders in the netherlands: About one in a million. *Mult. Scler. J. Exp. Transl. Clin.* **2016**, *2*, 2055217315625652. [CrossRef] [PubMed]

65. Houzen, H.; Kondo, K.; Niino, M.; Horiuchi, K.; Takahashi, T.; Nakashima, I.; Tanaka, K. Prevalence and clinical features of neuromyelitis optica spectrum disorders in northern japan. *Neurology* **2017**, *89*, 1995–2001. [CrossRef] [PubMed]

66. Hor, J.Y.; Lim, T.T.; Chia, Y.K.; Ching, Y.M.; Cheah, C.F.; Tan, K.; Chow, H.B.; Arip, M.; Eow, G.B.; Easaw, P.E.S.; et al. Prevalence of neuromyelitis optica spectrum disorder in the multi-ethnic penang island, malaysia, and a review of worldwide prevalence. *Mult. Scler. Relat. Disord.* **2018**, *19*, 20–24. [CrossRef] [PubMed]

67. Bukhari, W.; Prain, K.M.; Waters, P.; Woodhall, M.; O'Gorman, C.M.; Clarke, L.; Silvestrini, R.A.; Bundell, C.S.; Abernethy, D.; Bhuta, S.; et al. Incidence and prevalence of nmosd in australia and new zealand. *J. Neurol. Neurosurg. Psychiatry* **2017**, *88*, 632–638. [CrossRef] [PubMed]

68. Sepulveda, M.; Aldea, M.; Escudero, D.; Llufriu, S.; Arrambide, G.; Otero-Romero, S.; Sastre-Garriga, J.; Romero-Pinel, L.; Martinez-Yelamos, S.; Sola-Valls, N.; et al. Epidemiology of nmosd in catalonia: Influence of the new 2015 criteria in incidence and prevalence estimates. *Mult. Scler.* **2017**, *24*, 1843–1851. [CrossRef] [PubMed]

69. Holroyd, K.B.; Aziz, F.; Szolics, M.; Alsaadi, T.; Levy, M.; Schiess, N. Prevalence and characteristics of transverse myelitis and neuromyelitis optica spectrum disorders in the united arab emirates: A multicenter, retrospective study. *Clin. Exp. Neuroimmunol.* **2018**, *9*, 155–161. [CrossRef]

70. Mori, M.; Kuwabara, S.; Paul, F. Worldwide prevalence of neuromyelitis optica spectrum disorders. *J. Neurol. Neurosurg. Psychiatry* **2018**, *89*, 555–556. [CrossRef]

71. Kim, S.H.; Mealy, M.A.; Levy, M.; Schmidt, F.; Ruprecht, K.; Paul, F.; Ringelstein, M.; Aktas, O.; Hartung, H.P.; Asgari, N.; et al. Racial differences in neuromyelitis optica spectrum disorder. *Neurology* **2018**, *91*, e2089–e2099. [CrossRef]

72. Kitley, J.; Leite, M.I.; Nakashima, I.; Waters, P.; McNeillis, B.; Brown, R.; Takai, Y.; Takahashi, T.; Misu, T.; Elsone, L.; et al. Prognostic factors and disease course in aquaporin-4 antibody-positive patients with neuromyelitis optica spectrum disorder from the united kingdom and japan. *Brain J. Neurol.* **2012**, *135*, 1834–1849. [CrossRef] [PubMed]

73. Sepulveda, M.; Armangue, T.; Sola-Valls, N.; Arrambide, G.; Meca-Lallana, J.E.; Oreja-Guevara, C.; Mendibe, M.; Alvarez de Arcaya, A.; Aladro, Y.; Casanova, B.; et al. Neuromyelitis optica spectrum disorders: Comparison according to the phenotype and serostatus. *Neurol. Neuroimmunol. Neuroinflamm.* **2016**, *3*, e225. [CrossRef] [PubMed]

74. McKeon, A.; Lennon, V.A.; Lotze, T.; Tenenbaum, S.; Ness, J.M.; Rensel, M.; Kuntz, N.L.; Fryer, J.P.; Homburger, H.; Hunter, J.; et al. Cns aquaporin-4 autoimmunity in children. *Neurology* **2008**, *71*, 93–100. [CrossRef] [PubMed]

75. Matiello, M.; Kim, H.J.; Kim, W.; Brum, D.G.; Barreira, A.A.; Kingsbury, D.J.; Plant, G.T.; Adoni, T.; Weinshenker, B.G. Familial neuromyelitis optica. *Neurology* **2010**, *75*, 310–315. [CrossRef] [PubMed]

76. Matsushita, T.; Matsuoka, T.; Isobe, N.; Kawano, Y.; Minohara, M.; Shi, N.; Nishimura, Y.; Ochi, H.; Kira, J. Association of the hla-dpb1*0501 allele with anti-aquaporin-4 antibody positivity in japanese patients with idiopathic central nervous system demyelinating disorders. *Tissue Antigens* **2009**, *73*, 171–176. [CrossRef] [PubMed]

77. Wang, H.; Dai, Y.; Qiu, W.; Zhong, X.; Wu, A.; Wang, Y.; Lu, Z.; Bao, J.; Hu, X. Hla-dpb1 0501 is associated with susceptibility to anti-aquaporin-4 antibodies positive neuromyelitis optica in southern han chinese. *J. Neuroimmunol.* **2011**, *233*, 181–184. [CrossRef] [PubMed]

78. Blanco, Y.; Ercilla-Gonzalez, G.; Llufriu, S.; Casanova-Estruch, B.; Magraner, M.J.; Ramio-Torrenta, L.; Mendibe-Bilbao, M.M.; Ucles-Sanchez, A.J.; Casado-Chocan, J.L.; Lopez de Munain, A.; et al. hla-drb1 typing in caucasians patients with neuromyelitis optica. *Rev. De Neurol.* **2011**, *53*, 146–152.

79. Pandit, L.; Malli, C.; D'Cunha, A.; Mustafa, S. Human leukocyte antigen association with neuromyelitis optica in a south indian population. *Mult. Scler.* **2015**, *21*, 1217–1218. [CrossRef]

80. Deschamps, R.; Paturel, L.; Jeannin, S.; Chausson, N.; Olindo, S.; Bera, O.; Bellance, R.; Smadja, D.; Cesaire, D.; Cabre, P. Different hla class ii (drb1 and dqb1) alleles determine either susceptibility or resistance to nmo and multiple sclerosis among the french afro-caribbean population. *Mult. Scler.* **2011**, *17*, 24–31. [CrossRef]

81. Zephir, H.; Fajardy, I.; Outteryck, O.; Blanc, F.; Roger, N.; Fleury, M.; Rudolf, G.; Marignier, R.; Vukusic, S.; Confavreux, C.; et al. Is neuromyelitis optica associated with human leukocyte antigen? *Mult. Scler.* **2009**, *15*, 571–579. [CrossRef]

82. Popescu, B.F.; Lennon, V.A.; Parisi, J.E.; Howe, C.L.; Weigand, S.D.; Cabrera-Gomez, J.A.; Newell, K.; Mandler, R.N.; Pittock, S.J.; Weinshenker, B.G.; et al. Neuromyelitis optica unique area postrema lesions: Nausea, vomiting, and pathogenic implications. *Neurology* **2011**, *76*, 1229–1237. [CrossRef] [PubMed]

83. Dubey, D.; Pittock, S.J.; Krecke, K.N.; Flanagan, E.P. Association of extension of cervical cord lesion and area postrema syndrome with neuromyelitis optica spectrum disorder. *JAMA Neurol.* **2017**, *74*, 359–361. [CrossRef] [PubMed]

84. Kremer, L.; Mealy, M.; Jacob, A.; Nakashima, I.; Cabre, P.; Bigi, S.; Paul, F.; Jarius, S.; Aktas, O.; Elsone, L.; et al. Brainstem manifestations in neuromyelitis optica: A multicenter study of 258 patients. *Mult. Scler.* **2014**, *20*, 843–847. [CrossRef] [PubMed]

85. Jarius, S.; Wildemann, B. Aquaporin-4 antibodies (nmo-igg) as a serological marker of neuromyelitis optica: A critical review of the literature. *Brain Pathol.* **2013**, *23*, 661–683. [CrossRef] [PubMed]

86. Marignier, R.; Bernard-Valnet, R.; Giraudon, P.; Collongues, N.; Papeix, C.; Zephir, H.; Cavillon, G.; Rogemond, V.; Casey, R.; Frangoulis, B.; et al. Aquaporin-4 antibody-negative neuromyelitis optica: Distinct assay sensitivity-dependent entity. *Neurology* **2013**, *80*, 2194–2200. [CrossRef] [PubMed]

87. Pittock, S.J.; Lennon, V.A.; Bakshi, N.; Shen, L.; McKeon, A.; Quach, H.; Briggs, F.B.; Bernstein, A.L.; Schaefer, C.A.; Barcellos, L.F. Seroprevalence of aquaporin-4-igg in a northern california population representative cohort of multiple sclerosis. *JAMA Neurol.* **2014**, *71*, 1433–1436. [CrossRef] [PubMed]

88. Waters, P.; Reindl, M.; Saiz, A.; Schanda, K.; Tuller, F.; Kral, V.; Nytrova, P.; Sobek, O.; Nielsen, H.H.; Barington, T.; et al. Multicentre comparison of a diagnostic assay: Aquaporin-4 antibodies in neuromyelitis optica. *J. Neurol. Neurosurg. Psychiatry* **2016**, *87*, 1005–1015. [CrossRef] [PubMed]

89. Andersson, M.; Alvarez-Cermeno, J.; Bernardi, G.; Cogato, I.; Fredman, P.; Frederiksen, J.; Fredrikson, S.; Gallo, P.; Grimaldi, L.M.; Gronning, M.; et al. Cerebrospinal fluid in the diagnosis of multiple sclerosis: A consensus report. *J. Neurol. Neurosurg. Psychiatry* **1994**, *57*, 897–902. [CrossRef]

90. Jarius, S.; Ruprecht, K.; Wildemann, B.; Kuempfel, T.; Ringelstein, M.; Geis, C.; Kleiter, I.; Kleinschnitz, C.; Berthele, A.; Brettschneider, J.; et al. Contrasting disease patterns in seropositive and seronegative neuromyelitis optica: A multicentre study of 175 patients. *J. Neuroinflamm.* **2012**, *9*, 14. [CrossRef]

91. Kim, S.M.; Kim, S.J.; Lee, H.J.; Kuroda, H.; Palace, J.; Fujihara, K. Differential diagnosis of neuromyelitis optica spectrum disorders. *Ther. Adv. Neurol. Disord.* **2017**, *10*, 265–289. [CrossRef]

92. Flanagan, E.P.; Weinshenker, B.G.; Krecke, K.N.; Lennon, V.A.; Lucchinetti, C.F.; McKeon, A.; Wingerchuk, D.M.; Shuster, E.A.; Jiao, Y.; Horta, E.S.; et al. Short myelitis lesions in aquaporin-4-igg-positive neuromyelitis optica spectrum disorders. *JAMA Neurol.* **2015**, *72*, 81–87. [CrossRef] [PubMed]

93. Pittock, S.J.; Weinshenker, B.G.; Lucchinetti, C.F.; Wingerchuk, D.M.; Corboy, J.R.; Lennon, V.A. Neuromyelitis optica brain lesions localized at sites of high aquaporin 4 expression. *Arch. Neurol.* **2006**, *63*, 964–968. [CrossRef] [PubMed]

94. Matthews, L.; Marasco, R.; Jenkinson, M.; Kuker, W.; Luppe, S.; Leite, M.I.; Giorgio, A.; De Stefano, N.; Robertson, N.; Johansen-Berg, H.; et al. Distinction of seropositive nmo spectrum disorder and ms brain lesion distribution. *Neurology* **2013**, *80*, 1330–1337. [CrossRef] [PubMed]

95. Kim, H.J.; Paul, F.; Lana-Peixoto, M.A.; Tenembaum, S.; Asgari, N.; Palace, J.; Klawiter, E.C.; Sato, D.K.; de Seze, J.; Wuerfel, J.; et al. Mri characteristics of neuromyelitis optica spectrum disorder: An international update. *Neurology* **2015**, *84*, 1165–1173. [CrossRef] [PubMed]

96. Jurynczyk, M.; Tackley, G.; Kong, Y.; Geraldes, R.; Matthews, L.; Woodhall, M.; Waters, P.; Kuker, W.; Craner, M.; Weir, A.; et al. Brain lesion distribution criteria distinguish ms from aqp4-antibody nmosd and mog-antibody disease. *J. Neurol. Neurosurg. Psychiatry* **2017**, *88*, 132–136. [CrossRef]

97. Kira, J.I. Unexpected exacerbations following initiation of disease-modifying drugs in neuromyelitis optica spectrum disorder: Which factor is responsible, anti-aquaporin 4 antibodies, b cells, th1 cells, th2 cells, th17 cells, or others? *Mult. Scler.* **2017**, *23*, 1300–1302. [CrossRef] [PubMed]

98. Kleiter, I.; Gahlen, A.; Borisow, N.; Fischer, K.; Wernecke, K.D.; Wegner, B.; Hellwig, K.; Pache, F.; Ruprecht, K.; Havla, J.; et al. Neuromyelitis optica: Evaluation of 871 attacks and 1,153 treatment courses. *Ann. Neurol.* **2016**, *79*, 206–216. [CrossRef] [PubMed]

99. Weinshenker, B.G. What is the optimal sequence of rescue treatments for attacks of neuromyelitis optica spectrum disorder? *Ann. Neurol.* **2016**, *79*, 204–205. [CrossRef]

100. Wingerchuk, D.M.; Weinshenker, B.G. Neuromyelitis optica. *Curr. Treat. Options Neurol.* **2008**, *10*, 55–66. [CrossRef]

101. Kim, S.H.; Hyun, J.W.; Kim, H.J. Individualized b cell-targeting therapy for neuromyelitis optica spectrum disorder. *Neurochem. Int.* **2018**, in press. [CrossRef]

102. Paul, F.; Murphy, O.; Pardo, S.; Levy, M. Investigational drugs in development to prevent neuromyelitis optica relapses. *Expert Opin. Investig. Drugs* **2018**, *27*, 265–271. [CrossRef] [PubMed]

103. Kelly, R.J.; Hochsmann, B.; Szer, J.; Kulasekararaj, A.; de Guibert, S.; Roth, A.; Weitz, I.C.; Armstrong, E.; Risitano, A.M.; Patriquin, C.J.; et al. Eculizumab in pregnant patients with paroxysmal nocturnal hemoglobinuria. *N. Engl. J. Med.* **2015**, *373*, 1032–1039. [CrossRef] [PubMed]

104. McNamara, L.A.; Topaz, N.; Wang, X.; Hariri, S.; Fox, L.; MacNeil, J.R. High risk for invasive meningococcal disease among patients receiving eculizumab (soliris) despite receipt of meningococcal vaccine. *Am. J. Transplant. Off. J. Am. Soc. Transplant. Am. Soc. Transpl. Surg.* **2017**, *17*, 2481–2484. [CrossRef]

105. Traboulsee, A.; Greenberg, B.; Bennett, J.L.; Szczechowiski, L.; Fox, E.; Shkrobot, S.; Yamamura, T.; Terada, Y.; Kawata, Y.; Melia, A.; et al. A double-blind placebo-controlled study of satralizumab (sa 237), a recycling anti-il-6 receptor monoclonal antibody, as monotherapy for patients witn neuromyelitis optica spectrum disorder (nmosd). In Proceedings of the ECTRIMS, Berlin, Germany, 10–12 Octorber 2018. Poster 1278.

106. Steinman, L.; Bar-Or, A.; Behne, J.M.; Benitez-Ribas, D.; Chin, P.S.; Clare-Salzler, M.; Healey, D.; Kim, J.I.; Kranz, D.M.; Lutterotti, A.; et al. Restoring immune tolerance in neuromyelitis optica: Part i. *Neurol. Neuroimmunol. Neuroinflamm.* **2016**, *3*, e276. [CrossRef] [PubMed]

107. Brunner, C.; Lassmann, H.; Waehneldt, T.V.; Matthieu, J.M.; Linington, C. Differential ultrastructural localization of myelin basic protein, myelin/oligodendroglial glycoprotein, and 2′,3′-cyclic nucleotide 3′-phosphodiesterase in the cns of adult rats. *J. Neurochem.* **1989**, *52*, 296–304. [CrossRef]

108. Pham-Dinh, D.; Mattei, M.G.; Nussbaum, J.L.; Roussel, G.; Pontarotti, P.; Roeckel, N.; Mather, I.H.; Artzt, K.; Lindahl, K.F.; Dautigny, A. Myelin/oligodendrocyte glycoprotein is a member of a subset of the immunoglobulin superfamily encoded within the major histocompatibility complex. *Proc. Natl. Acad. Sci. USA* **1993**, *90*, 7990–7994. [CrossRef] [PubMed]

109. Gardinier, M.V.; Amiguet, P.; Linington, C.; Matthieu, J.M. Myelin/oligodendrocyte glycoprotein is a unique member of the immunoglobulin superfamily. *J. Neurosci. Res.* **1992**, *33*, 177–187. [CrossRef] [PubMed]

110. Berger, T.; Rubner, P.; Schautzer, F.; Egg, R.; Ulmer, H.; Mayringer, I.; Dilitz, E.; Deisenhammer, F.; Reindl, M. Antimyelin antibodies as a predictor of clinically definite multiple sclerosis after a first demyelinating event. *N. Engl. J. Med.* **2003**, *349*, 139–145. [CrossRef] [PubMed]

111. Reindl, M.; Linington, C.; Brehm, U.; Egg, R.; Dilitz, E.; Deisenhammer, F.; Poewe, W.; Berger, T. Antibodies against the myelin oligodendrocyte glycoprotein and the myelin basic protein in multiple sclerosis and other neurological diseases: A comparative study. *Brain J. Neurol.* **1999**, *122 Pt 11*, 2047–2056. [CrossRef]

112. Karni, A.; Bakimer-Kleiner, R.; Abramsky, O.; Ben-Nun, A. Elevated levels of antibody to myelin oligodendrocyte glycoprotein is not specific for patients with multiple sclerosis. *Arch. Neurol.* **1999**, *56*, 311–315. [CrossRef]

113. Markovic, M.; Trajkovic, V.; Drulovic, J.; Mesaros, S.; Stojsavljevic, N.; Dujmovic, I.; Mostarica Stojkovic, M. Antibodies against myelin oligodendrocyte glycoprotein in the cerebrospinal fluid of multiple sclerosis patients. *J. Neurol. Sci.* **2003**, *211*, 67–73. [CrossRef]

114. Gaertner, S.; de Graaf, K.L.; Greve, B.; Weissert, R. Antibodies against glycosylated native mog are elevated in patients with multiple sclerosis. *Neurology* **2004**, *63*, 2381–2383. [CrossRef] [PubMed]

115. Lindert, R.B.; Haase, C.G.; Brehm, U.; Linington, C.; Wekerle, H.; Hohlfeld, R. Multiple sclerosis: B- and t-cell responses to the extracellular domain of the myelin oligodendrocyte glycoprotein. *Brain J. Neurol.* **1999**, *122 Pt 11*, 2089–2100. [CrossRef]

116. Egg, R.; Reindl, M.; Deisenhammer, F.; Linington, C.; Berger, T. Anti-mog and anti-mbp antibody subclasses in multiple sclerosis. *Mult. Scler.* **2001**, *7*, 285–289. [CrossRef] [PubMed]

117. Kuhle, J.; Lindberg, R.L.; Regeniter, A.; Mehling, M.; Hoffmann, F.; Reindl, M.; Berger, T.; Radue, E.W.; Leppert, D.; Kappos, L. Antimyelin antibodies in clinically isolated syndromes correlate with inflammation in mri and csf. *J. Neurol.* **2007**, *254*, 160–168. [CrossRef] [PubMed]

118. Brilot, F.; Dale, R.C.; Selter, R.C.; Grummel, V.; Kalluri, S.R.; Aslam, M.; Busch, V.; Zhou, D.; Cepok, S.; Hemmer, B. Antibodies to native myelin oligodendrocyte glycoprotein in children with inflammatory demyelinating central nervous system disease. *Ann. Neurol.* **2009**, *66*, 833–842. [CrossRef] [PubMed]

119. Kitley, J.; Waters, P.; Woodhall, M.; Leite, M.I.; Murchison, A.; George, J.; Kuker, W.; Chandratre, S.; Vincent, A.; Palace, J. Neuromyelitis optica spectrum disorders with aquaporin-4 and myelin-oligodendrocyte glycoprotein antibodies: A comparative study. *JAMA Neurol.* **2014**, *71*, 276–283. [CrossRef] [PubMed]

120. Ramanathan, S.; Reddel, S.W.; Henderson, A.; Parratt, J.D.; Barnett, M.; Gatt, P.N.; Merheb, V.; Kumaran, R.Y.; Pathmanandavel, K.; Sinmaz, N.; et al. Antibodies to myelin oligodendrocyte glycoprotein in bilateral and recurrent optic neuritis. *Neurol. Neuroimmunol. Neuroinflamm.* **2014**, *1*, e40. [CrossRef]

121. Hoftberger, R.; Sepulveda, M.; Armangue, T.; Blanco, Y.; Rostasy, K.; Calvo, A.C.; Olascoaga, J.; Ramio-Torrenta, L.; Reindl, M.; Benito-Leon, J.; et al. Antibodies to mog and aqp4 in adults with neuromyelitis optica and suspected limited forms of the disease. *Mult. Scler.* **2015**, *21*, 866–874. [CrossRef]

122. Jarius, S.; Kleiter, I.; Ruprecht, K.; Asgari, N.; Pitarokoili, K.; Borisow, N.; Hummert, M.W.; Trebst, C.; Pache, F.; Winkelmann, A.; et al. Mog-igg in nmo and related disorders: A multicenter study of 50 patients. Part 3: Brainstem involvement—Frequency, presentation and outcome. *J. Neuroinflamm.* **2016**, *13*, 281. [CrossRef]

123. Spadaro, M.; Gerdes, L.A.; Krumbholz, M.; Ertl-Wagner, B.; Thaler, F.S.; Schuh, E.; Metz, I.; Blaschek, A.; Dick, A.; Bruck, W.; et al. Autoantibodies to mog in a distinct subgroup of adult multiple sclerosis. *Neurol. Neuroimmunol. Neuroinflamm.* **2016**, *3*, e257. [CrossRef] [PubMed]

124. Ramanathan, S.; Mohammad, S.; Tantsis, E.; Nguyen, T.K.; Merheb, V.; Fung, V.S.C.; White, O.B.; Broadley, S.; Lechner-Scott, J.; Vucic, S.; et al. Clinical course, therapeutic responses and outcomes in relapsing mog antibody-associated demyelination. *J. Neurol. Neurosurg. Psychiatry* **2018**, *89*, 127–137. [CrossRef] [PubMed]

125. Reindl, M.; Di Pauli, F.; Rostasy, K.; Berger, T. The spectrum of mog autoantibody-associated demyelinating diseases. *Nat. Rev. Neurol.* **2013**, *9*, 455–461. [CrossRef] [PubMed]

126. Kerlero de Rosbo, N.; Honegger, P.; Lassmann, H.; Matthieu, J.M. Demyelination induced in aggregating brain cell cultures by a monoclonal antibody against myelin/oligodendrocyte glycoprotein. *J. Neurochem.* **1990**, *55*, 583–587. [CrossRef] [PubMed]

127. Piddlesden, S.J.; Lassmann, H.; Zimprich, F.; Morgan, B.P.; Linington, C. The demyelinating potential of antibodies to myelin oligodendrocyte glycoprotein is related to their ability to fix complement. *Am. J. Pathol.* **1993**, *143*, 555–564. [CrossRef]

128. Bettelli, E.; Baeten, D.; Jager, A.; Sobel, R.A.; Kuchroo, V.K. Myelin oligodendrocyte glycoprotein-specific t and b cells cooperate to induce a devic-like disease in mice. *J. Clin. Investig.* **2006**, *116*, 2393–2402. [CrossRef] [PubMed]

129. Krishnamoorthy, G.; Lassmann, H.; Wekerle, H.; Holz, A. Spontaneous opticospinal encephalomyelitis in a double-transgenic mouse model of autoimmune t cell/b cell cooperation. *J. Clin. Investig.* **2006**, *116*, 2385–2392. [CrossRef]

130. Saadoun, S.; Waters, P.; Owens, G.P.; Bennett, J.L.; Vincent, A.; Papadopoulos, M.C. Neuromyelitis optica mog-igg causes reversible lesions in mouse brain. *Acta Neuropathol. Commun.* **2014**, *2*, 35. [CrossRef]

131. Sato, D.K.; Callegaro, D.; Lana-Peixoto, M.A.; Waters, P.J.; de Haidar Jorge, F.M.; Takahashi, T.; Nakashima, I.; Apostolos-Pereira, S.L.; Talim, N.; Simm, R.F.; et al. Distinction between mog antibody-positive and aqp4 antibody-positive nmo spectrum disorders. *Neurology* **2014**, *82*, 474–481. [CrossRef]

132. Jarius, S.; Ruprecht, K.; Kleiter, I.; Borisow, N.; Asgari, N.; Pitarokoili, K.; Pache, F.; Stich, O.; Beume, L.A.; Hummert, M.W.; et al. Mog-igg in nmo and related disorders: A multicenter study of 50 patients. Part 2: Epidemiology, clinical presentation, radiological and laboratory features, treatment responses, and long-term outcome. *J. Neuroinflamm.* **2016**, *13*, 280. [CrossRef]

133. Jarius, S.; Paul, F.; Aktas, O.; Asgari, N.; Dale, R.C.; de Seze, J.; Franciotta, D.; Fujihara, K.; Jacob, A.; Kim, H.J.; et al. Mog encephalomyelitis: International recommendations on diagnosis and antibody testing. *J. Neuroinflamm.* **2018**, *15*, 134. [CrossRef] [PubMed]

134. Chalmoukou, K.; Alexopoulos, H.; Akrivou, S.; Stathopoulos, P.; Reindl, M.; Dalakas, M.C. Anti-mog antibodies are frequently associated with steroid-sensitive recurrent optic neuritis. *Neurol. Neuroimmunol. Neuroinflamm.* **2015**, *2*, e131. [CrossRef] [PubMed]

7

Kappa Free Light Chains and IgG Combined in a Novel Algorithm for the Detection of Multiple Sclerosis

Monika Gudowska-Sawczuk [1,*], **Joanna Tarasiuk** [2], **Alina Kułakowska** [2], **Jan Kochanowicz** [2] and **Barbara Mroczko** [1,3]

[1] Department of Biochemical Diagnostics, Medical University of Bialystok, Waszyngtona 15A St., 15-269 Bialystok, Poland; mroczko@umb.edu.pl

[2] Department of Neurology, Medical University of Bialystok, M. Skłodowskiej—Curie 24A St., 15-276 Bialystok, Poland; amirtarasiuk@wp.pl (J.T.); alakul@umb.edu.pl (A.K.); kochanowicz@vp.pl (J.K.)

[3] Department of Neurodegeneration Diagnostics, Medical University of Bialystok, Waszyngtona 15A St., 15-269 Bialystok, Poland

* Correspondence: monika.gudowska-sawczuk@umb.edu.pl;

Abstract: Background: It is well known that the cerebrospinal fluid (CSF) concentrations of free light chains (FLC) and immunoglobulin G (IgG) are elevated in multiple sclerosis patients (MS). Therefore, in this study we aimed to develop a model based on the concentrations of free light chains and IgG to predict multiple sclerosis. We tried to evaluate the diagnostic usefulness of the novel κIgG index and λIgG index, here presented for the first time, and compare them with the κFLC index and the λFLC index in multiple sclerosis patients. Methods: CSF and serum samples were obtained from 76 subjects who underwent lumbar puncture for diagnostic purposes and, as a result, were divided into two groups: patients with multiple sclerosis ($n = 34$) and patients with other neurological disorders (control group; $n = 42$). The samples were analyzed using turbidimetry and isoelectric focusing. The κIgG index, λIgG index, κFLC index, and λFLC index were calculated using specific formulas. Results: The concentrations of CSF κFLC, CSF λFLC, and serum κFLC and the values of κFLC index, λFLC index, and κIgG index were significantly higher in patients with multiple sclerosis compared to controls. CSF κFLC concentration and the values of κFLC index, λFLC index, and κIgG index differed in patients depending on their pattern type of oligoclonal bands. κFLC concentration was significantly higher in patients with pattern type 2 and type 3 in comparison to those with pattern type 1 and type 4. The κFLC index, λFLC index, and κIgG index were significantly higher in patients with pattern type 2 in comparison to those with pattern type 4. The κFLC index and κIgG index were significantly higher in patients with pattern type 2 in comparison to those with pattern type 1, and in patients with pattern type 3 compared to those with pattern type 4. The κIgG index was markedly elevated in patients with pattern type 3 compared to those with pattern type 1. In the total study group, κFLC, λFLC, κFLC index, λFLC index, κIgG index, and λIgG index correlated with each other. The κIgG index showed the highest diagnostic power (area under the curve, AUC) in the detection of multiple sclerosis. The κFLC index and κIgG index showed the highest diagnostic sensitivity, and the κIgG index presented the highest ability to exclude multiple sclerosis. Conclusion: This study provides novel information about the diagnostic significance of four markers combined in the κIgG index. More investigations in larger study groups are needed to confirm that the κIgG index can reflect the intrathecal synthesis of immunoglobulins and may improve the diagnosis of multiple sclerosis.

Keywords: multiple sclerosis; diagnostic markers; immunoglobulins; kappa; free light chains

1. Introduction

Multiple sclerosis (MS) is a common neuroinflammatory and neurodegenerative disorder of the central nervous system (CNS) [1]. The etiology of multiple sclerosis is still unknown. However, the major pathology is mediated by an auto-reactive immune process of multifocal myelin destruction throughout the CNS. Prompt and accurate diagnosis is particularly important for the clinical management of patients, since disease-modifying therapies are the most effective at the early stage of the disease [2,3]. A perfect biomarker should allow the early diagnosis of a disease, aid in determining the prognosis of a disease, and be rapid and easily testable. Currently, there is no specific test for the diagnosis of multiple sclerosis. According to the 2017 revisions of the McDonald diagnostic criteria for MS, the diagnosis of this disease is based on clinical symptoms, imaging by MRI technology, and laboratory testing including cerebrospinal fluid (CSF) examination [4].

The main feature of multiple sclerosis consists of abnormalities of the cellular and humoral immune system. Combined actions of B cells and T cells play a role in the full development of demyelination and in the secretion of immunoglobulins. Therefore, in more than 90% of patients, an elevated level of immunoglobulins synthesized in the intrathecal space can be observed, and IgG oligoclonal bands (OCBs) are detected in the CSF. However, there is a proportion of subjects, i.e., patients presenting with their first episode of multiple sclerosis, whose results of oligoclonal bands are negative. On the other hand, increased intrathecal immunoglobulin synthesis may occur also in other inflammatory CNS disorders, and therefore, this test is not specific for MS [5–8].

It is well known that human immunoglobulins are composed of two heavy and two light chains. There are two types of light chains, kappa (κ) and lambda (λ), that are produced by B lymphocytes during the synthesis of immunoglobulins. Physiologically, an excess of light chains is normally produced. These light chains that are not combined with heavy chains are called free light chains (FLC). It has been proven that B cell abnormalities are associated with disorders leading to an abnormal concentration of free light chains [9,10]. Therefore, in this study we aimed to develop a model based on free light chains and other available laboratory data to predict multiple sclerosis. We tried to evaluate the diagnostics usefulness of the novel κIgG index and λIgG index and compare them to the already known κFLC index and λFLC index used for the assessment of patients with MS.

2. Material and Methods

2.1. Subjects

This study was approved by the Bioethical Committee of the Medical University of Bialystok. Informed consent was obtained from all individuals included in the study. The patients were admitted to the Department of Neurology at the Medical University of Bialystok and underwent lumbar puncture for diagnostic purposes. Paired CSF and serum samples from the patients were collected between 2018 and 2020. The tested group consisted of 76 patients with neurological disorders who were divided into 2 subgroups: relapsing–remitting MS patients ($n = 34$) and a control group ($n = 42$) (Figure 1). All MS patients included in the study were in the process of receiving an MS diagnosis. They had a history of one clinical attack, and there was no evidence of dissemination in time according to magnetic resonance imaging (MRI). Finally, after CSF analysis which revealed OCBs presence, they were diagnosed with relapsing–remitting multiple sclerosis according to MacDonald criteria 2017 [4]. The degree of neurological impairment in patients diagnosed with multiple sclerosis from whom CSF was obtained was evaluated using the expanded disability status scale [11]. All evaluations rated between 1 and 2 points, indicating an early stage of the disease. All MS patients were not treated with any disease-modifying drugs or glucocorticosteroids at the time of lumbar puncture. The control group (29 females and 13 males; age range: 18–78 years) included patients eventually diagnosed with multifocal vascular lesions of the CNS ($n = 18$), discopathy ($n = 6$), idiopathic cephalgia ($n = 9$), dementia ($n = 3$), idiopathic (Bell's) facial nerve palsy ($n = 3$), epilepsy ($n = 1$), herpetic encephalitis ($n = 1$), hydrocephalus ($n = 1$). Out of 34 patients with multiple sclerosis, 31 had OCBs in the CSF but not in serum (pattern type 2), and 3 had OCBs in CSF and serum, with additional OCBs in the CSF (pattern type 3). Out of 42 patients in the control group, 21 had no bands in CSF and serum (pattern type 1), 4 had pattern type 3, 16 had identical OCBs in CSF and serum (pattern type 4), and 1 had monoclonal bands in CSF and serum (pattern type 5).

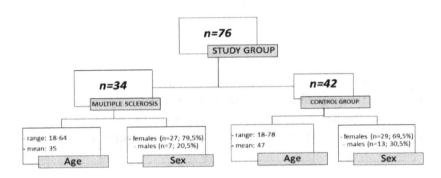

Figure 1. Characteristics of the study group.

2.2. Sample Collection

CSF specimens were collected from each patient by lumbar puncture. The samples were collected into polypropylene tubes, centrifuged, aliquoted, and frozen at −80 °C until assayed. Venous blood samples were collected and centrifuged to separate the serum. The serum samples were aliquoted and frozen at −80 °C until assayed.

IgG oligoclonal bands determination in human CSF and serum was performed at the time of diagnosis using isoelectric focusing on agarose gel. Each patient's serum and CSF samples were analyzed in parallel, in order to compare the IgG distribution. According to the manufacturer's instructions, the assay includes two steps. Firstly, we performed isoelectrofocusing on agarose gel to fractionate the proteins in the CSF and serum med. Secondly, we carried out immunofixation with peroxidase-labelled anti-IgG antiserum to detect IgG oligoclonal bands and demonstrate the distribution of IgG in both fluids (Hydragel 3 CSF Isofocusing; Hydrasys; Sebia). The concentrations of κFLC, λFLC, albumin, IgG, IgM, and IgA in CSF and serum were measured according to the turbidimetric method (Optilite; The Binding Site). The κIgG index, λIgG index, κFLC index, and λFLC index were calculated according to the following formulas: $\dfrac{\text{CSF } \kappa\text{FLC} \left(\frac{mg}{L}\right)/\text{serum } \kappa\text{FLC}\left(\frac{mg}{L}\right)}{\text{CSF IgG} \left(\frac{mg}{L}\right)/\text{serum IgG}\left(\frac{g}{L}\right)} \times 100$, $\dfrac{\text{CSF } \lambda\text{FLC} \left(\frac{mg}{L}\right)/\text{serum } \lambda\text{FLC}\left(\frac{mg}{L}\right)}{\text{CSF IgG} \left(\frac{mg}{L}\right)/\text{serum IgG}\left(\frac{g}{L}\right)} \times 100$, $\dfrac{\text{CSF } \kappa\text{FLC}\left(\frac{mg}{L}\right)/\text{serum } \kappa\text{FLC}\left(\frac{mg}{L}\right)}{\text{CSF albumin}\left(\frac{mg}{L}\right)/\text{serum albumin}\left(\frac{mg}{L}\right)}$ and $\dfrac{\text{CSF } \lambda\text{FLC}\left(\frac{mg}{L}\right)/\text{serum } \lambda\text{FLC}\left(\frac{mg}{L}\right)}{\text{CSF albumin}\left(\frac{mg}{L}\right)/\text{serum albumin}\left(\frac{mg}{L}\right)}$, respectively. In cases of FLCs concentrations below the lower limit of detection, we used the corresponding detection limit (CSF κFLC, 0.30 mg/L, CSF λFLC, 0.65 mg/L). Intrathecal synthesis was also evaluated using albumin, IgG, IgA, and IgM quotients (Q_{Alb}, Q_{IgG}, Q_{IgA}, Q_{IgM}, respectively).

2.3. Statistical Analysis

Data were stored and analyzed in Statistica 13.3. Differences between the multiple sclerosis and the control group were evaluated by Mann–Whitney U test. To test the hypothesis about the differences between subgroups, ANOVA rank Kruskal–Wallis test was performed. The post-hoc test was applied to determine which groups were different. We considered p-values < 0.05 as statistically significant. The diagnostic performance of each test was calculated as sensitivity, specificity, positive predictive value (PPV), negative predictive value (NPV), and accuracy (ACC). We used the area under the receiver operating characteristic (AUC ROC) curve to determine the optimal cut-off value and to calculate the diagnostic performance of the tests.

3. Results

The results of routine laboratory tests for patients with MS and the control group are presented in Table 1. Statistically significant differences between MS and controls in the Mann–Whitney U test were observed for the concentration of serum albumin and serum and CSF IgM and the values of Q_{IgM} and Q_{IgG} ($p = 0.010$; $p = 0.047$; $p = 0.003$; $p = 0.002$; $p = 0.002$, respectively).

3.1. CSF and Serum Concentrations of κFLC and λFLC

We determined the concentrations of κFLC and λFLC in the CSF and serum. κFLC and λFLC concentrations in the CSF and serum κFLC concentration were markedly elevated in MS patients (3.050 mg/L, 2.050 mg/L, 13.480 mg/L, respectively) compared to controls (0.310 mg/L, $p < 0.001$; 0.720 mg/L, $p = 0.017$; 16.265 mg/L, $p = 0.019$, respectively), while the concentration of serum λFLC did not differ between MS patients (11.715 mg/L) and controls (13.220 mg/L. $p = 0.066$). Furthermore, the concentrations of κFLC in the CSF differed depending on the types of OCB patterns (ANOVA rang Kruskal–Wallis test: $p < 0.001$, H = 36.472). Post-hoc analysis revealed that the CSF concentrations of κFLC were significantly lower in patients with pattern type 1 (0.300 mg/L) and type 4 (0.936 mg/L) of OCBs in comparison with those with pattern type 2 (2.905 mg/L; $p < 0.001$, $p = 0.002$, respectively) and type 3 (4.400 mg/L; $p = 0.002$, $p = 0.030$, respectively). There were no significant differences in CSF κFLC concentrations between patients with OCB pattern type 2 and type 3 ($p = 1.000$). The concentrations of serum κFLC and λFLC as well as CSF λFLC were similar in all patients irrespective of their OCB pattern type.

3.2. Values of κFLC Index, λFLC Index, κIgG Index, and λIgG Index

The values of κFLC index, λFLC index, κIgG index, and λIgG index are presented in Table 2. The values of κFLC index, λFLC index, and κIgG index were significantly higher in patients with multiple sclerosis compared to controls, but there were no differences in the λIgG index between the tested groups (Figure 2). The values of κFLC index, λFLC index, and κIgG index differed depending on the OCB pattern type ($p < 0.001$, H = 25.593; $p = 0.010$, H = 11.355; $p < 0.001$, H = 29.608). Post-hoc analysis revealed that the values of the κFLC index and κIgG index were significantly higher in patients with pattern type 2 (median: 58.551, 5.063) in comparison with those with pattern type 1 (5.933, 0.987; $p < 0.001$ for both) and type 4 (4.166, 0.636; $p < 0.001$ for both). The λFLC index was significantly elevated in patients with pattern type 2 (35.065) in comparison with those with pattern type 4 (7.208, $p = 0.013$). There were also differences in the κFLC index and κIgG index values between patients with pattern type 3 (56.172; 4.503) and those with pattern type 4 ($p = 0.034$; $p = 0.029$, respectively). In addition, the κIgG index was markedly elevated in patients with pattern type 3 compared with those with pattern type 1 ($p = 0.033$). There were no significant differences in the λIgG index between patients with different OCB types ($p = 0.106$, H = 6.123).

Table 1. Results of laboratory tests for patients with multiple sclerosis and the control group.

					Variable Tested Median (Min–Max Values)							
	Albumin S [g/L]	Albumin CSF [mg/L]	Q_{Alb}	IgG S [g/L]	IgG CSF [mg/L]	Q_{IgG}	IgM S [g/L]	IgM CSF [mg/L]	Q_{IgM}	IgA S [g/L]	IgA CSF [mg/L]	Q_{IgA}
Multiple Sclerosis (n = 34)	43.90 * (33.70–57.40)	187.95 (20.60–487.70)	4.80 (2.77–16.31)	10.72 (6.35–1320.00)	43.19 (3.37–20.47)	5.06 * (2.41–18.60)	1.57 * (0.57–360.00)	1.53 * (0.31–9.43)	1.05 (0.3–4.41)	2.18 (0.81–263.00)	3.47 (0.92–24.20)	1.67 (0.72–15.28)
Control group (n = 42)	40.00 (17.8–53.90)	196.45 (16.5–815.00)	5.95 (2.15–20.99)	10.00 (4.95–1150.00)	26.65 (2.14–151.72)	3.12 (1.07–19.50)	1.19 (0.35–249.00)	0.58 (0.11–103.00)	0.52 (0.12–8.95)	2.28 (0.02–434.00)	3.84 (0.88–37.20)	1.59 (0.45–15.44)
p-value	0.010 *	0.368	0.123	0.541	0.071	0.002 *	0.047 *	0.004 *	0.002 *	0.965	0.952	0.673

S, serum; CSF, cerebrospinal fluid; *, significant differences in comparison to the controls.

Table 2. Values of κFLC index, λFLC index, κIgG index, and λIgG index in multiple sclerosis patients and control group and their diagnostic significance.

	Median	Min	Max	Cut-off from the ROC	Sensitivity [%]	Specificity [%]	PPV [%]	NPV [%]	ACC	AUC
				κFLC-index						
MS (n = 34)	59.338 *	4.466	623.565	9.417	93.50	68.30	79.20	69.00	79.20	**0.866**
C (n = 42)	6.196	0.912	91.081							
				λFLC-index						
MS (n = 34)	35.070 *	6.336	792.533	21.446	71.90	64.30	60.50	75.00	67.60	**0.693**
C (n = 42)	14.450	1.015	157.741							
				κIgG-index						
MS (n = 34)	5.660 *	0.751	16.400	1.929	90.30	80.50	77.80	91.70	84.70	**0.871**
C (n = 42)	0.956	0.216	9.581							
				λIgG-index						
MS (n = 34)	3.571	0.330	10.374	3.161	65.6	71.4	63.6	73.2	68.9	**0.632**
C (n = 42)	1.974	0.241	35.665							

MS, multiple sclerosis; C, control group; FLC, free light chains; ROC, receiver operating characteristic; PPV, positive predictive value; NPV, negative predictive value; ACC, accuracy; AUC, area under the ROC; *, significant differences in comparison to the control group.

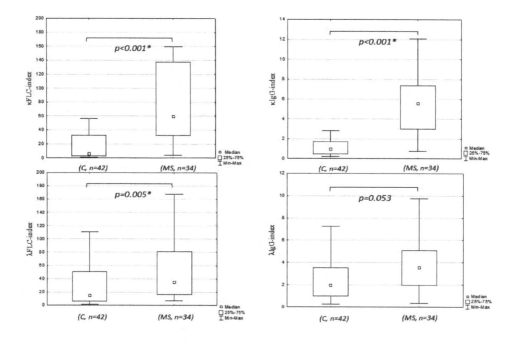

Figure 2. κFLC index, λFLC index, κIgG index, and λIgG index in the study groups. C, control group; MS, multiple sclerosis; *, significant differences in comparison to the controls.

3.3. Correlations of CSF κFLC, CSF λFLC, κFLC Index, λFLC Index, κIgG Index, and λIgG Index with Other Parameters Reflecting Pathological Processes in the CNS

The correlations between CSF κFLC, CSF λFLC, κFLC index, λFLC index, κIgG index, and λIgG index with other parameters reflecting pathological processed in the CNS are presented in Table 3. Sprearman's rank correlation test demonstrated that in the total study group, κFLC, λFLC, κFLC-index, λFLC index, κIgG index, and λIgG index correlated with each other. The CSF concentrations of κFLC and the values of the λIgG index were significantly associated with Q_{IgG}. CSF κFLC, CSF λFLC, and κFLC index correlated with Q_{IgM} values, while Q_{IgA} was associated with the values of κIgG index and λIgG index. Furthermore, we observed a negative correlation of Q_{Alb} and patients' age with κFLC index, λFLC index, κIgG index, and λIgG index.

Table 3. Spearman's correlations between tested variables in the total study group.

Total Study Group (n = 76)	Age	Q_Alb	Q_IgG	Q_IgM	Q_IgA	CSF κ	CSF λ	κFLC–Index	λFLC–Index	κIgG–Index	λIgG–Index
Q_Alb											
r	0.403		0.648	0.268	0.778	−0.120	0.049	−0.253	−0.244	−0.472	−0.433
p	<0.005 *		<0.005 *	0.030 *	<0.005 *	0.316	0.678	0.032 *	0.036 *	<0.005 *	<0.005 *
Q_IgG											
r	0.01	0.648		0.553	0.678	0.405	0.208	−0.197	−0.028	0.034	−0.296
p	0.936	<0.005 *		<0.005 *	<0.005 *	<0.005 *	0.076	0.097	0.81	0.776	0.010 *
Q_IgM											
r	−0.121	−0.268	0.553		0.547	0.425	0.302	0.333	0.164	0.231	0.015
p	0.331	0.030 *	<0.005 *		<0.005 *	0.005 *	0.013 *	0.007 *	0.185	0.064	0.907
Q_IgA											
r	0.253	0.778	0.678	0.547		0.01	0.078	−0.034	−0.101	−0.273	−0.335
p	0.031 *	<0.005 *	<0.005 *	<0.005 *		0.936	0.512	0.779	0.397	0.021 *	0.004 *
CSF κ											
r	−0.309	−0.120	0.405	0.424	0.01		0.661	0.802	0.515	0.843	0.372
p	0.007	0.316	<0.005 *	<0.005 *	0.936		<0.005 *	<0.005 *	<0.005 *	<0.005 *	0.001 *
CSF λ											
r	−0.138	0.049	0.208	0.302	0.078	−0.126		0.536	0.72	0.557	0.686
p	0.236	0.678	0.08	0.013	0.512	<0.005 *		<0.005 *	<0.005 *	<0.005 *	<0.005 *
κFLC index											
r	−0.459	−0.253	0.207	0.333	−0.034	0.802	0.536		0.784	0.866	0.495
p	<0.005 *	0.032	0.081	0.007 *	0.779	<0.005 *	<0.005 *		<0.005 *	<0.005 *	<0.005 *
λFLC index											
r	−0.369	−0.244	−0.030	0.164	−0.101	0.371	0.72	0.784		0.659	0.809
p	<0.005 *	0.040 *	0.81	0.185	0.397	<0.005 *	<0.005 *	<0.005 *		<0.005 *	<0.005 *
κIgG index											
r	−0.472	−0.472	0.034	0.231	−0.273	0.843	0.557	0.867	0.659		0.647
p	<0.005 *	<0.005 *	0.776	0.064	0.020 *	<0.005 *	<0.005 *	<0.005 *	<0.005 *		<0.005 *
λIgG index											
r	−0.388	0.432	−0.296	0.015	−0.335	0.372	0.686	0.495	0.809	0.647	
p	<0.005 *	<0.005 *	−0.010 *	0.907	<0.005 *	0.001 *	<0.005 *	<0.005 *	<0.005 *	<0.005 *	

* Statistically significant ($p < 0.05$).

3.4. Diagnostic Power of κFLC Index, λFLC Index, κIgG Index, and λIgG Index

The diagnostic usefulness of κFLC index, λFLC index, κIgG index, and λIgG index in multiple sclerosis is presented in Table 2. The κFLC index and κIgG index showed a very high ability to detect MS (sensitivity > 90.00% for both) in comparison to the λFLC index (sensitivity, 71.90%) and the λIgG index (sensitivity, 65.60%). The κIgG index showed the highest ability to exclude multiple sclerosis, with 80.50% specificity and 91.70% negative predictive value. The κIgG index presented the highest diagnostic power (AUC) in the detection of multiple sclerosis in comparison to the λIgG index, κFLC index, and λFLC index (Figure 3).

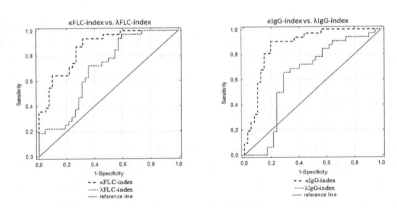

Figure 3. ROC curves for κFLC index, λFLC index, κIgG index, and λIgG index in multiple sclerosis.

4. Discussion

Multiple sclerosis is an inflammatory neurodegenerative disease characterized by intrathecal IgG synthesis. The detection by isoelectric focusing methods of oligoclonal IgG bands in parallel cerebrospinal fluid and serum samples is actually the gold standard for multiple sclerosis diagnosis [3,12]. However, there are some limitations of OCBs detection, such as still indefinite number of bands in the CSF without corresponding bands in serum defining positive results [13]. OCBs determination is not specific for multiple sclerosis, because the elevated intrathecal synthesis of IgG may occur in other CNS disorders [14]. In addition, OCBs are found in the CSF of about 90% of patients with multiple sclerosis, which means that there is always a group of MS patients without CSF bands [15]. Also, another problem is that isoelectric focusing methods are laborious and often difficult [16]. Taking all this into account, we believe that there is a need to find an additional indicator that can be used to diagnose multiple sclerosis. Therefore, in this study, we tried to define a novel diagnostic model using routinely available laboratory test results to predict multiple sclerosis in patients with symptoms of neurological disorders.

Firstly, we showed that the mean concentrations of κFLC and λFLC in the CSF and of serum κFLC are markedly elevated in patients with multiple sclerosis. Clearly, these changes in free light chains concentrations may originate from increased synthesis of immunoglobulins, a phenomenon firstly observed in the 1970s–1980s [17,18], or from the fact that light chains are synthesized at a speed more than twice higher compared to fully formed A, M, and G immunoglobulins [19]. Our results are totally consistent with the results obtained by other researchers [20–25]. Additionally, our study revealed that the CSF concentrations of κFLC were significantly increased in patients with OCB pattern types 2 and 3, which confirmed intrathecal immunoglobulins synthesis. This may suggest that the concentrations of FLCs in the CSF are highly sensitive and specific for the diagnosis of multiple sclerosis. Our findings of increased free light chains are consistent with those of other studies and support the inclusion of free light chains in our algorithm.

Many studies on the prediction of multiple sclerosis have been published in the past few years. Some studies have proposed a model based on κFLCs and albumin concentrations [16,17,22,23]. Presslauer et al. were the first scientists who developed a formula for the κFLC index and tried to evaluate its diagnostic significance. An index using a cut-off value ≥ 5.9 showed higher sensitivity for the diagnosis of multiple sclerosis than OCBs (96% vs. 80%, respectively) [16]. In our study, using the cut-off proposed by Presslauer et al., the κFLC index showed identical sensitivity with that previously reported, but the specificity for our patients' group was lower (46.3% vs. 86.0%). Therefore, for further analysis, we decided to use the best cut-off form the ROC. When we used a κFLC index value ≥ 9.4, we achieved a similar sensitivity, but the specificity was still lower than in Presslauer et al. study and equaled 68%. On the other hand, this index value was lower than the cut-off published by Menendez-Valladares et al., which was >10.62 and associated with higher specificity [21]. Despite the differences in the cut-off values and specificity, authors unanimously say that the κFLC index has high sensitivity and probably would avoid OCBs determination in most of patients with suspected multiple sclerosis.

It is well known that the CSF concentrations of FLCs and IgG are increased in patients with multiple sclerosis. The concentrations of free light chains and IgG have been used for the diagnosis of multiple sclerosis but never combined in a single algorithm. Our study was conducted to develop a new simple model for MS diagnosis using routine laboratory tests to predict this disease in a group of patients with neurological disorders. In our study, these variables were used together for the first time to create the novel κIgG index and λIgG index. We compared the already investigated κFLC index and λFLC index with panels named κIgG-index and λIgG-index combined of FLCs and IgG concentrations. The findings of our study confirmed significant differences in the values of κIgG index and λIgG index between multiple sclerosis patients and individuals with other neurological disorders. We denoted about a 9,5-fold difference of median κIgG index and a 2,4-fold difference of median λIgG index in multiple sclerosis patients in comparison to controls. Moreover, it is important to recognize that our model was developed considering different types of OCBs. Differentiation according to OCBs was chosen because clinically, patients with OCB pattern type 2 are almost always classified as multiple sclerosis patients. We observed that the κIgG index was significantly higher in patients with pattern type 2 in comparison with those with pattern type 1 and type 4. Additionally, only the values of the κIgG index were markedly higher in patients with pattern type 3 than in those with pattern type 4 and type 1, which does not exclude multiple sclerosis. In general, the κIgG index showed higher diagnostic significance compared with the λIgG index. The main factor causing this is probably the dominance of κ free light chains in humans (the normal total κFLC/λFLC ratio is approximately 2:1) [26]. These results indicate that the algorithm combining κFLC with IgG is more valid to evaluate the intrathecal synthesis of immunoglobulins in patients with neurological system disorders than other known algorithms.

5. Conclusions

In conclusion, we showed that a novel, simple κIgG index consisting of four variables combined together (serum κFLC, CSF κFLC, serum IgG, and CSF IgG) can predict the intrathecal synthesis of immunoglobulins and may serve as an additional, potential diagnostic marker for the diagnosis of multiple sclerosis, with a high degree of diagnostic sensitivity and accuracy. The main strength of our study is the use of readily available routine laboratory diagnostics tests. In addition, we examined a group of well-characterized patients including 45% multiple sclerosis patients and 55% controls. The control group in this study was highly heterogeneous; however, the purpose of this study was to determine the value of the κIgG index in the differentiation of multiple sclerosis from other neurological disorders. It is very important to differentiate multiple sclerosis from other neurological diseases, because they often require different treatments. While this study provides novel information about the diagnostic significance of four combined markers in the κIgG-index, in the context of practicality, further studies are required to determine the appropriateness of using the κIgG index as a diagnostic tool for multiple sclerosis in a clinical setting. Studies on larger samples should be performed to validate the quality and precision of the κIgG index. To our knowledge, there are no other studies combining FLCs with IgG concentrations, but we cautiously suggest that, in the future, this parameter could be determined as a complementary diagnostic element to oligoclonal bands determination.

Author Contributions: M.G.-S. and B.M. produced the idea of the study. M.G.-S. and B.M. contributed to research design and measurement of the tested proteins. J.T., A.K., and J.K. were involved in sample collection. All authors analyzed the data. M.G.-S. and B.M. coordinated project funding. All authors have read and agreed to the published version of the manuscript.

Acknowledgments: M.G.-S. has received consultation honorarium from Roche. B.M. has received consultation and/or lecture honoraria from Abbott, Wiener, Roche, Cormay, and Biameditek.

References

1.   Amato, M.P.; Prestipino, E.; Bellinvia, A.; Niccolai, C.; Razzolini, L.; Pastò, L.; Fratangelo, R.; Tudisco, L.; Fonderico, M.; Goretti, B.; et al. Cognitive impairment in multiple sclerosis: An exploratory analysis of environmental and lifestyle risk factors. *PLoS ONE* **2019**, *14*, e0222929. [CrossRef] [PubMed]

2.   Lutton, J.D.; Winston, R.; Rodman, T.C. Multiple sclerosis: Etiological mechanisms and future directions. *Exp. Biol. Med.* **2004**, *229*, 12–20. [CrossRef] [PubMed]

3.   Wootla, B.; Eriguchi, M.; Rodriguez, M. Is multiple sclerosis an autoimmune disease? *Autoimmune Dis.* **2012**, *2012*, 969657. [CrossRef] [PubMed]

4.   Thompson, A.J.; Banwell, B.L.; Barkhof, F. Diagnosis of multiple sclerosis: 2017 revisions of the McDonald criteria. *Lancet Neurol.* **2018**, *17*, 162–173. [CrossRef]

5.   Link, H.; Huang, Y.M. Oligoclonal bands in multiple sclerosis cerebrospinal fluid: An update on methodology and clinical usefulness. *J. Neuroimmunol.* **2006**, *180*, 17–28. [CrossRef]

6.   Giles, P.D.; Wroe, S.J. Cerebrospinal fluid oligoclonal IgM in multiple sclerosis: Analytical problems and clinical limitations. *Ann. Clin. Biochem.* **1990**, *27*, 199–207. [CrossRef]

7.   Puthenparampil, M.; Altinier, S.; Stropparo, E.; Zywicki, S.; Poggiali, D.; Cazzola, C.; Toffanin, E.; Ruggero, S.; Gallo, P.; Plebani, M.; et al. Intrathecal K free light chain synthesis in multiple sclerosis at clinical onset associates with local IgG production and improves the diagnostic value of cerebrospinal fluid examination. *Mult. Scler. Relat. Disord.* **2018**, *25*, 241–245. [CrossRef]

8.   McLaughlin, K.A.; Wucherpfennig, K.W. B cells and autoantibodies in the pathogenesis of multiple sclerosis and related inflammatory demyelinating diseases. *Adv. Immunol.* **2008**, *98*, 121–149. [CrossRef]

9.   Wang, X.; Xu, K.; Chen, S.; Li, Y.; Li, M. Role of Interleukin-37 in Inflammatory and Autoimmune Diseases. *Iran J. Immunol.* **2018**, *15*, 165–174. [CrossRef]

10. Janeway, C. Chapter 3. Antigen Recognition by B-cell and T-cell Receptors. In *Immunobiology: The Immune System in Health and Disease*; Garland Science: New York, NY, USA, 2001.

11. Kurtzke, J.F. Rating neurologic impairment in multiple sclerosis: An expanded disability status scale (EDSS). *Neurology* **1983**, *33*, 1444–1452. [CrossRef]

12. Trbojevic-Cepe, M. Detection of Oligoclonal Ig Bands: Clinical Significance and Trends in Methodological Improvement. *EJIFCC* **2004**, *15*, 86–94. [PubMed]

13. Hegen, H.; Zinganell, A.; Auer, M.; Deisenhammer, F. The clinical significance of single or double bands in cerebrospinal fluid isoelectric focusing. A retrospective study and systematic review. *PLoS ONE* **2019**, *14*, e0215410. [CrossRef] [PubMed]

14. Deisenhammer, F.; Zetterberg, H.; Fitzner, B.; Zettl, U.K. The Cerebrospinal Fluid in Multiple Sclerosis. *Front. Immunol.* **2019**, *10*, 726. [CrossRef] [PubMed]

15. Imrell, K.; Landtblom, A.M.; Hillert, J.; Masterman, T. Multiple sclerosis with and without CSF bands: Clinically indistinguishable but immunogenetically distinct. *Neurology* **2006**, *67*, 1062–1064. [CrossRef] [PubMed]

16. Cornell, F.N. Isoelectric focusing, blotting and probing methods for detection and identification of monoclonal proteins. *Clin. Biochem. Rev.* **2009**, *30*, 123–130.

17. Bracco, F.; Gallo, P.; Menna, R.; Battistin, L.; Tavolato, B. Free light chains in the CSF in multiple sclerosis. *J. Neurol.* **1987**, *234*, 303–307. [CrossRef]

18. Vandvik, B. Oligoclonal IgG and free light chains in the cerebrospinal fluid of patients with multiple sclerosis and infectious diseases of the central nervous system. *Scand. J. Immunol.* **1977**, *6*, 913–922. [CrossRef]

19. Zemana, D.; Hradilek, P.; Kusnierova, P. Oligoclonal free light chains in cerebrospinal fluid as markers of intrathecal inflammation. Comparison with oligoclonal IgG. *Biomed. Pap. Med. Fac. Univ. Palacky Olomouc Czech Repub.* **2015**, *15*, 104–113. [CrossRef]

20. Presslauer, S.; Milosavljevic, D.; Brücke, T.; Bayer, P.; Hübl, W. Elevated levels of kappa free light chains in CSF support the diagnosis of multiple sclerosis. *J. Neurol.* **2008**, *255*, 1508–1514. [CrossRef]

21. Menéndez-Valladares, P.; García-Sánchez, M.I.; Cuadri Benítez, P.; Lucas, M.; Adorna Martínez, M.; Carranco Galán, V.; García De Veas Silva, J.L.; Bermudo Guitarte, C.; Izquierdo Ayuso, G. Free kappa light chains in cerebrospinal fluid as a biomarker to assess risk conversion to multiple sclerosis. *Mult. Scler. J. Exp. Transl. Clin.* **2015**, *1*. [CrossRef]

22. Duranti, F.; Pieri, M.; Centonze, D.; Buttari, F.; Bernardini, S.; Dessi, M. Determination of kappa FLC and kappa index in cerebrospinal fluid: A valid alternative to assess intrathecal immunoglobulin synthesis. *J. Neuroimmunol.* **2013**, *263*, 116–120. [CrossRef] [PubMed]

23. Presslauer, S.; Milosavljevic, D.; Huebl, W.; Parigger, S.; Schneider-Koch, G.; Bruecke, T. Kappa free light chains: Diagnostic and prognostic relevance in MS and CIS. *PLoS ONE* **2014**, *9*, e89945. [CrossRef] [PubMed]

24. Voortman, M.M.; Stojakovic, T.; Pirpamer, L.; Jehna, M.; Langkammer, C.; Scharnagl, H.; Reindl, M.; Ropele, S.; Enzinger, C.; Fuchs, S.; et al. Prognostic value of free light chains lambda and kappa in early multiple sclerosis. *Mult. Scler.* **2017**, *23*, 1496–1505. [CrossRef] [PubMed]

25. Sáez, M.S.; Rojas, J.I.; Lorenzón, M.V.; Sánchez, F.; Patrucco, L.; Míguez, J.; Azcona, C.; Sorroche, P.; Cristiano, E. Validation of CSF free light chain in diagnosis and prognosis of multiple sclerosis and clinically isolated syndrome: Prospective cohort study in Buenos Aires. *J. Neurol.* **2019**, *266*, 112–118. [CrossRef]

26. Katzmann, J.A.; Clark, R.J.; Abraham, R.S.; Bryant, S.; Lymp, J.F.; Bradwell, A.R.; Kyle, R.A. Serum reference intervals and diagnostic ranges for free kappa and free lambda immunoglobulin light chains: Relative sensitivity for detection of monoclonal light chains. *Clin. Chem.* **2002**, *48*, 1437–1444. [CrossRef]

8

Multiple Sclerosis in a Multi-Ethnic Population in Houston, Texas: A Retrospective Analysis

Vicki Mercado [1,2,3], Deepa Dongarwar [3], Kristen Fisher [4], Hamisu M. Salihu [5], George J. Hutton [6] and Fernando X. Cuascut [3,6,*]

[1] Immunology and Microbiology Graduate Program, Baylor College of Medicine, Houston, TX 77030, USA; Vicki.Mercado@bcm.edu

[2] Medical Scientist Training Program, Baylor College of Medicine, Houston, TX 77030, USA

[3] Center of Excellence in Health Equity, Training and Research Program, Baylor College of Medicine, Houston, TX 77030, USA; deepa.dongarwar@bcm.edu

[4] Texas Children Hospital, Blue Bird Circle Clinic for Multiple Sclerosis, Houston, TX 77030, USA; Kristen.Fisher@bcm.edu

[5] Department of Family & Community Medicine, Baylor College of Medicine, Houston, TX 77030, USA; hamisu.salihu@bcm.edu

[6] Baylor College of Medicine, Maxine Mesinger Multiple Sclerosis Center, Houston, TX 77030, USA; ghutton@bcm.edu

* Correspondence: Fernando.Cuascut@bcm.edu

Abstract: Multiple Sclerosis (MS) is a progressive neurodegenerative disease that affects more than 2 million people worldwide. Increasing knowledge about MS in different populations has advanced our understanding of disease epidemiology and variation in the natural history of MS among White and minority populations. In addition to differences in incidence, African American (AA) and Hispanic patients have greater disease burden and disability in earlier stages of disease compared to White patients. To further characterize MS in AA and Hispanic populations, we conducted a retrospective chart analysis of 112 patients treated at an MS center in Houston, Texas. Here, we describe similarities and differences in clinical presentation, MRI findings, treatment regimens, disability progression, and relapse rate. While we found several similarities between the groups regarding mean age, disability severity, and degree of brain atrophy at diagnosis, we also describe a few divergences. Interestingly, we found that patients who were evaluated by a neurologist at symptom onset had significantly decreased odds of greater disability [defined as Expanded Disability Status Scale (EDSS) > 4.5] at last presentation compared to patients who were not evaluated by a neurologist (OR: 0.04, 95% CI: 0.16–0.9). We also found that active smokers had significantly increased odds of greater disability both at diagnosis and at last clinical encounter compared to nonsmokers (OR: 2.44, 95% CI: 1.10–7.10, OR= 2.44, 95% CI: 1.35–6.12, $p = 0.01$, respectively). Additionally, we observed significant differences in treatment adherence between groups. Assessment of the degree of brain atrophy and progression over time, along with an enumeration of T1, T2, and gadolinium-enhancing brain lesions, did not reveal differences across groups.

Keywords: multiple sclerosis; MS; disparities; minority populations

1. Introduction

Multiple Sclerosis (MS) is an autoimmune inflammatory demyelinating condition that affects more than 2 million people worldwide [1,2]. A recent study estimates that in 2017, nearly 1 million adults had MS in the United States [1]. MS leads to an accumulation of disability over time, although disease-modifying therapies (DMT) may lessen long-term disability severity in most patients [3]. MS is considered a heterogeneous disease thought to result from a complex interaction among genetic predisposition, sex, and environment [4]. Increasing evidence suggests that racial disparities are important factors that may explain differences in the disease course, prevalence, incidence, and outcomes [5–8]. Despite comprising 13.4% and 18.3% of the American population, African-Americans (AA) and Hispanics, respectively, remain largely underrepresented and understudied in clinical trials [9–11]. Fortunately, an accumulating body of work characterizes MS in diverse populations. This development could improve our understanding of disease course and epidemiology and uncover disparities across various racial/ethnic groups. Better understanding disparities in MS clinical course and outcomes will allow for the development of more effective disease management in patients of diverse backgrounds.

Historically, it had been widely accepted that MS incidence was higher in the White population compared to the AA population [12]. However, population-based cohort studies have challenged this paradigm. A 2013 retrospective cohort study found that AA had a 47% increased risk of MS compared to Whites [13]. Disparities in MS clinical course in minority populations also encompass disability progression, disease burden, symptom presentation, and relapse rates. AA and Hispanics with MS have a higher disease burden and more severe disability in earlier stages of disease than White patients [10,14–16]. Additionally, AA patients commonly have multi-symptomatic presentation and early motor system involvement [14,17]. AA also experience inadequate recovery from symptoms and have shorter intervals between clinical attacks [7,8]. Furthermore, amongst MS individuals admitted to US nursing homes, AA patients are younger and more disabled than White patients [18]. Studies comparing MRI findings between AA and White patients revealed that the former show an increased degree of T2 hyperintense lesions and T1 hypointense lesions, which correlate with greater MS-related disability [19].

Clinical data for MS in the Hispanic population is comparatively limited. The few studies on Hispanics suggest a more rapid disability accumulation over time compared to White patients [20–22]. Interestingly, Hispanics were found to have a 50% decreased risk of developing MS compared to Whites [13]. However, several studies concur that Hispanics may have an earlier age of disease onset compared with other patient cohorts [13,20]. Hispanics and AA with MS are less likely than their White counterparts to visit a neurologist or MS specialist for disease management and have decreased rates of DMT usage due to noncompliance or inappropriate understanding of the treatment plan [23,24]. DMTs are critical for effective management and reduction of long-term disability in MS patients. In assessing these data, it is essential to consider that the Hispanic population is multiethnic and diverse. Other compounding factors that should be considered include socioeconomic status, place of birth, age of migration to the US, health literacy, systemic biases and systematic racism in healthcare, and access to care [5,20,25].

Much of our understanding of MS manifestation and clinical course in minority populations have come from a limited set of studies. Clinical trials on DMTs mostly lack data for minorities despite mounting evidence that these groups are at higher risk for a more aggressive disease course [26]. Approximately only 1% of the MS literature focuses on minority populations [10]. The purpose of this study was to address this lack of information by describing the clinical presentation, MRI findings, treatment regimens, disability progression, and relapse patterns in a racially and ethnically diverse population of MS patients in Houston, Texas. Given that the data for this study were collected from a clinic that predominantly serves patients of low socioeconomic status (SES), this study captures ethnic and racial disparities in MS among patients with a similar SES, potentially decreasing the possible effects of confounding factors. This study is critical and timely because it adds to an emerging literature that explores disparity in MS disease progression in AA and Hispanic MS patients compared to their White counterparts.

2. Patients and Methods

2.1. Study Design and Setting

Subjects were identified by a retrospective chart review of patients treated at the Smith Clinic Multiple Sclerosis Center. Smith clinic is a unique center that is part of a network that specifically cares for underserved and low socio-economic groups in Harris County, which includes the city of Houston. Additionally, Harris County is the third most populous county in the US. The majority of the patient population seen in the clinic are Non-Hispanic Black (NH-Black) or of Hispanic descent, and Mexicans constitute the majority of the Hispanic population served at the clinic. There is also a small percentage of Non-Hispanic White (NH-White) patients seen in the clinic. For the purposes of this study we are using the terms NH-Black and NH-White to account for the racial diversity of Hispanics seen in our clinic. Patients are attended to irrespective of insurance status or ability to pay.

2.2. Cohort Identification and Selection

Information from all patients who visited Smith clinic from March 2019 to March 2020 was identified through chart review and included in this retrospective study. All patients with a diagnosis of Relapsing Remitting MS (RRMS), Secondary Progressive MS (SPMS), or Primary Progressive MS (PPMS) were included.

2.3. Outcome Measurements

The following pre-selected information was abstracted for each patient: year and age of first symptoms, age at diagnosis, the amount of time that elapsed between onset of symptoms and diagnosis, disease subtype, estimated Expanded Disability Status Scale (EDSS) at diagnosis and last encounter, Disease Modifying Therapy (DMT) history (adverse reactions, relapses, and changes in immunomodulatory therapy), radiological findings, number of clinical relapses, smoking status, and autoimmune comorbidities. Escalation therapies included Glatiramer Acetate, Interferons, Teriflunomide, Dimethyl Fumarate and Fingolimod. High efficacy therapies included Rituximab, Ocrelizumab, Alemtuzumab and Natalizumab. Symptoms at disease onset were recorded and included motor, sensory, cerebellar, brainstem, bowel, and bladder function among others.

2.4. Data Collection and Management

Two neurologists extracted patient data from medical records and the study protocol was approved by an Institutional Review Board. Information from the most recent clinical encounter and from the clinical encounter at diagnosis was included. The EDSS at presentation was estimated based on the first documented neurologic examination by a neurologist and was not indicative of the maximal neurologic deficit during the demyelinating episode that led to the diagnosis. Severe disability was defined as an estimated EDSS score > 4.5. MRI interpretations were collected from radiology reports. Lesion quantification and atrophy scoring were extracted directly from radiology reports and raw images were not independently interpreted by the neurologists gathering the data. A relapse was defined as a new, documented, neurological complaint lasting more than 24 h with objective findings in the documented neurological exam, or a follow-up MRI showing new enhancing lesions.

2.5. Statistical Analysis

The statistical analyses were performed using R (version 3·6·1, Vienna, Austria) and RStudio (Version 1·2·5001, Boston, MA, USA). Based on the race and ethnicity information of the patients, we created a composite variable called 'race/ethnicity' and categorized the responses as Non-Hispanic (NH) White, NH-Black, Hispanic and 'others'. We conducted descriptive statistics on patient socio-demographic and disease characteristics stratified by race/ethnicity. We conducted Fisher's exact tests (for categorical variables) and ANOVA (for continuous variables). We examined the usage and impact of DMTs across racial/ethnic groups. We also examined various markers of disease progression including lesions and atrophy in the brain as well as the thoracic and cervical spine stratified by race/ethnicity using Fisher's exact test. Applying adjusted Exact logistic regression models, we evaluated the association between various patient characteristics and a high EDSS score (EDSS > 4.5). Models were adjusted for different covariates based on the literature and context, along with experts' recommendations. All analyses were based on two-tailed probabilities with a type 1 error rate set at 5%.

3. Results

Data from a total of 114 patients were analyzed in this study. Two patients were excluded due to a substantial amount of missing information. Of the included 112 patients, most were diagnosed with Relapsing Remitting MS (RRMS). About 73% of NH-White, 92% of NH-Black, and 95% of Hispanic patients had RRMS, whereas only 18% of NH-White, 5% of NH-Black, and 2.5% of Hispanic patients were diagnosed with Primary Progressive MS (PPMS) (Table 1). One Hispanic patient had a diagnosis of SPMS. There were no significant differences among the groups with regard to MS type at diagnosis ($p = 0.1859$), or smoking status ($p = 0.3079$). All groups had a similar female to male ratio, with a greater proportion of female MS patients (Table 1, $p = 0.3675$). Average age at diagnosis ($p = 0.9918$) and mean time to diagnosis ($p = 0.9934$) were also similar across all groups (Table 1). Interestingly, between the groups, we found significant differences in the percentage of patients who were adherent or experienced relapse while on escalation or high efficacy therapies. Specifically, 63.2% of NH-White, 73% of NH-Black, and 61.8% of Hispanic patients were adherent to escalation therapy (Table 1, $p = 0.0252$). 100% of NH-White, 84.2% of NH-Black, and 50% of Hispanic patients were adherent to high efficacy therapy (Table 1, $p = 0.0252$). 26.3% of NH-White, 31.1% of NH-Black, and 36.4% of Hispanic patients relapsed while on escalation therapy (Table 1, $p = 0.000151$). 0% of NH-White, 10.5% of NH-Black, and 0% of Hispanic patients relapsed while on high efficacy therapy (Table 1, $p = 0.00015$). Of note, one of the reasons for relapse includes non-adherence; thus interpretation of relapse data must consider the adherence percentages presented.

Notably, only 28% of the NH-Black population had received an evaluation by a neurologist at symptom onset, whereas 53% of Hispanic and 45% of NH-White patients had, although this was not statistically significant (Table 1, $p = 0.1778$). In this cohort, there were no statistically significant differences in receipt of a medical evaluation at symptom onset; 63–70% of patients from all groups were able to access medical evaluation. Additionally, NH-White, NH-Black and Hispanic patients exhibited no differences in symptoms at diagnosis or mean EDSS score at diagnosis and last encounter (Table 2). There was a significant difference in the percentage of patients with severe disability (EDSS score > 4.5) at diagnosis and at last encounter; 14.3% of NH-White MS patients had severe disability at diagnosis compared to 50% of NH-Black and 31.6% of Hispanic patients (Table 2, $p < 0.001$). This was also true at last encounter with 32.5% of NH-White, 45.5% of NH-Black and 41% of Hispanic MS patients with severe disability at their most recent clinical visit (Table 2, $p < 0.001$).

Assessment of degree of brain atrophy and progression over time revealed that NH-White, NH-Black and Hispanic patients in this cohort had a similar degree of brain atrophy at diagnosis and over time (Figure 1). Enumeration of T1, T2, and gadolinium-enhancing brain lesions at diagnosis also showed no significant differences between the groups (data not shown). Spinal atrophy and quantity of T2 and gadolinium-enhancing lesions in the spine at diagnosis and at last presentation were also similar between groups (Figure 2).

Table 1. Diagnosis Characteristics of patients with MS stratified by race/ethnicity.

Characteristics	NH-White (n = 11)	NH-Black (n = 61)	Hispanic (n = 40)	p Value
Multiple Sclerosis (MS) type at diagnosis				p = 0.1859
Relapsing remitting MS	82%	95%	95%	
Primary progressive MS	18%	5%	2.5%	
Secondary progressive MS	0%	0%	2.5%	
Mean Age at diagnosis (years)	39.9 (11.3)	36.7 (11.4)	32.4 (11.5)	p = 0.9918
Female/Male ratio	1.70/1	2.33/1	1.22/1	p = 0.3765
Active smokers	55%	44%	30%	p = 0.3079
Mean time from symptom onset to diagnosis (months)	30.8 (38.9)	32.9 (32.1)	13.7 (15.4)	p = 0.9934
Medical Evaluation at symptom onset	64%	63%	70%	p = 0.8597
Neurological Evaluation at symptom onset	45%	28%	53%	p = 0.1778
Adherence (Adherence/Ever used)				p = 0.0252
Escalation therapy	63.2%	73%	61.8%	
High efficacy therapy	100%	84.2%	50%	
Relapse (Relapse/Ever used)				p = 0.00015
Escalation therapy	26.3%	31.1%	36.4%	
High efficacy therapy	0%	10.5%	0%	

EDSS score at diagnosis and EDSS score at last clinical visit were compared within each group. Standard deviation is shown in parentheses. $p = 0.4253$ (NH-Black), $p = 0.1757$ (Hispanic), $p = 0.0324$ (NH-White), (paired sample t-test). For adherence and relapse data, chi-squared test and Fisher's-exact test were used respectively. Escalation therapies included Glatiramer Acetate, Interferons, Teriflunomide, Dimethyl Fumarate and Fingolimod. High efficacy therapies included Rituximab, Ocrelizumab, Alemtuzumab and Natalizumab.

Table 2. Clinical characteristics of MS patients by race/ethnicity.

Clinical Characteristics	NH-White (n = 11)	NH-Black (n = 61)	Hispanic (n = 40)	p Value
EDSS scores				
Mean EDSS score at diagnosis (SD)	2.6 (2.1)	2.2 (1.1)	3.8 (1.9)	p = 0.9328
Mean EDSS score at last presentation (SD)	2.9 (2.8)	4.2 (2.9)	3.8 (2.3)	p = 0.9950
Severe disability at diagnosis (EDSS > 4.5)	14.3%	50%	31.6%	p = < 0.001
Severe disability at last presentation (EDSS > 4.5)	32.5%	45.5%	41%	p = < 0.001
Symptoms at Presentation				p = 0.1473
Motor	72.7%	57.4%	47.5%	
Brainstem	27.3%	24.9%	25%	
Cerebellar	27.3%	37.7%	37.5%	
Gait	27.3%	26.2%	15%	
Sensory	72.7%	37.7%	52.5%	
Visual	9.1%	27.9%	30%	
Cognitive	9.1%	9.8%	5%	
Other or unknown	36.4%	18.1%	15%	

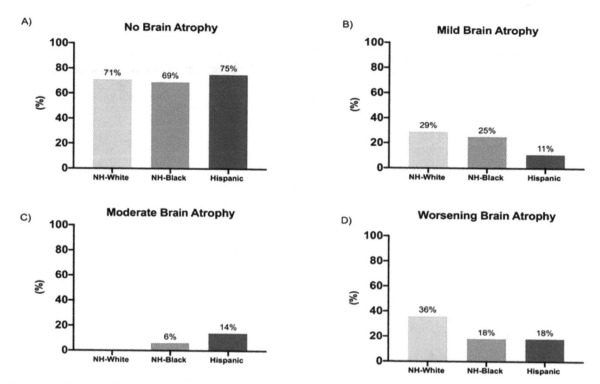

Figure 1. Degree of brain atrophy at diagnosis and worsening of brain atrophy from diagnosis to most recent MRI scan. Presented as the total percentage of each group, is the proportion of patients who had none (**A**), mild (**B**), or moderate (**C**) brain atrophy at the time of diagnosis, as well as the proportion of patients who had increased brain atrophy in their most recent MRI scan compared to diagnosis (**D**). Only patients who had MRI scans on file were included in this analysis. $p = 0.5155$ for comparison between degree of brain atrophy (none, mild, moderate) (Fisher's exact). $p = 0.3387$ for comparison of total percentage of patients who had worsening brain atrophy on most recent MRI compared to diagnosis (Fisher's exact).

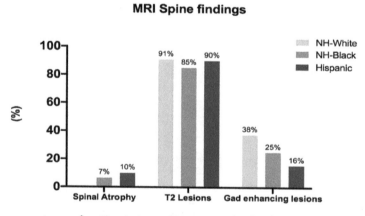

Figure 2. The total percentage of patients in each group who had spinal atrophy, T2, or gadolinium-enhancing lesions in the spine as determined by MRI findings at diagnosis. Only patients who had MRI scans on file were included in this analysis. $p = 0.6974$, $p = 0.5128$, $p = 0.2957$ for comparison of total percentage of patients in each group that had spinal atrophy, spinal T2 lesions, and spinal gadolinium-enhancing lesions respectively (Fisher's exact).

Patient usage of escalation or high efficacy therapies did not significantly impact the patient's likelihood of having an EDSS score > 4.5 at last clinical encounter after adjustment for adherence, smoking, race, age, prior exposure to escalation therapies, and EDSS at diagnosis (Table 3). Active smokers were 2.44 times as likely to have an EDSS score > 4.5 at their last clinical encounter compared to non-smokers after adjustment for age and race (OR: 2.44, 95% CI: 1.36–6.12, $p = 0.01$) (Table 3).

Interestingly, after adjustment for race and age, patients who were evaluated by a neurologist at diagnosis had significantly lower adjusted odds of an EDSS score > 4.5 at last presentation compared to patients who were not evaluated by a neurologist (OR: 0.40, 95% CI: 0.16–0.90, $p = 0.04$) (Table 3).

Table 3. Association between various patient characteristics and high EDSS score (>4.5) at last presentation.

High EDSS Score at Last Presentation		
	OR	p-Value
Usage of escalation therapies [a]		
No	reference	
Yes	1.60 (0.45–6.14)	0.48
Usage of high efficacy therapies [b]		
No	reference	
Yes	2.64 (0.87–8.33)	0.09
Smoker [c]		
No	reference	
Yes	2.44 (1.36–6.12)	0.01
Medical evaluation by Neurologist [c]		
No	reference	
Yes	0.40 (0.16–0.90)	0.04
Adherence to DMT [c]		
Yes	reference	
No	0.73 (0.31–1.62)	0.43
Time to diagnosis [c]		
<=12 months	reference	
>12 months	1.73 (0.75–4.01)	0.2

[a] adjusted for adherence, smoking, race and age and EDSS at diagnosis; [b] adjusted for prior exposure to escalation therapies, adherence, smoking, race, age and EDSS at diagnosis; [c] adjusted for age and race.

Active smokers were 2.79 times as likely to have an EDSS score > 4.5 at diagnosis compared to non-smokers after adjustment for age and race (OR: 2.79, 95% CI: 1.10–7.10, $p = 0.01$) (Table 4). There was no significant association between time to diagnosis and having a high EDSS score at diagnosis (Table 4). There were no significant differences in total relapse occurrence for patients on escalation therapy vs. high efficacy therapy for each racial/ethnic group (data not shown). Of 24 NH-white patients, 19 had ever used escalation therapy, and 5 had used high efficacy therapy. Of 93 NH-Black patients, 74 had used escalation therapy, and 19 had used high efficacy therapy. For the Hispanic patients group of 63 patients, 55 had ever used escalation therapy while 18 had documented high efficacy therapy use. We found no differences between the groups concerning the usage of escalation vs. high efficacy therapies.

Table 4. Association between various patient characteristics and high EDSS score at diagnosis (>4.5).

High EDSS Score at Diagnosis		
	OR	p-Value
Smoker [c]		
No	reference	
Yes	2.79 (1.10–7.10)	0.01
Time to diagnosis [c]		
<=12 months	reference	
>12 months	1.15 (0.46–2.83)	0.77

[c] adjusted for age and race.

4. Discussion

The goal of this retrospective cohort study was to describe MS patient characteristics in a multi-ethnic population in Houston and compare findings between racial/ethnic groups. Our study demonstrates several racial/ethnic similarities and a few differences in multiple sclerosis presentation and disease course. We found that the groups had a similar mean age at diagnosis, mean EDSS score at diagnosis and last presentation, and a similar degree of brain and spinal atrophy at diagnosis as well. MRI spinal findings were also comparable between NH-White, Black and Hispanic groups. The average time from symptom onset to diagnosis, and overall symptom presentation, were also similar between the groups. The clinic that these patients were treated at is a hub for the underserved and low socioeconomic communities. Thus, we suspect that many of the patients in this cohort were of a similar socioeconomic background, which undoubtedly can influence disease manifestation and outcomes. It is plausible that these similar environmental factors, along with the small sample size may explain the many similarities detected between the groups. However, further studies are required to evaluate this hypothesis.

Interestingly, after adjustment for race and age, patients who were evaluated by a neurologist at diagnosis had 60% lower odds (OR = 0.40, 95% CI: 0.16–0.90) of an EDSS score > 4.5 at last presentation compared to patients who were evaluated by a non-neurology specialist. This suggests a logical protective effect of treatment by a neurologist at symptom onset and highlights the importance of access to treatment for all patients. Indeed, a national descriptive study found that people with MS who saw a neurologist were more likely to receive appropriate DMT treatment and see rehabilitation and urologist specialists compared to people who saw other providers [27]. A 2017 study on racial disparities in neurologic health care access revealed that Black patients were 30% less likely to see an outpatient neurologist and were more likely to be cared for in the emergency department compared to their White counterparts [23]. Similarly, Hispanic patients were 40% less likely to see an outpatient neurologist compared to NH-Whites [23].

We found that actively smoking patients were 2.44 times as likely (95% CI: 1.36–6.12) to have severe disability at diagnosis and at the last clinic follow up. A recent systematic review and meta-analysis found evidence supporting the causal involvement of smoking in the development and progression of MS [28]. Altogether, these data suggest that smoking prevention and cessation education programs and early intervention by a neurologist should be implemented to achieve optimal MS care in diverse patient populations.

Consistent with published reports, a greater proportion of NH-Black patients had early severe disability (defined in our study as an estimated EDSS score > 4.5) when compared to NH-White and Hispanic patients [29,30]. In our present study, treatment modality did not impact the risk of having an estimated EDSS score > 4.5 at the last visit. Nonetheless, we observed a trend towards a higher relapse rate in escalation therapies vs. high efficacy therapies, especially in NH-Blacks. We also observed significant differences in adherence between the groups. Interestingly, a greater percentage of NH-Black patients relapsed while on high efficacy therapy compared to Hispanic patients, despite having greater adherence. Other studies have found that NH-Black patients treated with interferons experienced more relapses and new MS lesions on T2-weighted brain magnetic imaging than NH-Whites [31]. However, further studies on the interaction between race/ethnicity and DMT response for MS are necessary.

Several studies have shown that African Americans have significantly higher CNS lesion burden, more frequent relapses, worse ambulatory disability, worse post-relapse recoveries, and higher overall disability at diagnosis [5,10,19,29]. Overall, our findings did not confirm these prior observations and we believe that the similar socioeconomic background of this patient cohort, along with the small sample size, may have contributed to this. Nevertheless, it is evident that further studies are needed to investigate the various environmental and social factors contributing to divergent MS clinical course outcomes between diverse populations.

Limitations of this study include its retrospective nature, the variable periods of follow-up and the selection of therapy by the treating physician (nonrandomized). The study was also constrained by a small sample size, which could have induced a type 2 error leading to the inability to reject the null hypothesis in some of our comparisons. Additionally, our interpretation of the relapse data is limited because one of the possible reasons for relapse is non-adherence. Thus, relapse data are not corrected for the degree of non-adherence and should be assessed accordingly. Lastly, it is important to note that we did not analyze the imaging data ourselves. Instead, we collected information from MRI reports. Often, the number of lesions was documented as a range, thereby limiting data precision. Moreover, the atrophy measurements were subjective rather than objective quantification, and some patients were missing MRI information at diagnosis (e.g., performed at a different institution). These limitations may have impacted the capability to show radiological differences at presentation between groups.

Our study is important because it adds to emerging literature describing disease characteristics in minority populations with MS. The disparities in MS progression, onset, and disease course warrants further study. Of 60,000 published articles on MS, only 113 focused on NH-Black and only 23 focused on Hispanic American patients with MS as of 2014 [10]. This demonstrates a need for studies that are intentionally inclusive of these populations. Since 2014, there has been a modest but steady increase in studies focused on these populations. There is a clear disparity in MS treatment access for patients from different racial and ethnic backgrounds. Drivers of disparity are often comprised of complex interactions among factors such as socioeconomic status, access to healthcare and wellness resources (clinics, hospitals, grocery stores, fitness centers), systemic racism and biases in healthcare, and limited health literacy. This systemic web of disparity can be challenging to disentangle, but understanding it is necessary for improving the care of minority patients with MS.

Future prospective randomized controlled trials in different racial/ethnic groups with MS are essential to better understand the disease progression, management and treatment outcomes for diverse patient populations.

Author Contributions: Conceptualization, F.X.C. and G.J.H.; methodology D.D.; software, D.D.; validation, F.X.C. and V.M.; formal analysis, D.D.; writing—original draft preparation, V.M., D.D., K.F. and F.X.C.; writing—review and editing, H.M.S and G.J.H.; supervision, H.M.S. All authors have read and agreed to the published version of the manuscript.

References

1. Wallin, M.T.; Culpepper, W.J.; Campbell, J.D.; Nelson, L.M.; Langer-Gould, A.; Marrie, R.A.; Cutter, G.R.; Kaye, W.E.; Wagner, L.; Tremlett, H.; et al. The prevalence of MS in the United States: A population-based estimate using health claims data. *Neurology* **2019**, *92*, 1029–1040. [CrossRef] [PubMed]

2. Wallin, M.T.; Culpepper, W.J.; Nichols, E.; Bhutta, Z.A.; Gebrehiwot, T.T.; Hay, S.I.; Khalil, I.A.; Krohn, K.J.; Liang, X.; Naghavi, M.; et al. Global, regional, and national burden of multiple sclerosis 1990–2016: A systematic analysis for the Global Burden of Disease Study 2016. *Lancet Neurol.* **2019**, *18*, 269–285. [CrossRef]

3. Freedman, M.S. Present and emerging therapies for multiple sclerosis. *Contin. Lifelong Learn. Neurol.* **2013**, *19*, 968–991. [CrossRef] [PubMed]

4. Muñoz-Culla, M.; Irizar, H.; Otaegui, D. The genetics of multiple sclerosis: Review of current and emerging candidates. *Appl. Clin. Genet.* **2013**, *6*, 63–73. [CrossRef]

5. Amezcua, L.; McCauley, J.L. Race and ethnicity on MS presentation and disease course. *Mult. Scler. J.* **2020**, *26*, 561–567. [CrossRef]

6. Wallin, M.T.; Culpepper, W.J.; Coffman, P.; Pulaski, S.; Maloni, H.; Mahan, C.M.; Haselkorn, J.K.; Kurtzke, J.F.; Veterans Affairs Multiple Sclerosis Centres of Excellence Epidemiology Group. The Gulf War era multiple sclerosis cohort: Age and incidence rates by race, sex and service. *Brain* **2012**, *135*, 1778–1785. [CrossRef]

7. Amezcua, L.; Rivas, E.; Joseph, S.; Zhang, J.; Liu, L. Multiple Sclerosis Mortality by Race/Ethnicity, Age, Sex, and Time Period in the United States, 1999–2015. *Neuroepidemiology* **2018**, *50*, 35–40. [CrossRef]

8. Rivas-Rodríguez, E.; Amezcua, L. Ethnic Considerations and Multiple Sclerosis Disease Variability in the United States. *Neurol. Clin.* **2018**, *36*, 151–162. [CrossRef]

9. U.S. Census Bureau QuickFacts: United States. Available online: https://www.census.gov/quickfacts/fact/table/US/PST045219#qf-headnote-a (accessed on 4 September 2020).

10. Khan, O.; Williams, M.J.; Amezcua, L.; Javed, A.; Larsen, K.E.; Smrtka, J.M. Multiple Sclerosis in US Minority Populations Clinical Practice Insights. *Neurol Clin Pr.* **2015**, *5*, 132–142. [CrossRef]

11. Diaz, V. Encouraging participation of minorities in research studies. *Ann. Fam. Med.* **2012**, *10*, 372–373. [CrossRef]

12. Rosati, G. The prevalence of multiple sclerosis in the world: An update. *Neurol. Sci.* **2001**, *22*, 117–139. [CrossRef] [PubMed]

13. Langer-Gould, A.; Brara, S.M.; Beaber, B.E.; Zhang, J.L. Incidence of multiple sclerosis in multiple racial and ethnic groups. *Neurology* **2013**, *80*, 1734–1739. [CrossRef] [PubMed]

14. Kister, I.; Chamot, E.; Bacon, J.H.; Niewczyk, P.M.; De Guzman, R.A.; Apatoff, B.; Coyle, P.; Goodman, A.D.; Gottesman, M.; Granger, C.; et al. Rapid disease course in African Americans with multiple sclerosis. *Neurology* **2010**, *75*, 217–223. [CrossRef] [PubMed]

15. Marrie, R.A.; Cutter, G.; Tyry, T.; Vollmer, T.; Campagnolo, D. Does multiple sclerosis-associated disability differ between races? *Neurology* **2006**, *66*, 1235–1240. [CrossRef] [PubMed]

16. Weinstock-Guttman, B.; Jacobs, L.D.; Brownscheidle, C.M.; Baier, M.; Rea, D.F.; Apatoff, B.R.; Blitz, K.M.; Coyle, P.K.; Frontera, A.T.; Goodman, A.D.; et al. Multiple sclerosis characteristics in African American patients in the New York State Multiple Sclerosis Consortium. *Mult. Scler.* **2003**, *9*, 293–298. [CrossRef] [PubMed]

17. Cree, B.A.C.; Khan, O.; Bourdette, D.; Goodin, D.S.; Cohen, J.A.; Marrie, R.A.; Glidden, D.; Weinstock-Guttman, B.; Reich, D.; Patterson, N.; et al. Clinical Characteristics of African Americans vs Caucasian Americans with Multiple Sclerosis. *Neurology* **2004**, *63*, 2039–2045. [CrossRef] [PubMed]

18. Buchanan, R.J.; Wang, S.; Huang, C.; Graber, D. Profiles of nursing home residents with multiple sclerosis using the minimum data set. *Mult. Scler.* **2001**, *7*, 189–200. [CrossRef]

19. Howard, J.; Battaglini, M.; Babb, J.S.; Arienzo, D.; Holst, B. MRI Correlates of Disability in African-Americans with Multiple Sclerosis. *PLoS ONE* **2012**, *7*, e43061. [CrossRef]

20. Amezcua, L.; Lund, B.T.; Weiner, L.P.; Islam, T. Multiple sclerosis in Hispanics: A study of clinical disease expression. *Mult. Scler.* **2011**, *17*, 1010–1016. [CrossRef]

21. Hadjixenofontos, A.; Beecham, A.H.; Manrique, C.P.; Pericak-Vance, M.A.; Tornes, L.; Ortega, M.; Rammohan, K.W.; McCauley, J.L.; Delgado, S.R. Clinical expression of multiple sclerosis in Hispanic whites of primarily Caribbean ancestry. *Neuroepidemiology* **2015**, *44*, 62–268. [CrossRef]

22. Ventura, R.E.; Antezana, A.O.; Bacon, T.; Kister, I. Hispanic Americans and African Americans with multiple sclerosis have more severe disease course than Caucasian Americans. *Mult. Scler.* **2017**, *23*, 1554–1557. [CrossRef] [PubMed]

23. Saadi, A.; Himmelstein, D.U.; Woolhandler, S.; Mejia, N.I. Racial disparities in neurologic health care access and utilization in the United States. *Neurology* **2017**, *88*, 2268–2275. [CrossRef] [PubMed]

24. Shabas, D.; Heffner, M. Multiple sclerosis management for low-income minorities. *Mult. Scler. J.* **2005**, *11*, 635–640. [CrossRef] [PubMed]

25. Langille, M.M.; Islam, T.; Burnett, M.; Amezcua, L. Clinical Characteristics of Pediatric-Onset and Adult-Onset Multiple Sclerosis in Hispanic Americans. *J. Child Neurol.* **2016**, *31*, 1068–1073. [CrossRef]

26. Avasarala, J. FDA-approved drugs for multiple sclerosis have no efficacy or disability data in non-Caucasian patients. *CNS Spectr.* **2019**, *24*, 279–280. [CrossRef]

27. Minden, S.L.; Hoaglin, D.C.; Hadden, L.; Frankel, D.; Robbins, T.; Perloff, J. Access to and utilization of neurologists by people with multiple sclerosis. *Neurology* **2008**, *70*, 1141–1149. [CrossRef]

28. Degelman, M.L.; Herman, K.M. Smoking and multiple sclerosis: A systematic review and meta-analysis using the Bradford Hill criteria for causation. *Mult. Scler. Relat. Disord.* **2017**, *17*, 207–216. [CrossRef]

29. Dong, D.; Carlson, J.; Ruberwa, J.; Snihur, T.; Al-Obaidi, N.; Bustillo, J. Unmasking the Masquerader: A Delayed Diagnosis of MS and Its 4.5 Years of Implications in an Older African American Male. *Case Rep. Med.* **2019**. [CrossRef]

30. Naismith, R.T.; Trinkaus, K.; Cross, A.H. Phenotype and prognosis in African-Americans with multiple sclerosis: A retrospective chart review. *Mult. Scler.* **2006**, *12*, 775–781. [CrossRef]

31. Cree, B.A.C.; Al-Sabbagh, A.; Bennett, R.; Goodin, D. Response to interferon beta-1a treatment in African American multiple sclerosis patients. *Arch. Neurol.* **2005**, *62*, 1681–1683. [CrossRef]

9

Molecular Interventions towards Multiple Sclerosis Treatment

Athanasios Metaxakis [1], Dionysia Petratou [1] and Nektarios Tavernarakis [1,2,*]

[1]   Institute of Molecular Biology and Biotechnology, Foundation for Research and Technology Hellas, Nikolaou
       Plastira 100, 70013 Heraklion, Greece; thanos_metaxakis@imbb.forth.gr (A.M.);
       dipetratou@imbb.forth.gr (D.P.)

[2]   Department of Basic Sciences, Faculty of Medicine, University of Crete, 71110 Heraklion, Greece

*   Correspondence: tavernarakis@imbb.forth.gr;

Abstract: Multiple sclerosis (MS) is an autoimmune life-threatening disease, afflicting millions of people worldwide. Although the disease is non-curable, considerable therapeutic advances have been achieved through molecular immunotherapeutic approaches, such as peptides vaccination, administration of monoclonal antibodies, and immunogenic copolymers. The main aims of these therapeutic strategies are to shift the MS-related autoimmune response towards a non-inflammatory T helper 2 (Th2) cells response, inactivate or ameliorate cytotoxic autoreactive T cells, induce secretion of anti-inflammatory cytokines, and inhibit recruitment of autoreactive lymphocytes to the central nervous system (CNS). These approaches can efficiently treat autoimmune encephalomyelitis (EAE), an essential system to study MS in animals, but they can only partially inhibit disease progress in humans. Nevertheless, modern immunotherapeutic techniques remain the most promising tools for the development of safe MS treatments, specifically targeting the cellular factors that trigger the initiation of the disease.

Keywords: B cell receptor; delivery methods; immunotherapy; monoclonal antibodies; multiple sclerosis; T cell receptor; tolerance; vaccine

1. Introduction

Multiple sclerosis (MS) is the commonest inflammatory autoimmune disorder of the central nervous system (CNS), progressively leading to demyelination, neurodegeneration, and neuronal disability [1–3]. MS globally affects more than 2.5 million people and it often afflicts young people, mainly women [4,5]. Despite the availability of a large arsenal of putative therapeutic approaches, numerous studies in animal model systems, and clinical trials, MS is still non-curable. As a result, the average life expectancy of MS patients is shorter by 5 to 10 years [6].

Inflammatory lesions at the CNS, generated by autoreactive lymphocytes, are suggested to underlie the pathophysiology of the disease, which results in neuronal demyelination and damage. Genetic and environmental factors influence MS susceptibility: Family history, single nucleotide polymorphisms, Epstein–Barr virus (EBV) infection, smoking, obesity, and vitamin D shortage are associated with MS development [7–11]. Patients experience relapsing-remitting phases of the disease, which are followed, even years later, by a progressive phase, accompanied by neurodegeneration [12,13]. MS symptomatology largely varies among patients, including sensory disturbances, cognitive defects, loss of vision, weakness, bladder dysfunction and neurological disability among others [14,15].

Therapeutic strategies against MS have been mainly relied on immune function suppressors, such as glucocorticoids, methotrexate, and antihistamines, which non-specifically reduce immune activity. These strategies have been enforced in recent years by the usage of antibodies against proinflammatory mediators [16]. However, this approach has severe side effects and dangers for patients, since the general inhibition of immune responses risks the development of infections and tumors. Hence, modern therapeutic approaches must aim at disease-modifying interventions that will counteract specifically the excessive immune response against self-antigens. Administration of self-antigens, an intervention that has been successfully applied in other autoimmune diseases and has been shown to eliminate the autoimmune response, is a widely accepted methodology to achieve this [17]. A major drawback of this technique is the poor targeting of CNS by the exogenously supplied antigens, for their inability to cross the brain–blood barrier and increased degradation. As such, the improvement of delivery methods used to protect and adequately transfer self-antigens to the inflammation sites has been an intriguing research field [18]. Nevertheless, a prerequisite for the success of this approach is that the epitope of the self-antigen is known. This is not true in the case of MS yet, although proteins within the myelin sheath have been suggested to be promising candidates [19,20]. Consequently, much research effort must be invested before modern immunomodulatory approaches can assure the cure of MS.

Recent experimental studies and clinical trials show that modern immunotherapeutic techniques have the potential to treat MS with less or no side effects in the future. Extensive work in mammalian model organisms has given insights into the mechanisms of the disease development and efficiency of several drugs in animals and humans. Indeed, novel drugs, such as Glatiramer acetate (Copaxone), a random sequence of four synthetic polypeptides with similar immunogenic properties to myelin protein, are currently being used against MS with very promising results [21]. In this review, we discuss antigen-specific and cell-specific immunotherapeutic approaches, applications of monoclonal antibodies against MS, anti-inflammatory strategies, peptide delivery methodologies and biological mechanisms that can serve as targets for the development of adjunctive MS treatments.

2. Immunotherapeutic Approaches

2.1. Antigen-Specific Immunotherapy (ASI)

Antigen-specific immunotherapy (ASI) is a promising strategy to treat MS with the least possible side effects. It was firstly introduced several decades ago, when Leonard Noon suppressed conjunctival sensitivity to grass pollen through prophylactic inoculation with grass pollen extracts [22]. His work paved the way for the first clinical trial of allergen immunotherapy a few decades later [23,24]. Allergen immunotherapy is based on the prevention of immune over-reaction against an allergen when repetitive doses of the latest are supplied to the organism. Repeated exposure to increasing amounts of an allergen results in altered cytokine production and shifts the immune response from a T helper 2 (Th2) to a T helper 1 (Th1) response, and also in the activation of regulatory T cells (Tregs) that secrete interleukin (IL)-10 and transforming growth factor (TGF)-β [25].

Contrary to allergic responses, where Th2 immune responses prevail, in autoimmune diseases, the prevalent responses are Th1 and Th17 against self-antigens. ASI for MS aims to induce Tregs in order to promote autoantigen-specific tolerance. The elimination of pathogenic Th1 and Th17 cells or the inhibition of the autoantigen-specific T cells-induced immune response might be the treatment for MS. Through repeated exposure to antigens, both allergen immunotherapy and ASI aim to promote self-tolerance [26].

Inspired by the progress in allergen immunotherapy, researchers have aimed at treating MS through the administration of self-peptides, which are expected to mimic the immunogenicity of self-antigens. This technique is called 'peptide vaccination' and promises to eliminate the antigen-specific attack without diminishing the organism's immune capacity against other threats. The most successful peptide vaccines applied so far are fractions of myelin proteins, such as myelin basic protein (MBP), myelin oligodendrocyte glycoprotein (MOG), and proteolipid protein (PLP) [27]. These antigens have been used to induce autoimmune encephalomyelitis (EAE) in mouse models, a widely accepted inflammatory model used to study MS. Several trials of myelin self-antigen peptide vaccines have cured EAE to a lesser or greater extent. Vaccination of an immunodominant epitope of myelin basic protein (MBP) (peptide 87–99), shown to be recognized and attacked by the T cell receptor (TCR), prevented and treated EAE, while it reduced tumor necrosis factor (TNF)-alpha and interferon (IFN)-gamma production, two determinant cytokines in the pathogenesis of EAE and MS [28]. More MBP peptides are shown to be immunogenic, and upon vaccination, they can mildly or strongly counteract EAE pathogenesis [29]. Myelin PLP (peptide 139–151) peptides can also prevent or treat EAE in animals [30,31]. A peptide from another myelin protein, the myelin oligodendrocyte glycoprotein (MOG) (peptide 35–55), can inhibit EAE development in mice [32,33], similarly to peptides derived from proteolipid protein (PLP) [34,35]. Hence, promising results from animal model systems have recommended peptide vaccination as a featured strategy to counteract MS.

In humans, two promising vaccination-based clinical trials with myelin peptides were safe and well tolerated by MS patients. Moreover, vaccination suppressed autoreactive responses and IFN-gamma production, while it significantly improved clinical disease measures. The activation of Langerhans cells and generation of IL-10-secreting cells are suggested to underlie these effects [36,37]. *Chataway et al.* showed that a mixture of peptides derived from MBP (peptide ATX-MS-1467) was safe and well tolerated by MS patients, while it improved radiographic activity in magnetic resonance imaging (MRI) [38]. *Crowe et al.* used a fragment of MBP (peptide 83–99) to induce immune responses and enhance anti-inflammatory cytokine secretion from T lymphocytes that cross-react with MBP [39]. Similarly, subcutaneous administration of a mixture of three MBP peptides (peptides 46-64, 124–139, and 147-170), termed Xemys, in MS patients was safe, while treatment decreased the cytokines monocyte chemoattractant protein-1, macrophage inflammatory protein-1β, and IL-7 and -2 levels, thus indicating reduced inflammation. However, clinical parameters were not significantly changed in patients [40]. In another scheme, researchers vaccinated MS patients with autologous peripheral blood mononuclear cells, chemically coupled with seven myelin peptides. Administration of antigen-coupled cells did not cause adverse effects, it was well tolerated and patients exhibited decreased antigen-specific T cell responses after treatment [41].

Contrary to the above, some studies show that peptide vaccination can have severe side effects and few clinical trials have not been completed for safety reasons. In two studies, MBP peptide 83–99 not only did not improve the disease state of MS [42], but even aggravated it, with few patients having exacerbations of MS [20]. Furthermore, administration of myelin epitopes has raised safety concerns of anaphylaxis [43–45]. In conclusion, specific attention should be paid to the adverse effects of peptides vaccination and future studies must identify the factors underlying the diversity of evoked responses in MS patients. Genomic profiling of MS patients that develop such effects can indicate factors that underlie the toxicity of this approach and indicate complementary treatments to reduce side effects. Moreover, trials with novel immunogenic peptides and further experimentation on the timing and dosage of vaccination can improve the efficiency and reduce the adverse effects of peptides vaccination.

Another immunotherapy technique that has been applied to induce self-tolerance in MS patients is the administration of genetically engineered DNA that encodes human MBP protein (BHT-3009). Experiments with animals clearly highlighted the potential of DNA vaccination as a safe and efficient technique at inducing regulatory T cells and EAE inhibition in animals. Its application in MS patients was safe and well tolerated, thus offering an alternative to peptide vaccination in terms of safety. Moreover, it decreased the proliferation of IFN-gamma-producing myelin-reactive T cells, the number of myelin-specific autoantibodies in the cerebrospinal fluid, and MRI-measured disease activity, while it increased the antigen-specific tolerance to myelin-specific B and T cells [46–49]. Nevertheless, no significant clinical improvements in the disease development were observed in these trials.

2.2. Cell-specific Immunotherapy

T cell vaccination is another immunotherapeutic approach, which is aimed at reducing or inactivating pathogenic T cells that maintain an autoimmune attack on myelin in MS. T cells' reaction is believed to be the initial step that drives the pathogenesis of MS [50]. In this technique, autologous myelin-reactive T cells are isolated and inactivated prior to their administration to MS patients.

Initial trials clearly showed safety and encouraging effects from T cell vaccination [51]. In a matched trial, MS patients were vaccinated with irradiated MBP-reactive T cells. Vaccinated patients with relapsing-remitting disease phases experienced a remarkable decrease in disease exacerbations and a five-fold lower increase in brain lesion size, compared to controls [52]. In three cases, however, T cell vaccine aggravated brain lesions and worsened relapses, a condition accompanied by reactivation of circulating MBP-reactive T cells. *Zhang et al.* showed that inhibition of MBP-reactive T cells was correlated with a 40% reduction in the rate of disease relapses, while brain lesion activity in vaccinated patients was stabilized [53]. This trial revealed that repetitive T cell vaccinations are needed to hamper the reappearance of myelin-reactive T cell clones.

Alternative T cell vaccination schemes use mixtures of inactivated autoreactive T cells, selected with more than one myelin peptides. In one trial, T cells activated with synthetic MBP and MOG peptides were administered in MS patients, with no adverse effects being reported. Patients exhibited stabilized neurological symptoms and vaccination reduced active brain lesions both in number and size [54,55]. Tcelna (formerly known as Tovaxin) is a T cell vaccine containing T cell populations selected with peptides derived from MBP, PLP, and MOG. In a double-blind trial involving a restricted number of MS patients, vaccination did not cause adverse effects and showed mild clinical efficacy [56]. More studies are required to properly evaluate the potency of Tcelna to treat MS.

Another suggested methodology to inhibit the autoimmune response in MS is via the elimination of dendritic cells, which play a major role in inflammation induction. Dendritic cells are the most efficient antigen-presenting cells (APCs) of the immune system and they have a particular role in the stimulation of naïve T cells. They regulate T cell differentiation and priming, secrete proinflammatory cytokines, orchestrate the immune response against self-antigens, and initiate chronic inflammation and loss of tolerance [57]. Dendritic cells respond occasionally to a specific antigen, in a manner dependent on the tissue environment. Tolerance-inducing (Tolerogenic) dendritic cells are dendritic cells with immunosuppressive properties, elicited by the induction of T cell anergy, T cell apoptosis, regulatory T cell activity, and production of anti-inflammatory cytokines [58]. In vitro treatment of monocyte-derived dendritic cells with vitamin D3 causes T cell hyporesponsiveness to myelin [19,59]. MOG 40–55 peptide-treated tolerogenic cells that were administered in mice preventively or after EAE induction reduced incidence of the disease or improved its clinical features, respectively [60]. Several trials in humans show that the technique is safe in patients with other autoimmune diseases [19]. Recently, engineered dendritic cells, loaded with specific antigens, were used to induce tolerance in MS patients. Therapy was safe and well tolerated; it increased IL-10 levels and the number of regulatory T cells, indicating that antigen-specific tolerance can be, at least partially, induced with this approach [61].

2.3. Cell Receptor-Specific Immunotherapy

A similar approach to cell-specific immunotherapy is T cell receptor-specific immunotherapy. Here, fragments of the T cell receptor (TCR) from pathogenic T cell clones are used as peptide vaccines, in order to activate immune responses against TCR-expressing T cells. TCR is a protein complex that recognizes antigens bound to major histocompatibility complex (MHC) molecules. Different TCRs can be specific for the same antigen, while more than one antigen peptides can be recognized by the same TCR [62].

Vaccination of rats with a synthetic TCR V-region peptide conferred resistance to subsequent induction of EAE [63]. According to the study, T cells specific for the TCR peptide weakened the immune attack to the encephalitogenic epitope. Furthermore, *Offner et al.* showed that TCR vaccination can not only prevent EAE but also cure it. When a TCR-V beta 8-39-59 peptide was injected into rats with EAE, disease symptoms were alleviated and recovery from the disease was fast [64].

To test safety and immunogenicity of TCR vaccines in humans, *Bourdette et al.* intradermally injected MS patients with two synthetic TCR peptides (TCR peptides V beta 5.2, 39-59 and V beta 6.1, 39-59). Low doses of the TCR vaccine caused no side effects, restricted spectrum immunosuppression, generated TCR peptide-specific T cells, and reduced MBP-specific T cells [65]. In a subsequent trial,

TCR vaccination enhanced TCR-reactive T cells, reduced the MBP response against MBP antigen, stabilized clinical features, and caused no adverse effects to MS patients [66]. In support, TCR-specific Th2 cells inhibit the MBP-specific Th1 response in vitro through the release of IL-10, and a triplicate TCR vaccine (BV5S2, BV6S5, and BV13S1 peptides) increases the numbers of circulating IL-10-secreting T cells, reactive to the TCR peptides, in MS patients [67].

Together with pathogenic T cells, autoreactive B cells are involved in MS induction. Hence, the B cell receptor (BCR) can be used as a vaccine as well. Single-cell sequencing and phage display libraries of B cells derived from MS patients have been performed to identify BCR structures involved in MS autoimmunity [68–70]. *Gabibov et al.* showed that, antibodies induced against Epstein–Barr virus latent membrane protein 1 (LMP1) potentially react with MBP. This suggests that natural molecular reactivity might underlie MS induction and raises questions about the causal link between virus infection and MS development. Recently, antibody engineering techniques have allowed for the targeting of BCR with toxins, resulting in the cell death of pathogenic B cells [29,71,72]. This makes BCR-specific immunotherapy an alternative, although still at a preliminary state, approach to treat MS.

2.4. Monoclonal Antibodies (MABs)

The usage of monoclonal antibodies is another encouraging molecular therapy against MS, for their high specificity and high efficacy. Several ones have been approved for MS treatment [73,74]. Natalizumab, an adhesion molecule inhibitor, was the first MAB to be approved in 2004 [75]. It is a recombinant humanized MAB that binds integrin α-4 on the surface of activated inflammatory lymphocytes and monocytes. This inhibits the interaction of integrin a-4 with vascular cell adhesion molecule-1 (VCAM-1) on endothelial cells and consequently circulation into the CNS. Clinical trials show that it is safe, well tolerated, and efficient, since it reduces the risk of sustained progression of disability and MS relapses [76]. Ocrelizumab and Rituximab are MABs that target CD20 protein on B lymphocytes. They have been shown to reduce the rates of disease activity and disease progression [77, 78]. Ofatumumab also binds on CD20, albeit at a different epitope, and its administration in MS patients reduces new MRI-detected lesions by 99% [79]. Another MAB, Opicinumab, has been designed to repair and enhance re-myelination of lesions in MS patients. Opicinumab is a fully humanized MAB that targets and inactivates leucine rich repeat and immunoglobin-like domain-containing protein 1 (LINGO-1), a transmembrane signaling protein that inhibits the differentiation of oligodendrocytes and myelination. Hence, it is potentially a promising tool to induce re-myelination in MS patients and alleviate disease symptoms. It has been tested in mice and in humans, where it increases myelination and re-myelination in MS patients [80,81]. Alemtuzumab is a humanized monoclonal antibody, approved in several countries for the treatment of relapsing-remitting MS. It targets CD52 antigen on lymphocytes, resulting in their depletion [82]. Hence, monoclonal antibodies are very promising tools for MS therapy for their safety, specificity, and efficacy but also for the various cellular procedures they can target to reduce autoimmunity and its clinical consequences.

2.5. HLA Antagonistic Co-polymers

Synthetic materials (copolymers) can mimic the immunogenic properties of endogenous proteins and compete with them for binding to HLA class II molecules. Glatiramer acetate (Copaxone or GA) is a random polymer of four amino acids (L-alanine, L-glutamic acid, L-lysine, and L-tyrosine) that effectively treats experimental encephalomyelitis and reduces relapses in MS patients [83–85]. GA is suggested to specifically inhibit the production of myelin-reactive antibodies, by directly acting on APCs. This modifies them into non-inflammatory type II cells. APCs-mediated presentation of GA to CD8+ and CD4+ T cells results in the generation of CD4+ regulatory T cells and immune response deviation towards Th2 responses [86,87]. A second generation of polymers has been synthesized with stronger binding activities on HLA molecules compared to GA. They have been successfully used to suppress EAE in mice [88]. In transgenic mice with human HLA-DR-TCR, poly(VWAK)n copolymers are shown to induce T cells' anergy, while poly(FYAK)n copolymers induce Th2 cells that secrete anti-inflammatory cytokines [29]. Hence, they can serve as alternative tools for shifting the immune response towards Th2 activation in MS patients.

3. Delivery Methods of Immunotherapeutic Factors

A key point for the successful implementation of immunotherapy treatment is the efficacy of the delivery methodology. Oral, skin, parenteral, intramuscular, intravenous, and intra-peritoneal routes are mainly used with various delivery vehicles. These vehicles must enhance the tolerance of immunomodulatory molecules against the harsh intra-organismal environment and advance their efficacy to overcome the brain–blood barrier. Synthetic polymers, such as poly lactide-co-glycolide (PLGA), polyethylene glycol (PEG), and polymethylmethacrylate (PMMA), are easily synthesized and modified, capable of transferring sufficient amounts of immunotherapeutic molecules and facilitating their gradual release [18]. Permeability is decreased when electrically charged nanoparticles are used, such as orally administrated polyethylene imine-based nanoparticles and thiol-modified Eudragit polymers (polymethacrylates) [89,90]. Transgenic plant delivery is another technique that takes advantage of the protective effect of the plant cell wall, especially for delivery through the gastrointestinal tract [91,92]. Nanoemulsions, small colloidal particles, provide a high encapsulation efficiency [93], while phosphatidylserine-liposomes have been efficiently used to reduce EAE severity in mice [94]. Much attention has been paid to lipid-based nanocarriers, such as nanoemulsions, nanoliposomes, solid lipid nanoparticles (SLNs), and nanostructured lipid carriers (NLCs), which are suggested to be efficient for brain targeting. NLCs have been reported to be very safe and stable, with a high encapsulation efficiency [95,96]. A major challenge in the field of immunotherapy treatment is the improvement of delivery methods so that immunotherapeutic molecules can be transferred more efficiently through the brain–blood barrier. This will improve the therapeutic efficiency, reduce side effects, and decrease the number of administration procedures. More selective delivery to the CNS can be achieved through the covalent tethering of delivery molecules with ligands capable of overcoming the brain–blood barrier, the use of fusion antibodies that target specific lymphocytes, and of liposomes that intrinsically tend to reach inflammation sites.

Therapeutic treatments for MS target lymphocyte subpopulations, specific for autoreactive response towards the myelin sheath. Tolerogenic DCs, myelin peptide and DNA vaccines, TCR peptides and GA lead to the activation of Th2 cells, through Tregs. Subsequent release of IL-10 leads to the inhibition of Th1 cells. DMF acts on HCAR2, found on dendritic cells, to induce Th2 cells. Toxins targeting BCRs lead to the elimination of pathogenic B cells. Fingolimod blocks the circulation of mature lymphocytes through S1PR, and Teriflunomide and Mitoxantrone inhibit T and B cell proliferation. Anti-CD 20 and anti-CD 52 antibodies deplete CD 20+ and CD 52+ lymphocytes. Tolerogenic TCs block MBP-reactive T and B cells. Natalizumab binds to α 4 β 1 integrin on activated T and B cells and prevent their interaction with VCAM-1. Opicinumab promotes the differentiation of oligodendrocyte precursor cells by inactivating LINGO-1. Abbreviations: Antigen Presenting Cell (APC), Blood–Brain Barrier (BBB), B Cell Receptor (BCR), cluster of differentiation 52/20 (CD52/20), Dendritic Cells (DCs), DMF (Dimethyl Fumarate), Glatiramer Acetate (GA), hydroxycarboxylic acid receptor 2 (HCAR2), Interferon (IFN), Interleukin (IL), Immunoglobin-like domain-containing protein 1 (LINGO-1), MBP (Myelin Binding Protein), MMF (Monomethyl Fumarate), Multiple Sclerosis (MS), Sphingosine-1-phosphate receptor (S1PR), TCR (T cell Receptor), T helper 2 cell (Th2), T helper 1 cell (Th1), T Cell Receptor (TCR), T regulatory cells (Tregs), TCs (T cells), vascular cell adhesion molecule-1 (VCAM-1). (Table 1).

Table 1. Overview of medical treatments for multiple sclerosis.

Treatment	Mode of Action	MS Type	Study Format (Number of Participants)	Clinical Outcomes	Adverse Effects	Administration Route	References
Interferons							
Interferon-β1a *	reduces immature-transitional B cell subset/plasmablasts ratio, increases CD27 and CD27+IgM+ memory B cell subsets, enhances Tregs	RRMS	case-control study/multicenter, open-label, prospective clinical trial, phase 4 (96)	reduction in relapse rates, reduction in MRI measurement of disease, well tolerated	flu-like symptoms, asthenia, fever, malaise, fatigue, local pain at the injection site	intramuscular injection	[97,98]
Interferon-β1b *	reduces neuron inflammation	RRMS	multicenter, randomized, double-blind, placebo-controlled trial (372)	reduced ARR, and MRI lesions	lymphopenia, skin reactions to injection, flu-like symptoms, fever, chills, myalgia, sweating, malaise	subcutaneous injection	[99,100]
Peptides							
Myelin peptides (MOG1-20, MOG35-55, MBP13-32, MBP83-99, MBP111-129, MBP146-170, PLP139-154)	myelin peptide coupled autologous peripheral blood mononuclear cells, slightly increase T regulatory cells	RRMS SPMS	open-label, single-center, dose-escalation study, phase 1 trial (9)	safe and well tolerated	metallic flavor during infusion and IARs (diarrhea, headache, diverticulitis of sigma, neck pain, vision disturbance, dysesthesia, cold, gastric pain)	infusion	[41]
Peptide vaccines							
NBI-5788	altered MBP83-99 peptide, induces Th2-like cells APL-reactive	PPMS SPMS RRMS	multicenter phase 1 trial (11)	induced NBI-5788 responsive T cells, no clinical exacerbations	-	subcutaneous infusion	[39]
Xemys	mannosylated liposomes encapsulating MBP peptides, increases TNF-α, cytokine's levels normalization	RRMS SPMS	phase 1 trial (18)/phase 1, open-label, dose-escalating, proof-of-concept study (20)	increased TNF-α serum levels, safe and well tolerated	injection site reaction, rhinitis, general weakness	subcutaneous infusion	[40,101]
peptides MBP85-99, MOG35-55, and PLP139-155	induce T regs producing IL-10, reduce IFN-γ and TGF-β	RRMS	double-blind, placebo-controlled cohort study (30)	reduced GdE lesions and ARR	local skin reaction (redness, itching), upper respiratory tract infection, lacrimation	transdermally, with skin patch	[36,37]
ATX-MS-1467	peptide mixture of MBP derived epitopes, induces MBP tolerance and IL-10 secreting T regs	RMS	multicenter, phase 1b (43), phase 2a, multicenter, single-arm trial (37)	reduced GdE lesions	erythema, induration, pain, pruritus, hemorrhage, alopecia, diarrhea	intradermal/ subcutaneous injection	[38,102]
DNA vaccine							
BHT-3009	decreases T cells	RRMS	randomized, multicenter, double-blind, placebo-controlled dose escalation, phase 1/2 trial (30)/randomized, placebo-controlled, phase 2 trial (289)	reduced GdE lesions, reduced myelin-specific autoantibodies, safe and well tolerated	infections, musculoskeletal, urinary, gastrointestinal psychiatric, respiratory effects (IARs)	intramuscular injections	[47,48]

Table 1. *Cont.*

Treatment	Mode of Action	MS Type	Study Format (Number of Participants)	Clinical Outcomes	Adverse Effects	Administration Route	References
TCR vaccines							
TCR V beta 5.2, 39-59 and V beta 6.1, 39-59	induce T regs	PMS	dose escalation study (11)	induced T cell immunity to synthetic peptides, safe	skin hypersensitivity reaction to the injection, no side effects or broad immunosuppression	intradermal injection	[65,103]
vβ5.2-38-58	induce Th2 cells and inhibits MBP-specific Th1 cells	PMS	double-blind (23)	induced T cell immunity to synthetic peptides, attenuated disease progression	no side effects or broad immunosuppression	intradermal injection	[66]
BV5S2, BV6S5 and BV13S1	induce IL-10 secreting T cells	RRM PMS	single-arm, open-label study (23)	induced T cell immunity to synthetic peptides, stabilized disease, improved FoxP3 expression, safe	no side effects	intramuscular injection	[67]
Monoclonal antibodies							
Natalizumab *	anti-a4-integrin Ab, prevents leukocytes crossing BBB	early RRMS	controlled, non-randomized trial (34)/multicenter, observational, open-label, single-arm, phase 4 study (222)	reduced relapse rates, MRI lesions and progression of disability, improvement in information processing speed, NEDA, SDMT and MSIS-29 physical, psychological and quality-of-life	suicide attempt, acute kidney injury, anaphylactic reactions, bronchial obstruction, clostridium difficile colitis, conversion disorder, hydronephrosis, hyperkaliemia, hypotension, ileus, melanoma recurrent, migraine	intravenous infusion	[104,105]
		SPMS	randomized, double-blind, placebo-controlled, phase 3 trial (889), open-label extension (291)	reduced progression of disability, improved ARR and MRI measurements, well tolerated	urinary tract infection, nasopharyngitis, fall, MS relapse, headache, fatigue, upper respiratory tract infection, back pain, arthralgia, pain in hands and feet, muscular weakness (IARs)	intravenous infusion	[106]
Opicinumab	anti-LINGO-1 Ab, allows oligodendricy maturation	RRMS SPMS	double-blind, dose-ranging, proof-of-concept, phase 2b study (418)/phase 1, randomized, multiple ascending dose study	primary endpoint was not met, inverted U-shaped dose-response	unaffected immune function	intravenous infusion	[81,107]
Alemtuzumab*	anti-CD52 IgG Ab, depletes circulating T and B lymphocytes	RRMS	rater-masked, randomized, controlled phase 3 trial (667)	reduced ARR, stabilized disability levels, improved clinical and MRI outcomes, reduced brain volume loss	infections, thyroid-associated adverse events, thrombocytopenia IARs (headache, pyrexia, rash, bradycardia, insomnia, erythema, nausea, Urticaria, pruritus, abdominal pain, fatigue, dyspnea, flushing)	intravenous infusion	[108]
Ofatumumab	anti-CD20, cytotoxic to B lymphocytes	RRMS	randomized, double-blind, placebo-controlled, phase 2 study (36)/randomized, double-blind, phase 2b study (232)	decreased new MRI lesions, safe	rash, erythema, upper respiratory tract infection, viral infection, throat irritation, headache, fatigue, back pain, flushing, injection related reactions	subcutaneous injection	[79,109]

Table 1. *Cont.*

Treatment	Mode of Action	MS Type	Study Format (Number of Participants)	Clinical Outcomes	Adverse Effects	Administration Route	References
Rituximab	selective depletion of CD20+ B lymphocytes	PMS	single-center, open-label trial (8)/retrospective, uncontrolled, observational, multicenter study (822)	reduced peripheral B cells, CSF B cells and CXCL-13 levels, increased BAFF levels/ lower EDSS score, delayed CDP	IARs (lower extremity paresthesia), lower extremity spasticity or weakness, fatigue, fever, rigors/ infections (respiratory, intestinal), disorders (cardiac, respiratory, neuronal, immune) and IARs (malaise, headache, chills, nausea)	intrathecal infusion	[110,111]
		RRMS	blind, single-center, phase 2 trial (30)	reduced relapses and GdE lesions	IARs (fever, chills, flushing, itching of body or throat, and/or diarrhea, shortness of breath), urinary tract infections, thigh pain, upper respiratory tract infection, bronchitis, hand tendonitis, dizziness	intravenous infusion	[112]
		PPMS SPMS	multicenter, prospective, open-label phase 1b trial (23)/randomized, double-blind, placebo-controlled, multicenter, phase 2/3 trial (439)	well tolerated and feasible, reduced GdE lesions, delayed CDP	IARs (vertigo, nausea), infections, paresthesia, fall, nervous system disorders, fever, fatigue, meningitis/IARs (nausea, fatigue, chills, pyrexia, headache, dizziness, throat irritation, pharyngolaryngeal pain, pruritus, rash, flushing, hypotension), pneumonia, bronchitis	intravenous or intrathecal infusion	[113,114]
Ocrelizumab*	anti-CD20 Ab, depletes circulating CD20+ B cells	RMS PPMS	randomized, double-blind, active-controlled, phase 3 trials (1651), randomized, parallel-group, double-blind, placebo- controlled, phase 3 study (725)	reduced new and GdE lesions, improved ARR, disability progression, and MRI outputs	IARs (pruritus, rash, throat irritation, flushing, urticaria, oropharyngeal pain, headache, tachycardia, pyrexia, nausea, hypo-, hyper-tension, myalgia, dizziness, fatigue)	intravenous infusion	[115,116]
		PPMS	randomized, double-blind, placebo-controlled, phase 3 trial (732)	reduced risk of Upper Extremity disability progression, enhanced NEPAD, reduced brain volume loss	IARs (upper respiratory tract infections, oral herpes infections, pruritus, rash, throat irritation, flushing)	intravenous infusion	[117,118]
HLA antagonistic co-polymers							
Glatiramer acetate *	increases Tregs to suppress inflammatory response	RRMS	randomized, placebo-controlled, double-blind study (251), open-label study (208)	reduced relapse rate, reduced GdE and new lesions	IARs (flushing, anxiety, dyspnea)	subcutaneous injection	[119]

Table 1. *Cont.*

Treatment	Mode of Action	MS Type	Study Format (Number of Participants)	Clinical Outcomes	Adverse Effects	Administration Route	References
Sphingosine-1-phosphate receptor modulators							
Fingolimod *	structural analogue of sphingosine, anti-inflammatory, impairs cytotoxic CD8 T cells function	RRMS	prospective observational study (60)	higher retention rate, increased satisfaction at MSQ, reduced dGM volume loss, ARR and EDSS	influenza-like illness, pain in extremity, headache, anxiety, depression, nasopharyngitis, hypoesthesia, arthralgia, dizziness, fatigue, rash, urinary tract infection, abdominal pain, hypertension, lymphopenia	oral	[120,121]
Other inhibitors							
Teriflunomide *	DHODH inhibitor, reduces proliferation of T- and B-cells	RMS	prospective, single-arm, open-label, phase 4 real-world study (1000)/randomized, double-blind, placebo-controlled, phase 3 trial (168)/multicenter, multinational, randomized, double-blind, parallel-group, placebo-controlled, phase 3 study (2251)	well tolerated, improved MRI outcomes, reduced ARR and CDW, improved TSQM scores, stabilized disability measures, improved cognition and quality of life measures	neutropenia, hair thinning, diarrhea, nausea, headache, urinary tract infection, increased alanine aminotransferase, nasopharyngitis, fatigue, paresthesia	oral	[122–124]
T cell vaccination							
MBP-reactive T cells	deplete circulating MBP-reactive T cells.	RRMSSPMS	pilot, controlled (8)/preliminary open label study (54)	safe and well tolerated, improved MRI outcome, reduced relapse rates	no adverse effects, skin infection	subcutaneous injection	[52,53]
MBB-, MOG-reactive T cells	deplete circulating MBP-, MOG-reactive T cells.	RRMS	20	improved MRI outcome	no adverse effects, skin infection	S subcutaneous injection	[55]
MBB-, MOG-, PLP-reactive T cells/ Tovaxin	deplete circulating MBP-, MOG-, PLP-reactive T cells.	RRMSSPMS	open-label dose escalation study (16)/randomized, double-blind trial, phase 2 study (26)	well tolerated, reduced EDSS, ARR and 10 min walking time, stabilized MRI lesions, improved EDSS and MSIS-29	relapse of MS, pain in extremity, IARs (injection site pain, erythema, inflammation, pruritus), unrelated to TCV administration (anemia, intestinal obstruction, pneumonia, carpal tunnel syndrome, headache, respiratory distress, infections)	Subcutaneous injection	[54,56]

Table 1. *Cont.*

Treatment	Mode of Action	MS Type	Study Format (Number of Participants)	Clinical Outcomes	Adverse Effects	Administration Route	References
Dendritic cell vaccination							
peptide loaded cells	increase T regulatory cells and IL-10 levels	RRMS SPMS PPMS	open-label, single-center, multiple ascending-dose, phase 1b trial (12)	well tolerated, stabilized disease progress	headache, leg pain, cold, palpitations, influenza (and unrelated to TCV administration)	intravenous	[61]
Esters							
Dimethyl Fumarate *	fumaric acid ester, modulates CD4(+) cells, M2 monocytes and B-cells, induction of antioxidant response	RRMS	randomized, double-blind, placebo controlled, phase 3 trial (213)/open-label, observational, phase 4 study (1105)	decreased EDSS, GdE and new lesions, reduced ARR, improved treatment satisfaction and quality of life measures	flushing, nausea, abdominal pain, diarrhea, gastrointestinal events, nasopharyngitis, infections, cardiovascular, skin and hepatic events, pruritus, rash, headache, fall, lymphopenia, breast cancer, MS relapse	oral delayed release	[125,126] -
Other Immunomodulators							
Mitoxantrone *	a synthetic anthracenedione, inhibits T-cell, B-cell and macrophage proliferation	SPMS RRMS PRMS	multicenter, prospective, open-label, observational, phase 4 study (509)	reduced GdE lesions and relapse rate, improved EDSS	congestive heart failure, leukemia, amenorrhea, decreased ejection fraction, urinary tract infection	intravenous infusion	[127]

Table 1. The main MS treatments are summarized. Some of them are approved while others are still under clinical trial. Their mode of action and outcomes of some indicative clinical trials are tabulated. With asterisk (*) are indicated the MS medications approved by the FDA. Abbreviations: Antibody (Ab), Altered Peptide Ligand (APL), Annualized Relapse Rate (ARR), B-cell Activating Factor (BAFF), Blood-Brain Barrier (BBB), Confirmed Disability Progression (CDP), Confirmed Disability Worsening (CDW), CerebroSpinal Fluid (CSF), C-X-C motif chemokinebinding Ligand-13 (CXCL-13), DiHydro-Orotate DeHydrogenase (DHODH), deep Gray Matter (dGM), Expanded Disability Status Scale (EDSS), Gadolinium-Enhanced (GdE), Infusion-Associated Reactions (IARs), InterLeukin (IL), InterFeroN (IFN), Leucine rich repeat and Immunoglobulin-like domain-containing protein 1 (LINGO-1), Myelin Basic Protein (MBP), myelin oligodendrocyte glycoprotein (MOG), Modified Fatigue Impact Scale (MFIS), Mental Health Inventory (MHI), Medication Satisfaction Questionnaire (MSQ), Multiple Sclerosis (MS), No Evidence of Disease Activity (NEDA), No Evidence of Progression or active Disease (NEPAD), proteolipid protein (PLP), Primary Progressive Multiple Sclerosis (PPMS), Relapsing Multiple Sclerosis (RMS), Relapsing-Remitting Multiple Sclerosis (RRMS), Sphingosine-1-phosphate receptor (S1PR), Symbol Digit Modalities Test (SDMT), Secondary Progressive Multiple Sclerosis (SPMS), T-helper-2 cell (Th2), T Cell Receptor (TCR), Transforming Growth Factor beta (TGF-β), T regulatory cells (Tregs), Treatment Satisfaction Questionnaire for Medication Version 1.4 (TSQM 1.4).

4. Conclusions

Researchers in the field of MS treatment have been trying to cure the disease via the elimination of CNS inflammation, elicited by the MS-related autoimmune response. Different applied strategies include the deviation of the immune response towards non-inflammatory Th2 activation, inactivation or amelioration of cytotoxic autoreactive T cells, induction of anti-inflammatory cytokines' secretion, inhibition of inflammatory cytokines, blockage of autoreactive-lymphocytes' recruitment to the CNS, and enhancement of myelination mechanisms (Figure 1). Several drugs have been tested so far in clinical trials, some of which can reduce relapses and symptoms in MS patients (Table 1), thus significantly improving their quality of life. However, none of them can cure MS. Despite the success of allergen immunotherapy in treating allergies, ASI has not displayed great achievements so far as a putative MS treatment. Reasons underlying this might be the difficulty in the identification of the self-antigens that trigger autoimmunity, the inability of regulatory T cells to suppress cytokine production under inflammatory conditions, the different immune players participating in allergies compared to MS (e.g., IgE antibodies, Th2 responses), and also the route, dosage, and timing used for ASI treatments [128]. Nevertheless, more than 10 drugs are currently being used against the secondary progressive form of MS, characterized by the relapsing-remitting phases, significantly reducing the frequency of relapses and disease symptoms [14]. These drugs are either immunosuppressants (such as Natalizumab, Ocrelizumab, Fingolimod, Alemtuzumab) or immunomodulatory (such as Interferon beta, GA, Teriflunomide, Mitoxantrone, Dimethylfumarate). Fingolimod reduces the number of circulating mature lymphocytes [129], Teriflunomide and Mitoxantrone are inhibitors of lymphocytes proliferation and the secretion of cytokines [130,131], while Dimethylfumarate (DMF), used for psoriasis treatment, shifts the Th1 and Th17 immune responses to Th2 [132]. However, these drugs do not cure the primary progressive form of MS, they must be repetitively supplied to the MS patients, and they can have adverse effects. As such, more selective and efficient drugs are required to assure safe treatment of MS in the future.

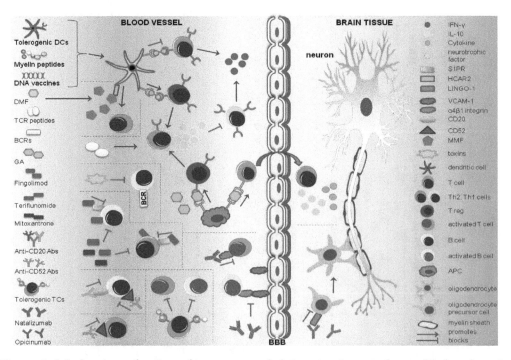

Figure 1. Mechanism of action of immunomodulatory treatments for multiple sclerosis.

Basic research on the mechanisms that underlie MS can reveal novel targets for monoclonal antibodies, identify the specific self-antigens that trigger autoimmunity, and characterize the types of lymphocytes that participate in the inflammatory reaction, so that antigen and cell-specific immunotherapies expand and become more precise. In addition, the identification of novel carriers or ligands that, upon conjugation, will lead these immunotherapeutic molecules to the CNS inflammatory sites can improve the efficiency of treatments. It is also important to clarify the role of Epstein–Barr virus infection on MS development and their possible association, which might give further insights into the disease etiology and treatment. Improved delivery of therapeutic molecules is another challenge of research in MS, which can be achieved through the generation of fusions between the therapeutic molecules and peptide leaders that will efficiently guide them to the inflammation sites in the brain [133]. Recently, a fusion protein of an NOD-like receptor family member X1 (NLRX1) and blood–brain barrier-permeable peptide dNP2 treated experimental autoimmune encephalomyelitis in mice [134] and a peptide that selectively recognizes the CNS was used for targeted drug delivery to the CNS in mice [135]. Genome-wide DNA sequencing analysis of MS patients is another approach that can advance our knowledge on the disease etiology and on MS patients' responses to medical treatments; it can reveal genes that make people more susceptible to MS and identify the reasons why specific drug treatments have adverse effects in some patients. In this case, the proper therapy could be administrated to patients that have certain genetic profiles, so that adverse effects of MS therapy could be minimized. Furthermore, drugs that enhance myelination, such as metformin [136], growth factors shown to regulate inflammation [137], and hormones known to affect autoimmunity [138] can offer new perspectives into the development of novel complementary treatments of MS in the future.

Author Contributions: A.M. and D.P. summarized the literature, wrote the paper and created the initial figure and table. N.T. edited the paper, revised the figures and contributed to the writing. All authors have read and agreed to the published version of the manuscript.

References

1. Compston, A.; Coles, A. Multiple sclerosis. *Lancet* **2008**, *372*, 1502–1517. [CrossRef]

2. Dendrou, C.A.; Fugger, L.; Friese, M.A. Immunopathology of multiple sclerosis. *Nat. Rev. Immunol.* **2015**, *15*, 545–558. [CrossRef]

3. Grigoriadis, N.; van Pesch, V. A basic overview of multiple sclerosis immunopathology. *Eur. J. Neurol.* **2015**, *22* (Suppl. 2), 3–13. [CrossRef]

4. Koch-Henriksen, N.; Sorensen, P.S. The changing demographic pattern of multiple sclerosis epidemiology. *Lancet. Neurol.* **2010**, *9*, 520–532. [CrossRef]

5. Kurtzke, J.F. Epidemiology of multiple sclerosis. Does this really point toward an etiology? Lectio doctoralis. *Neurol. Sci.* **2000**, *21*, 383–403. [CrossRef]

6. GBD 2015 Disease and Injury Incidence and Prevalence Collaborators. Global, regional, and national incidence, prevalence, and years lived with disability for 310 diseases and injuries, 1990–2015: A systematic analysis for the global burden of disease study 2015. *Lancet* **2016**, *388*, 1545–1602. [CrossRef]

7. Sintzel, M.B.; Rametta, M.; Reder, A.T. Vitamin d and multiple sclerosis: A comprehensive review. *Neurol. Ther.* **2018**, *7*, 59–85. [CrossRef]

8. Oksenberg, J.R. Decoding multiple sclerosis: An update on genomics and future directions. *Expert Rev. Neurother.* **2013**, *13*, 11–19. [CrossRef]

9. Ascherio, A. Environmental factors in multiple sclerosis. *Expert Rev. Neurother.* **2013**, *13*, 3–9. [CrossRef]

10. Ramagopalan, S.V.; Dobson, R.; Meier, U.C.; Giovannoni, G. Multiple sclerosis: Risk factors, prodromes, and potential causal pathways. *Lancet. Neurol.* **2010**, *9*, 727–739. [CrossRef]

11. Hedstrom, A.K.; Baarnhielm, M.; Olsson, T.; Alfredsson, L. Tobacco smoking, but not swedish snuff use, increases the risk of multiple sclerosis. *Neurology* **2009**, *73*, 696–701. [CrossRef]

12. Bjartmar, C.; Wujek, J.R.; Trapp, B.D. Axonal loss in the pathology of ms: Consequences for understanding the progressive phase of the disease. *J. Neurol. Sci.* **2003**, *206*, 165–171. [CrossRef]

13. Lublin, F.D.; Reingold, S.C. Defining the clinical course of multiple sclerosis: Results of an international survey. National multiple sclerosis society (USA) advisory committee on clinical trials of new agents in multiple sclerosis. *Neurology* **1996**, *46*, 907–911. [CrossRef]

14. Huang, W.J.; Chen, W.W.; Zhang, X. Multiple sclerosis: Pathology, diagnosis and treatments. *Exp. Ther. Med.* **2017**, *13*, 3163–3166. [CrossRef]

15. de Sa, J.C.; Airas, L.; Bartholome, E.; Grigoriadis, N.; Mattle, H.; Oreja-Guevara, C.; O'Riordan, J.; Sellebjerg, F.; Stankoff, B.; Vass, K.; et al. Symptomatic therapy in multiple sclerosis: A review for a multimodal approach in clinical practice. *Ther. Adv. Neurol. Disord.* **2011**, *4*, 139–168. [CrossRef]

16. Ransohoff, R.M.; Hafler, D.A.; Lucchinetti, C.F. Multiple sclerosis-a quiet revolution. *Nat. Rev. Neurol.* **2015**, *11*, 134–142. [CrossRef]

17. Critchfield, J.M.; Racke, M.K.; Zuniga-Pflucker, J.C.; Cannella, B.; Raine, C.S.; Goverman, J.; Lenardo, M.J. T cell deletion in high antigen dose therapy of autoimmune encephalomyelitis. *Science* **1994**, *263*, 1139–1143. [CrossRef]

18. Shakya, A.K.; Nandakumar, K.S. Antigen-specific tolerization and targeted delivery as therapeutic strategies for autoimmune diseases. *Trends Biotechnol.* **2018**, *36*, 686–699. [CrossRef]

19. Willekens, B.; Cools, N. Beyond the magic bullet: Current progress of therapeutic vaccination in multiple sclerosis. *CNS Drugs* **2018**, *32*, 401–410. [CrossRef]

20. Bielekova, B.; Goodwin, B.; Richert, N.; Cortese, I.; Kondo, T.; Afshar, G.; Gran, B.; Eaton, J.; Antel, J.; Frank, J.A.; et al. Encephalitogenic potential of the myelin basic protein peptide (amino acids 83–99) in multiple sclerosis: Results of a phase ii clinical trial with an altered peptide ligand. *Nat. Med.* **2000**, *6*, 1167–1175. [CrossRef]

21. Schrempf, W.; Ziemssen, T. Glatiramer acetate: Mechanisms of action in multiple sclerosis. *Autoimmun. Rev.* **2007**, *6*, 469–475. [CrossRef]

22. Noon, L. Prophylactic inoculation against hay fever. *Int. Arch. Allergy Appl. Immunol.* **1953**, *4*, 285–288. [CrossRef]

23. Frankland, A.W.; Augustin, R. Prophylaxis of summer hay-fever and asthma: A controlled trial comparing crude grass-pollen extracts with the isolated main protein component. *Lancet* **1954**, *266*, 1055–1057. [CrossRef]

24. Freeman, J. " Rush " inoculation, with special reference to hay-fever treatment. *Lancet* **1930**, *215*, 744–747. [CrossRef]

25. Hochfelder, J.L.; Ponda, P. Allergen immunotherapy: Routes, safety, efficacy, and mode of action. *Immunotargets Ther.* **2013**, *2*, 61–71. [CrossRef]

26. Pozsgay, J.; Szekanecz, Z.; Sarmay, G. Antigen-specific immunotherapies in rheumatic diseases. *Nat. Rev. Rheumatol.* **2017**, *13*, 525–537. [CrossRef]

27. Hohlfeld, R.; Wekerle, H. Autoimmune concepts of multiple sclerosis as a basis for selective immunotherapy: From pipe dreams to (therapeutic) pipelines. *Proc. Natl. Acad. Sci. USA* **2004**, *101* (Suppl. 2), 14599–14606. [CrossRef]

28. Karin, N.; Mitchell, D.J.; Brocke, S.; Ling, N.; Steinman, L. Reversal of experimental autoimmune encephalomyelitis by a soluble peptide variant of a myelin basic protein epitope: T cell receptor antagonism and reduction of interferon gamma and tumor necrosis factor alpha production. *J. Exp. Med.* **1994**, *180*, 2227–2237. [CrossRef]

29. Stepanov, A.; Lomakin, Y.; Gabibov, A.; Belogurov, A. Peptides against autoimmune neurodegeneration. *Curr. Med. Chem.* **2017**, *24*, 1761–1771. [CrossRef]

30. Puentes, F.; Dickhaut, K.; Hofstatter, M.; Falk, K.; Rotzschke, O. Active suppression induced by repetitive self-epitopes protects against eae development. *PLoS ONE* **2013**, *8*, e64888. [CrossRef]

31. Metzler, B.; Wraith, D.C. Inhibition of experimental autoimmune encephalomyelitis by inhalation but not oral administration of the encephalitogenic peptide: Influence of mhc binding affinity. *Int. Immunol.* **1993**, *5*, 1159–1165. [CrossRef] [PubMed]

32. Tselios, T.; Aggelidakis, M.; Tapeinou, A.; Tseveleki, V.; Kanistras, I.; Gatos, D.; Matsoukas, J. Rational design and synthesis of altered peptide ligands based on human myelin oligodendrocyte glycoprotein 35–55 epitope: Inhibition of chronic experimental autoimmune encephalomyelitis in mice. *Molecules* **2014**, *19*, 17968–17984. [CrossRef] [PubMed]

33. Yeste, A.; Nadeau, M.; Burns, E.J.; Weiner, H.L.; Quintana, F.J. Nanoparticle-mediated codelivery of myelin antigen and a tolerogenic small molecule suppresses experimental autoimmune encephalomyelitis. *Proc. Natl. Acad. Sci. USA* **2012**, *109*, 11270–11275. [CrossRef] [PubMed]

34. Nicholson, L.B.; Greer, J.M.; Sobel, R.A.; Lees, M.B.; Kuchroo, V.K. An altered peptide ligand mediates immune deviation and prevents autoimmune encephalomyelitis. *Immunity* **1995**, *3*, 397–405. [CrossRef]

35. Kuchroo, V.K.; Greer, J.M.; Kaul, D.; Ishioka, G.; Franco, A.; Sette, A.; Sobel, R.A.; Lees, M.B. A single tcr antagonist peptide inhibits experimental allergic encephalomyelitis mediated by a diverse t cell repertoire. *J. Immunol.* **1994**, *153*, 3326–3336.

36. Walczak, A.; Siger, M.; Ciach, A.; Szczepanik, M.; Selmaj, K. Transdermal application of myelin peptides in multiple sclerosis treatment. *JAMA Neurol.* **2013**, *70*, 1105–1109. [CrossRef]

37. Jurynczyk, M.; Walczak, A.; Jurewicz, A.; Jesionek-Kupnicka, D.; Szczepanik, M.; Selmaj, K. Immune regulation of multiple sclerosis by transdermally applied myelin peptides. *Ann. Neurol.* **2010**, *68*, 593–601. [CrossRef]

38. Chataway, J.; Martin, K.; Barrell, K.; Sharrack, B.; Stolt, P.; Wraith, D.C. Effects of atx-ms-1467 immunotherapy over 16 weeks in relapsing multiple sclerosis. *Neurology* **2018**, *90*, e955–e962. [CrossRef]

39. Crowe, P.D.; Qin, Y.; Conlon, P.J.; Antel, J.P. Nbi-5788, an altered mbp83–99 peptide, induces a t-helper 2-like immune response in multiple sclerosis patients. *Ann. Neurol.* **2000**, *48*, 758–765. [CrossRef]

40. Lomakin, Y.; Belogurov, A., Jr.; Glagoleva, I.; Stepanov, A.; Zakharov, K.; Okunola, J.; Smirnov, I.; Genkin, D.; Gabibov, A. Administration of myelin basic protein peptides encapsulated in mannosylated liposomes normalizes level of serum tnf-alpha and il-2 and chemoattractants ccl2 and ccl4 in multiple sclerosis patients. *Mediat. Inflamm.* **2016**, *2016*, 2847232. [CrossRef]

41. Lutterotti, A.; Yousef, S.; Sputtek, A.; Sturner, K.H.; Stellmann, J.P.; Breiden, P.; Reinhardt, S.; Schulze, C.; Bester, M.; Heesen, C.; et al. Antigen-specific tolerance by autologous myelin peptide-coupled cells: A phase 1 trial in multiple sclerosis. *Sci. Transl. Med.* **2013**, *5*, 188ra175. [CrossRef] [PubMed]

42. Kappos, L.; Comi, G.; Panitch, H.; Oger, J.; Antel, J.; Conlon, P.; Steinman, L. Induction of a non-encephalitogenic type 2 t helper-cell autoimmune response in multiple sclerosis after administration of an altered peptide ligand in a placebo-controlled, randomized phase ii trial. The altered peptide ligand in relapsing ms study group. *Nat. Med.* **2000**, *6*, 1176–1182. [CrossRef] [PubMed]

43. Smith, C.E.; Eagar, T.N.; Strominger, J.L.; Miller, S.D. Differential induction of ige-mediated anaphylaxis after soluble vs. Cell-bound tolerogenic peptide therapy of autoimmune encephalomyelitis. *Proc. Natl. Acad. Sci. USA* **2005**, *102*, 9595–9600. [CrossRef]

44. Warren, K.G.; Catz, I.; Wucherpfennig, K.W. Tolerance induction to myelin basic protein by intravenous synthetic peptides containing epitope p85 vvhffkniivtp96 in chronic progressive multiple sclerosis. *J. Neurol. Sci.* **1997**, *152*, 31–38. [CrossRef]

45. Weiner, H.L.; Mackin, G.A.; Matsui, M.; Orav, E.J.; Khoury, S.J.; Dawson, D.M.; Hafler, D.A. Double-blind pilot trial of oral tolerization with myelin antigens in multiple sclerosis. *Science* **1993**, *259*, 1321–1324. [CrossRef]

46. Fissolo, N.; Montalban, X.; Comabella, M. DNA-based vaccines for multiple sclerosis: Current status and future directions. *Clin. Immunol.* **2012**, *142*, 76–83. [CrossRef]

47. Stuve, O.; Cravens, P.D.; Eagar, T.N. DNA-based vaccines: The future of multiple sclerosis therapy? *Expert Rev. Neurother.* **2008**, *8*, 351–360. [CrossRef]

48. Garren, H.; Robinson, W.H.; Krasulova, E.; Havrdova, E.; Nadj, C.; Selmaj, K.; Losy, J.; Nadj, I.; Radue, E.W.; Kidd, B.A.; et al. Phase 2 trial of a DNA vaccine encoding myelin basic protein for multiple sclerosis. *Ann. Neurol.* **2008**, *63*, 611–620. [CrossRef]

49. Bar-Or, A.; Vollmer, T.; Antel, J.; Arnold, D.L.; Bodner, C.A.; Campagnolo, D.; Gianettoni, J.; Jalili, F.; Kachuck, N.; Lapierre, Y.; et al. Induction of antigen-specific tolerance in multiple sclerosis after immunization with DNA encoding myelin basic protein in a randomized, placebo-controlled phase 1/2 trial. *Arch. Neurol.* **2007**, *64*, 1407–1415. [CrossRef]

50. Friese, M.A.; Schattling, B.; Fugger, L. Mechanisms of neurodegeneration and axonal dysfunction in multiple sclerosis. *Nat. Rev. Neurol.* **2014**, *10*, 225–238. [CrossRef]

51. Zhang, J.; Raus, J. T cell vaccination in multiple sclerosis: Hopes and facts. *Acta Neurol. Belg.* **1994**, *94*, 112–115.

52. Medaer, R.; Stinissen, P.; Truyen, L.; Raus, J.; Zhang, J. Depletion of myelin-basic-protein autoreactive t cells by t-cell vaccination: Pilot trial in multiple sclerosis. *Lancet* **1995**, *346*, 807–808. [CrossRef]

53. Zhang, J.Z.; Rivera, V.M.; Tejada-Simon, M.V.; Yang, D.; Hong, J.; Li, S.; Haykal, H.; Killian, J.; Zang, Y.C. T cell vaccination in multiple sclerosis: Results of a preliminary study. *J. Neurol.* **2002**, *249*, 212–218. [CrossRef]

54. Loftus, B.; Newsom, B.; Montgomery, M.; Von Gynz-Rekowski, K.; Riser, M.; Inman, S.; Garces, P.; Rill, D.; Zhang, J.; Williams, J.C. Autologous attenuated t-cell vaccine (tovaxin) dose escalation in multiple sclerosis relapsing-remitting and secondary progressive patients nonresponsive to approved immunomodulatory therapies. *Clin. Immunol.* **2009**, *131*, 202–215. [CrossRef]

55. Achiron, A.; Lavie, G.; Kishner, I.; Stern, Y.; Sarova-Pinhas, I.; Ben-Aharon, T.; Barak, Y.; Raz, H.; Lavie, M.; Barliya, T.; et al. T cell vaccination in multiple sclerosis relapsing-remitting nonresponders patients. *Clin. Immunol.* **2004**, *113*, 155–160. [CrossRef]

56. Karussis, D.; Shor, H.; Yachnin, J.; Lanxner, N.; Amiel, M.; Baruch, K.; Keren-Zur, Y.; Haviv, O.; Filippi, M.; Petrou, P.; et al. T cell vaccination benefits relapsing progressive multiple sclerosis patients: A randomized, double-blind clinical trial. *PLoS ONE* **2012**, *7*, e50478. [CrossRef]

57. Agrawal, A.; Agrawal, S.; Gupta, S. Role of dendritic cells in inflammation and loss of tolerance in the elderly. *Front. Immunol.* **2017**, *8*, 896. [CrossRef]

58. Raker, V.K.; Domogalla, M.P.; Steinbrink, K. Tolerogenic dendritic cells for regulatory t cell induction in man. *Front. Immunol.* **2015**, *6*, 569. [CrossRef] [PubMed]

59. Lee, W.P.; Willekens, B.; Cras, P.; Goossens, H.; Martinez-Caceres, E.; Berneman, Z.N.; Cools, N. Immunomodulatory effects of 1,25-dihydroxyvitamin d3 on dendritic cells promote induction of t cell hyporesponsiveness to myelin-derived antigens. *J. Immunol. Res.* **2016**, *2016*, 5392623. [CrossRef]

60. Mansilla, M.J.; Selles-Moreno, C.; Fabregas-Puig, S.; Amoedo, J.; Navarro-Barriuso, J.; Teniente-Serra, A.; Grau-Lopez, L.; Ramo-Tello, C.; Martinez-Caceres, E.M. Beneficial effect of tolerogenic dendritic cells pulsed with mog autoantigen in experimental autoimmune encephalomyelitis. *CNS Neurosci. Ther.* **2015**, *21*, 222–230. [CrossRef]

61. Zubizarreta, I.; Florez-Grau, G.; Vila, G.; Cabezon, R.; Espana, C.; Andorra, M.; Saiz, A.; Llufriu, S.; Sepulveda, M.; Sola-Valls, N.; et al. Immune tolerance in multiple sclerosis and neuromyelitis optica with peptide-loaded tolerogenic dendritic cells in a phase 1b trial. *Proc. Natl. Acad. Sci. USA* **2019**, *116*, 8463–8470. [CrossRef] [PubMed]

62. Sewell, A.K. Why must t cells be cross-reactive? *Nat. Rev. Immunol.* **2012**, *12*, 669–677. [CrossRef] [PubMed]

63. Vandenbark, A.A.; Hashim, G.; Offner, H. Immunization with a synthetic t-cell receptor v-region peptide protects against experimental autoimmune encephalomyelitis. *Nature* **1989**, *341*, 541–544. [CrossRef] [PubMed]

64. Offner, H.; Hashim, G.A.; Vandenbark, A.A. T cell receptor peptide therapy triggers autoregulation of experimental encephalomyelitis. *Science* **1991**, *251*, 430–432. [CrossRef]

65. Bourdette, D.N.; Whitham, R.H.; Chou, Y.K.; Morrison, W.J.; Atherton, J.; Kenny, C.; Liefeld, D.; Hashim, G.A.; Offner, H.; Vandenbark, A.A. Immunity to tcr peptides in multiple sclerosis. I. Successful immunization of patients with synthetic v beta 5.2 and v beta 6.1 cdr2 peptides. *J. Immunol.* **1994**, *152*, 2510–2519.

66. Vandenbark, A.A.; Chou, Y.K.; Whitham, R.; Mass, M.; Buenafe, A.; Liefeld, D.; Kavanagh, D.; Cooper, S.; Hashim, G.A.; Offner, H. Treatment of multiple sclerosis with t-cell receptor peptides: Results of a double-blind pilot trial. *Nat. Med.* **1996**, *2*, 1109–1115. [CrossRef]

67. Vandenbark, A.A.; Culbertson, N.E.; Bartholomew, R.M.; Huan, J.; Agotsch, M.; LaTocha, D.; Yadav, V.; Mass, M.; Whitham, R.; Lovera, J.; et al. Therapeutic vaccination with a trivalent t-cell receptor (tcr) peptide vaccine restores deficient foxp3 expression and tcr recognition in subjects with multiple sclerosis. *Immunology* **2008**, *123*, 66–78. [CrossRef]

68. Gabibov, A.G.; Belogurov, A.A., Jr.; Lomakin, Y.A.; Zakharova, M.Y.; Avakyan, M.E.; Dubrovskaya, V.V.; Smirnov, I.V.; Ivanov, A.S.; Molnar, A.A.; Gurtsevitch, V.E.; et al. Combinatorial antibody library from multiple sclerosis patients reveals antibodies that cross-react with myelin basic protein and ebv antigen. *FASEB J.* **2011**, *25*, 4211–4221. [CrossRef]

69. Lambracht-Washington, D.; O'Connor, K.C.; Cameron, E.M.; Jowdry, A.; Ward, E.S.; Frohman, E.; Racke, M.K.; Monson, N.L. Antigen specificity of clonally expanded and receptor edited cerebrospinal fluid b cells from patients with relapsing remitting ms. *J. Neuroimmunol.* **2007**, *186*, 164–176. [CrossRef]

70. Yu, X.; Gilden, D.H.; Ritchie, A.M.; Burgoon, M.P.; Keays, K.M.; Owens, G.P. Specificity of recombinant antibodies generated from multiple sclerosis cerebrospinal fluid probed with a random peptide library. *J. Neuroimmunol.* **2006**, *172*, 121–131. [CrossRef]

71. Stepanov, A.V.; Belogurov, A.A., Jr.; Ponomarenko, N.A.; Stremovskiy, O.A.; Kozlov, L.V.; Bichucher, A.M.; Dmitriev, S.E.; Smirnov, I.V.; Shamborant, O.G.; Balabashin, D.S.; et al. Design of targeted b cell killing agents. *PLoS ONE* **2011**, *6*, e20991. [CrossRef]

72. Madhumathi, J.; Verma, R.S. Therapeutic targets and recent advances in protein immunotoxins. *Curr. Opin. Microbiol.* **2012**, *15*, 300–309. [CrossRef] [PubMed]

73. Voge, N.V.; Alvarez, E. Monoclonal antibodies in multiple sclerosis: Present and future. *Biomedicines* **2019**, *7*, 20. [CrossRef]

74. Wootla, B.; Watzlawik, J.O.; Stavropoulos, N.; Wittenberg, N.J.; Dasari, H.; Abdelrahim, M.A.; Henley, J.R.; Oh, S.H.; Warrington, A.E.; Rodriguez, M. Recent advances in monoclonal antibody therapies for multiple sclerosis. *Expert Opin. Biol. Ther.* **2016**, *16*, 827–839. [CrossRef]

75. Yaldizli, O.; Putzki, N. Natalizumab in the treatment of multiple sclerosis. *Ther. Adv. Neurol. Disord.* **2009**, *2*, 115–128. [CrossRef]

76. Polman, C.H.; O'Connor, P.W.; Havrdova, E.; Hutchinson, M.; Kappos, L.; Miller, D.H.; Phillips, J.T.; Lublin, F.D.; Giovannoni, G.; Wajgt, A.; et al. A randomized, placebo-controlled trial of natalizumab for relapsing multiple sclerosis. *New Engl. J. Med.* **2006**, *354*, 899–910. [CrossRef]

77. Hauser, S.L.; Waubant, E.; Arnold, D.L.; Vollmer, T.; Antel, J.; Fox, R.J.; Bar-Or, A.; Panzara, M.; Sarkar, N.; Agarwal, S.; et al. B-cell depletion with rituximab in relapsing-remitting multiple sclerosis. *New Engl. J. Med.* **2008**, *358*, 676–688. [CrossRef]

78. Hauser, S.L.; Bar-Or, A.; Comi, G.; Giovannoni, G.; Hartung, H.P.; Hemmer, B.; Lublin, F.; Montalban, X.; Rammohan, K.W.; Selmaj, K.; et al. Ocrelizumab versus interferon beta-1a in relapsing multiple sclerosis. *New Engl. J. Med.* **2017**, *376*, 221–234. [CrossRef]

79. Sorensen, P.S.; Lisby, S.; Grove, R.; Derosier, F.; Shackelford, S.; Havrdova, E.; Drulovic, J.; Filippi, M. Safety and efficacy of ofatumumab in relapsing-remitting multiple sclerosis: A phase 2 study. *Neurology* **2014**, *82*, 573–581. [CrossRef]

80. Mi, S.; Miller, R.H.; Lee, X.; Scott, M.L.; Shulag-Morskaya, S.; Shao, Z.; Chang, J.; Thill, G.; Levesque, M.; Zhang, M.; et al. Lingo-1 negatively regulates myelination by oligodendrocytes. *Nat. Neurosci.* **2005**, *8*, 745–751. [CrossRef]

81. Mellion, M.; Edwards, K.R.; Hupperts, R.; Drulović, J.; Montalban, X.; Hartung, H.P.; Brochet, B.; Calabresi, P.A.; Rudick, R.; Ibrahim, A.; et al. Efficacy results from the phase 2b synergy study: Treatment of disabling multiple sclerosis with the anti-lingo-1 monoclonal antibody opicinumab (s33.004). *Neurology* **2017**, *88* (Suppl. 16).

82. Havrdova, E.; Horakova, D.; Kovarova, I. Alemtuzumab in the treatment of multiple sclerosis: Key clinical trial results and considerations for use. *Ther. Adv. Neurol. Disord.* **2015**, *8*, 31–45. [CrossRef] [PubMed]

83. Ford, C.; Goodman, A.D.; Johnson, K.; Kachuck, N.; Lindsey, J.W.; Lisak, R.; Luzzio, C.; Myers, L.; Panitch, H.; Preiningerova, J.; et al. Continuous long-term immunomodulatory therapy in relapsing multiple sclerosis: Results from the 15-year analysis of the us prospective open-label study of glatiramer acetate. *Mult. Scler.* **2010**, *16*, 342–350. [CrossRef] [PubMed]

84. Johnson, K.P.; Brooks, B.R.; Cohen, J.A.; Ford, C.C.; Goldstein, J.; Lisak, R.P.; Myers, L.W.; Panitch, H.S.; Rose, J.W.; Schiffer, R.B. Copolymer 1 reduces relapse rate and improves disability in relapsing-remitting multiple sclerosis: Results of a phase iii multicenter, double-blind placebo-controlled trial. The copolymer 1 multiple sclerosis study group. *Neurology* **1995**, *45*, 1268–1276. [CrossRef]

85. Arnon, R.; Teitelbaum, D.; Sela, M. Suppression of experimental allergic encephalomyelitis by cop1–relevance to multiple sclerosis. *Isr. J. Med Sci.* **1989**, *25*, 686–689.

86. Racke, M.K.; Lovett-Racke, A.E. Glatiramer acetate treatment of multiple sclerosis: An immunological perspective. *J. Immunol.* **2011**, *186*, 1887–1890. [CrossRef]

87. Ponomarenko, N.A.; Durova, O.M.; Vorobiev, I.I.; Belogurov, A.A., Jr.; Kurkova, I.N.; Petrenko, A.G.; Telegin, G.B.; Suchkov, S.V.; Kiselev, S.L.; Lagarkova, M.A.; et al. Autoantibodies to myelin basic protein catalyze site-specific degradation of their antigen. *Proc. Natl. Acad. Sci. USA* **2006**, *103*, 281–286. [CrossRef]

88. Fridkis-Hareli, M.; Santambrogio, L.; Stern, J.N.; Fugger, L.; Brosnan, C.; Strominger, J.L. Novel synthetic amino acid copolymers that inhibit autoantigen-specific t cell responses and suppress experimental autoimmune encephalomyelitis. *J. Clin. Investig.* **2002**, *109*, 1635–1643. [CrossRef]

89. Salvioni, L.; Fiandra, L.; Del Curto, M.D.; Mazzucchelli, S.; Allevi, R.; Truffi, M.; Sorrentino, L.; Santini, B.; Cerea, M.; Palugan, L.; et al. Oral delivery of insulin via polyethylene imine-based nanoparticles for colonic release allows glycemic control in diabetic rats. *Pharmacol. Res.* **2016**, *110*, 122–130. [CrossRef]

90. Sajeesh, S.; Vauthier, C.; Gueutin, C.; Ponchel, G.; Sharma, C.P. Thiol functionalized polymethacrylic acid-based hydrogel microparticles for oral insulin delivery. *Acta Biomater.* **2010**, *6*, 3072–3080. [CrossRef]

91. Posgai, A.L.; Wasserfall, C.H.; Kwon, K.C.; Daniell, H.; Schatz, D.A.; Atkinson, M.A. Plant-based vaccines for oral delivery of type 1 diabetes-related autoantigens: Evaluating oral tolerance mechanisms and disease prevention in nod mice. *Sci. Rep.* **2017**, *7*, 42372. [CrossRef] [PubMed]

92. Ma, S.; Huang, Y.; Yin, Z.; Menassa, R.; Brandle, J.E.; Jevnikar, A.M. Induction of oral tolerance to prevent diabetes with transgenic plants requires glutamic acid decarboxylase (gad) and il-4. *Proc. Natl. Acad. Sci. USA* **2004**, *101*, 5680–5685. [CrossRef] [PubMed]

93. Ma, Y.; Liu, D.; Wang, D.; Wang, Y.; Fu, Q.; Fallon, J.K.; Yang, X.; He, Z.; Liu, F. Combinational delivery of hydrophobic and hydrophilic anticancer drugs in single nanoemulsions to treat mdr in cancer. *Mol. Pharm.* **2014**, *11*, 2623–2630. [CrossRef] [PubMed]

94. Pujol-Autonell, I.; Mansilla, M.J.; Rodriguez-Fernandez, S.; Cano-Sarabia, M.; Navarro-Barriuso, J.; Ampudia, R.M.; Rius, A.; Garcia-Jimeno, S.; Perna-Barrull, D.; Martinez-Caceres, E.; et al. Liposome-based immunotherapy against autoimmune diseases: Therapeutic effect on multiple sclerosis. *Nanomed. (Lond.)* **2017**, *12*, 1231–1242. [CrossRef]

95. Teixeira, M.I.; Lopes, C.M.; Amaral, M.H.; Costa, P.C. Current insights on lipid nanocarrier-assisted drug delivery in the treatment of neurodegenerative diseases. *Eur. J. Pharm. Biopharm.* **2020**, *149*, 192–217. [CrossRef]

96. Agrawal, M.; Saraf, S.; Dubey, S.K.; Puri, A.; Patel, R.J.; Ajazuddin; Ravichandiran, V.; Murty, U.S.; Alexander, A. Recent strategies and advances in the fabrication of nano lipid carriers and their application towards brain targeting. *J. Control. Release* **2020**, *321*, 372–415. [CrossRef]

97. Ebrahimimonfared, M.; Ganji, A.; Zahedi, S.; Nourbakhsh, P.; Ghasami, K.; Mosayebi, G. Characterization of regulatory t-cells in multiple sclerosis patients treated with interferon beta-1a. *CNS Neurol. Disord. Drug Targets* **2018**, *17*, 113–118. [CrossRef]

98. Fernandez, O.; Arbizu, T.; Izquierdo, G.; Martinez-Yelamos, A.; Gata, J.M.; Luque, G.; de Ramon, E. Clinical benefits of interferon beta-1a in relapsing-remitting ms: A phase iv study. *Acta Neurol. Scand.* **2003**, *107*, 7–11. [CrossRef]

99. The IFNB multiple sclerosis study group. Interferon beta-1b is effective in relapsing-remitting multiple sclerosis, I. Clinical results of a multicenter, randomized, double-blind, placebo-controlled trial. *Neurology* **1993**, *43*, 655–661. [CrossRef]

100. Paty, D.W.; Li, D.K.; Ubc ms/mri study group; the ifnb multiple sclerosis study group. Interferon beta-1b is effective in relapsing-remitting multiple sclerosis. II. Mri analysis results of a multicenter, randomized, double-blind, placebo-controlled trial. *Neurology* **1993**, *43*, 662–667. [CrossRef]

101. Belogurov, A., Jr.; Zakharov, K.; Lomakin, Y.; Surkov, K.; Avtushenko, S.; Kruglyakov, P.; Smirnov, I.; Makshakov, G.; Lockshin, C.; Gregoriadis, G.; et al. Cd206-targeted liposomal myelin basic protein peptides in patients with multiple sclerosis resistant to first-line disease-modifying therapies: A first-in-human, proof-of-concept dose-escalation study. *Neurotherapeutics* **2016**, *13*, 895–904. [CrossRef]

102. De Souza, A.L.S.; Rudin, S.; Chang, R.; Mitchell, K.; Crandall, T.; Huang, S.; Choi, J.K.; Okitsu, S.L.; Graham, D.L.; Tomkinson, B.; et al. Atx-ms-1467 induces long-term tolerance to myelin basic protein in (dr2 x ob1)f1 mice by induction of il-10-secreting itregs. *Neurol. Ther.* **2018**, *7*, 103–128. [CrossRef] [PubMed]

103. Vandenbark, A.A. Tcr peptide vaccination in multiple sclerosis: Boosting a deficient natural regulatory network that may involve tcr-specific cd4+cd25+ treg cells. *Curr. Drug Targets. Inflamm. Allergy* **2005**, *4*, 217–229. [CrossRef]

104. Rorsman, I.; Petersen, C.; Nilsson, P.C. Cognitive functioning following one-year natalizumab treatment: A non-randomized clinical trial. *Acta Neurol. Scand.* **2018**, *137*, 117–124. [CrossRef]

105. Perumal, J.; Fox, R.J.; Balabanov, R.; Balcer, L.J.; Galetta, S.; Makh, S.; Santra, S.; Hotermans, C.; Lee, L. Outcomes of natalizumab treatment within 3 years of relapsing-remitting multiple sclerosis diagnosis: A prespecified 2-year interim analysis of strive. *BMC Neurol.* **2019**, *19*, 116. [CrossRef]

106. Kapoor, R.; Ho, P.R.; Campbell, N.; Chang, I.; Deykin, A.; Forrestal, F.; Lucas, N.; Yu, B.; Arnold, D.L.; Freedman, M.S.; et al. Effect of natalizumab on disease progression in secondary progressive multiple sclerosis (ascend): A phase 3, randomised, double-blind, placebo-controlled trial with an open-label extension. *Lancet. Neurol.* **2018**, *17*, 405–415. [CrossRef]

107. Ranger, A.; Ray, S.; Szak, S.; Dearth, A.; Allaire, N.; Murray, R.; Gardner, R.; Cadavid, D.; Mi, S. Anti-lingo-1 has no detectable immunomodulatory effects in preclinical and phase 1 studies. *Neurol. (R) Neuroimmunol. Neuroinflammation* **2018**, *5*, e417. [CrossRef] [PubMed]

108. Coles, A.J.; Twyman, C.L.; Arnold, D.L.; Cohen, J.A.; Confavreux, C.; Fox, E.J.; Hartung, H.P.; Havrdova, E.; Selmaj, K.W.; Weiner, H.L.; et al. Alemtuzumab for patients with relapsing multiple sclerosis after disease-modifying therapy: A randomised controlled phase 3 trial. *Lancet* **2012**, *380*, 1829–1839. [CrossRef]

109. Bar-Or, A.; Grove, R.A.; Austin, D.J.; Tolson, J.M.; VanMeter, S.A.; Lewis, E.W.; Derosier, F.J.; Lopez, M.C.; Kavanagh, S.T.; Miller, A.E.; et al. Subcutaneous ofatumumab in patients with relapsing-remitting multiple sclerosis: The mirror study. *Neurology* **2018**, *90*, e1805–e1814. [CrossRef]

110. Bhargava, P.; Wicken, C.; Smith, M.D.; Strowd, R.E.; Cortese, I.; Reich, D.S.; Calabresi, P.A.; Mowry, E.M. Trial of intrathecal rituximab in progressive multiple sclerosis patients with evidence of leptomeningeal contrast enhancement. *Mult. Scler. Relat. Disord.* **2019**, *30*, 136–140. [CrossRef]

111. Salzer, J.; Svenningsson, R.; Alping, P.; Novakova, L.; Bjorck, A.; Fink, K.; Islam-Jakobsson, P.; Malmestrom, C.; Axelsson, M.; Vagberg, M.; et al. Rituximab in multiple sclerosis: A retrospective observational study on safety and efficacy. *Neurology* **2016**, *87*, 2074–2081. [CrossRef] [PubMed]

112. Naismith, R.T.; Piccio, L.; Lyons, J.A.; Lauber, J.; Tutlam, N.T.; Parks, B.J.; Trinkaus, K.; Song, S.K.; Cross, A.H. Rituximab add-on therapy for breakthrough relapsing multiple sclerosis: A 52-week phase ii trial. *Neurology* **2010**, *74*, 1860–1867. [CrossRef] [PubMed]

113. Bergman, J.; Burman, J.; Gilthorpe, J.D.; Zetterberg, H.; Jiltsova, E.; Bergenheim, T.; Svenningsson, A. Intrathecal treatment trial of rituximab in progressive ms: An open-label phase 1b study. *Neurology* **2018**, *91*, e1893–e1901. [CrossRef] [PubMed]

114. Hawker, K.; O'Connor, P.; Freedman, M.S.; Calabresi, P.A.; Antel, J.; Simon, J.; Hauser, S.; Waubant, E.; Vollmer, T.; Panitch, H.; et al. Rituximab in patients with primary progressive multiple sclerosis: Results of a randomized double-blind placebo-controlled multicenter trial. *Ann. Neurol.* **2009**, *66*, 460–471. [CrossRef]

115. Mayer, L.; Kappos, L.; Racke, M.K.; Rammohan, K.; Traboulsee, A.; Hauser, S.L.; Julian, L.; Kondgen, H.; Li, C.; Napieralski, J.; et al. Ocrelizumab infusion experience in patients with relapsing and primary progressive multiple sclerosis: Results from the phase 3 randomized opera i, opera ii, and oratorio studies. *Mult. Scler. Relat. Disord.* **2019**, *30*, 236–243. [CrossRef]

116. Turner, B.; Cree, B.A.C.; Kappos, L.; Montalban, X.; Papeix, C.; Wolinsky, J.S.; Buffels, R.; Fiore, D.; Garren, H.; Han, J.; et al. Ocrelizumab efficacy in subgroups of patients with relapsing multiple sclerosis. *J. Neurol.* **2019**, *266*, 1182–1193. [CrossRef]

117. Fox, E.J.; Markowitz, C.; Applebee, A.; Montalban, X.; Wolinsky, J.S.; Belachew, S.; Fiore, D.; Pei, J.; Musch, B.; Giovannoni, G. Ocrelizumab reduces progression of upper extremity impairment in patients with primary progressive multiple sclerosis: Findings from the phase iii randomized oratorio trial. *Mult. Scler.* **2018**, *24*, 1862–1870. [CrossRef]

118. Montalban, X.; Hauser, S.L.; Kappos, L.; Arnold, D.L.; Bar-Or, A.; Comi, G.; de Seze, J.; Giovannoni, G.; Hartung, H.P.; Hemmer, B.; et al. Ocrelizumab versus placebo in primary progressive multiple sclerosis. *New Engl. J. Med.* **2017**, *376*, 209–220. [CrossRef]

119. Johnson, K.P.; Brooks, B.R.; Ford, C.C.; Goodman, A.; Guarnaccia, J.; Lisak, R.P.; Myers, L.W.; Panitch, H.S.; Pruitt, A.; Rose, J.W.; et al. Sustained clinical benefits of glatiramer acetate in relapsing multiple sclerosis patients observed for 6 years. Copolymer 1 multiple sclerosis study group. *Mult. Scler.* **2000**, *6*, 255–266. [CrossRef]

120. Ouspid, E.; Razazian, N.; Moghadasi, A.N.; Moradian, N.; Afshari, D.; Bostani, A.; Sariaslani, P.; Ansarian, A. Clinical effectiveness and safety of fingolimod in relapsing remitting multiple sclerosis in western iran. *Neurosciences (Riyadh)* **2018**, *23*, 129–134. [CrossRef]

121. Ntranos, A.; Hall, O.; Robinson, D.P.; Grishkan, I.V.; Schott, J.T.; Tosi, D.M.; Klein, S.L.; Calabresi, P.A.; Gocke, A.R. Fty720 impairs cd8 t-cell function independently of the sphingosine-1-phosphate pathway. *J. Neuroimmunol.* **2014**, *270*, 13–21. [CrossRef] [PubMed]

122. Coyle, P.K.; Khatri, B.; Edwards, K.R.; Meca-Lallana, J.E.; Cavalier, S.; Rufi, P.; Benamor, M.; Poole, E.M.; Robinson, M.; Gold, R. Teriflunomide real-world evidence: Global differences in the phase 4 teri-pro study. *Mult. Scler. Relat. Disord.* **2019**, *31*, 157–164. [CrossRef] [PubMed]

123. Miller, A.E.; Xu, X.; Macdonell, R.; Vucic, S.; Truffinet, P.; Benamor, M.; Thangavelu, K.; Freedman, M.S. Efficacy and safety of teriflunomide in asian patients with relapsing forms of multiple sclerosis: A subgroup analysis of the phase 3 tower study. *J. Clin. Neurosci.* **2019**, *59*, 229–231. [CrossRef] [PubMed]

124. Freedman, M.S.; Wolinsky, J.S.; Comi, G.; Kappos, L.; Olsson, T.P.; Miller, A.E.; Thangavelu, K.; Benamor, M.; Truffinet, P.; O'Connor, P.W. The efficacy of teriflunomide in patients who received prior disease-modifying treatments: Subgroup analyses of the teriflunomide phase 3 temso and tower studies. *Mult. Scler.* **2018**, *24*, 535–539. [CrossRef]

125. Saida, T.; Yamamura, T.; Kondo, T.; Yun, J.; Yang, M.; Li, J.; Mahadavan, L.; Zhu, B.; Sheikh, S.I. A randomized placebo-controlled trial of delayed-release dimethyl fumarate in patients with relapsing-remitting multiple sclerosis from east asia and other countries. *BMC Neurol.* **2019**, *19*, 5. [CrossRef]

126. Berger, T.; Brochet, B.; Brambilla, L.; Giacomini, P.S.; Montalban, X.; Vasco Salgado, A.; Su, R.; Bretagne, A. Effectiveness of delayed-release dimethyl fumarate on patient-reported outcomes and clinical measures in patients with relapsing-remitting multiple sclerosis in a real-world clinical setting: Protec. *Mult. Scler. J. Exp. Transl. Clin.* **2019**, *5*, 2055217319887191. [CrossRef]

127. Rivera, V.M.; Jeffery, D.R.; Weinstock-Guttman, B.; Bock, D.; Dangond, F. Results from the 5-year, phase iv renew (registry to evaluate novantrone effects in worsening multiple sclerosis) study. *BMC Neurol.* **2013**, *13*, 80. [CrossRef]

128. Hirsch, D.L.; Ponda, P. Antigen-based immunotherapy for autoimmune disease: Current status. *Immunotargets Ther.* **2015**, *4*, 1–11. [CrossRef]

129. Chiba, K.; Yanagawa, Y.; Masubuchi, Y.; Kataoka, H.; Kawaguchi, T.; Ohtsuki, M.; Hoshino, Y. Fty720, a novel immunosuppressant, induces sequestration of circulating mature lymphocytes by acceleration of lymphocyte homing in rats. I. Fty720 selectively decreases the number of circulating mature lymphocytes by acceleration of lymphocyte homing. *J. Immunol.* **1998**, *160*, 5037–5044.

130. Claussen, M.C.; Korn, T. Immune mechanisms of new therapeutic strategies in ms: Teriflunomide. *Clin. Immunol.* **2012**, *142*, 49–56. [CrossRef]

131. Fox, E.J. Mechanism of action of mitoxantrone. *Neurology* **2004**, *63*, S15–S18. [CrossRef] [PubMed]

132. Linker, R.A.; Gold, R. Dimethyl fumarate for treatment of multiple sclerosis: Mechanism of action, effectiveness, and side effects. *Curr. Neurol. Neurosci. Rep.* **2013**, *13*, 394. [CrossRef] [PubMed]

133. Lim, S.; Kim, W.J.; Kim, Y.H.; Lee, S.; Koo, J.H.; Lee, J.A.; Yoon, H.; Kim, D.H.; Park, H.J.; Kim, H.M.; et al. Dnp2 is a blood-brain barrier-permeable peptide enabling ctctla-4 protein delivery to ameliorate experimental autoimmune encephalomyelitis. *Nat. Commun.* **2015**, *6*, 8244. [CrossRef]

134. Koo, J.H.; Kim, D.H.; Cha, D.; Kang, M.J.; Choi, J.M. Lrr domain of nlrx1 protein delivery by dnp2 inhibits t cell functions and alleviates autoimmune encephalomyelitis. *Theranostics* **2020**, *10*, 3138–3150. [CrossRef] [PubMed]

135. Acharya, B.; Meka, R.R.; Venkatesha, S.H.; Lees, J.R.; Teesalu, T.; Moudgil, K.D. A novel cns-homing peptide for targeting neuroinflammatory lesions in experimental autoimmune encephalomyelitis. *Mol. Cell. Probes* **2020**, *51*, 101530. [CrossRef] [PubMed]

136. Sanadgol, N.; Barati, M.; Houshmand, F.; Hassani, S.; Clarner, T.; Shahlaei, M.; Golab, F. Metformin accelerates myelin recovery and ameliorates behavioral deficits in the animal model of multiple sclerosis via adjustment of ampk/nrf2/mtor signaling and maintenance of endogenous oligodendrogenesis during brain self-repairing period. *Pharmacol. Rep.* **2019**. [CrossRef]

137. Harada, M.; Kamimura, D.; Arima, Y.; Kohsaka, H.; Nakatsuji, Y.; Nishida, M.; Atsumi, T.; Meng, J.; Bando, H.; Singh, R.; et al. Temporal expression of growth factors triggered by epiregulin regulates inflammation development. *J. Immunol.* **2015**, *194*, 1039–1046. [CrossRef]

138. Severa, M.; Zhang, J.; Giacomini, E.; Rizzo, F.; Etna, M.P.; Cruciani, M.; Garaci, E.; Chopp, M.; Coccia, E.M. Thymosins in multiple sclerosis and its experimental models: Moving from basic to clinical application. *Mult. Scler. Relat. Disord.* **2019**, *27*, 52–60. [CrossRef]

10

Multiple Sclerosis: A Global Concern with Multiple Challenges in an Era of Advanced Therapeutic Complex Molecules and Biological Medicines

Victor M. Rivera

Department of Neurology, Baylor College of Medicine, Houston, TX 77030, USA; vrivera@bcm.edu;

Abstract: Multiple sclerosis (MS) has become a common neurological disorder involving populations previously considered to be infrequently affected. Genetic dissemination from high- to low-risk groups is a determining influence interacting with environmental and epigenetic factors, mostly unidentified. Disease modifying therapies (DMT) are effective in treating relapsing MS in variable degrees; one agent is approved for primary progressive disease, and several are in development. In the era of high-efficacy medications, complex molecules, and monoclonal antibodies (MAB), including anti-VLA4 (natalizumab), anti-CD52 (alemtuzumab), and anti-CD20 (ocrelizumab), obtaining NEDA (no evidence of disease activity) becomes an elusive accomplishment in areas of the world where access to MS therapies and care are generally limited. Countries' income and access to public MS care appear to be a shared socioeconomic challenge. This disparity is also notable in the utilization of diagnostic tools to adhere to the proposed elements of the McDonald Criteria. The impact of follow-on medications ("generics"); injectable non-biological complex drugs (NBCD), oral sphingosine-1-phosphate receptor modulators, and biosimilars (interferon 1-a and 1-b), utilized in many areas of the world, is disconcerting considering these products generally lack data documenting their efficacy and safety. Potential strategies addressing these concerns are discussed from an international point of view.

Keywords: multiple sclerosis; genetics; disease modifying therapies; generic medicines

---

1. Introduction

Multiple sclerosis (MS) is an inflammatory and demyelinating disease that manifests pathologically and clinically after the disruption of the dynamic equilibrium of brain plasticity enables the development of a chronic process affecting the central nervous system (CNS). Common association with comorbidities impacts the course of disease and quality of life of the individual. MS derives from a complex multifactorial etiological process where genetic and environmental agents decisively interact. Neuroinflammation associated to MS results in a constellation of clinical manifestations as well as mood disorders, depression, and anxiety in a large proportion of patients [1]. Persistent inflammation is also one of the causes of chronicity of disease and phenotype definition [2]. The disease may become neurodegenerative, progressive, and incapacitating in almost of half of the untreated population [3]. This outcome has been improved by early and effective use of disease modifying therapies (DMT [4]. The disease commonly affects white Caucasians, particularly people of Northern European ancestry and their descendants living in recognized high-risk areas of the world: Scandinavia and the British Islands, Canada, the U.S., Australia, and New Zealand. Nevertheless, MS is increasingly identified among populations who were considered uncommonly affected by the disease. This phenomenon is generally attributed to genetic dissemination from high- to low-risk groups owing to historical and political events favoring racial intermixing. This situation has apparently contributed to the increasing frequency of the disease among Latin American Mestizos and African Americans [5]. Similar observations apply to Māori people in New Zealand, whose present genetic make-up is described as of both European and aboriginal descent [6]. Higher MS frequency rates have been reported recently in Middle Eastern and North African countries [7,8], while in other areas of the world (Asia, South America), serial epidemiologic studies reveal a true augmentation in regional rates occurring over short periods of time [9,10]. Other factors contributing to the globalization of MS are exposure to changing environmental factors, improved medical education on the disease, increasing availability of neurologists in most areas the world, as well as magnetic resonance imaging (MRI) machines, and widespread public awareness, including locally developed patient support groups and coordinated international advocacy groups like the MS International Federation (MSIF, London).

The increasing presence of MS has resulted in serious challenges to providing adequate care and accessibility to therapies. The socioeconomic challenges posed by MS as a universal disease are emphasized in countries with economies in development, but it is also an important consideration in industrialized countries that theoretically have more advanced health systems.

From initial diagnosis to long-term management, MS is a very onerous and complicated medical condition. The disease exerts a substantial economic impact on health systems, particularly where therapeutic availability is compromised by technological limitations to fulfilling all necessary elements for diagnosis proposed by modern criteria. The impact of follow-on "generic" and biosimilar medications in some areas of the world deserves discussion in view of the lack of data substantiating their efficacy and safety profiles. These preoccupations are enhanced in many areas of the world where limited capabilities exist affecting their local licensing agencies in their ability to provide an objective, analytical, and educated approval process for complex therapeutic molecules.

This commentary addresses the concerns derived from the expanding global presence of MS, the unexpected consequences of the socioeconomic burden to MS communities, and the impact exerted in the different aspects of the disease, from adequate application of the elements of the current diagnostic criteria to access to care. Potential alleviating strategies are discussed.

2. The Global Emergence of MS

Following Jean Martin Charcot's papers on his lessons on "La Sclèrose en Plaque Disseminées" in 1868 [11], scholars in France and Europe utilized the modified denomination "Insular sclerosis of the Brain and Spinal Cord". The term "The Multiple Scleroses (as utilized in the paper) was first employed by the Philadelphia botanist Horatio Curtis Wood in 1878 [12] and adopted internationally since then as multiple sclerosis. For decades, European and American clinicians considered it as a "new" but rare neurological disease studied merely in the U.S. and Western Europe. The perception that MS was minimally or non-existent in places with non-Caucasian populations was reinforced by the 1970 observation from Alter and Olivares [13] on the prevalence in Mexico as "one of the lowest in the world" (1.6/100,000). During the last part of the 20th century and the first decades of the current epoch, epidemiologic studies have shown a notable increase in prevalence in Latin American countries [14], including Mexico [15], and the Middle East [16], while frequencies remain elevated in North America and some European countries. On the American continent, the increasing presence of the disease is now evident in populations that were hypothetically "resistant" to the disease. For five centuries, historical, sociopolitical, and migratory events favored the introduction of the European genetic risk into Native Americans (or Amerindians) and into Central and West African groups brought to the continent between the 16th and 19th centuries, resulting in the modern emergence of MS among the Latin American populations [17]. Mestizo groups constitute the most representative ethnic group in Latin America and form the largest minority in the U.S. ("Hispanics"). Studies consistently show these groups carry the inherited MS genetic European signature: HLA-DRB1*1501 [18,19]. On the other hand, the disease is rare, or practically non-existent, among non-mixed Amerindians [20]. The most plausible explanation for this phenomenon lies in the fact that Native Americans (across the continent) possess a predominantly Asian genetic makeup probably owed to the early peopling of the Americas.

Low prevalence continues to be reported among Chinese communities (5.2/100,000) [21], in Japan (3.9/100,000), and in Korea (3.5/100,000) [22,23]. Contrarily, Western Siberian populations have increased their prevalence in the last thirty years from 24 to 54/100,000 [24]. It is noted the Western Siberian MS patients are practically of European origin (white Caucasians). The disease however remains unreported among Yakuts and smaller Asiatic tribes [25]. At present, the MS prevalence in the Russian Federation is at a medium risk level (30–70/100,000) [26].

Despite epidemiologic methodological inconsistencies in acquiring data in the Middle East and nearby areas, current information shows frequencies fluctuating from low to high prevalence in this region [27]. Substantial MS prevalence has been noted in some countries, i.e., the United Arab Emirates 64.4/100,000 [28] and Iran 101.13/100,000 [29]. Observations in Kuwait show Palestinian emigres have a higher prevalence (23.8/100,000) in comparison to local Kuwaitis (9.5/100,000) [30]. Qatar reports a high MS concentration (64.57/100,000), also contributed in part by a large immigrant working force [31].

The highest prevalence rates are reported from the Scottish Northern Isles: the Orkney (402/100,000) and Shetland Islands (295/100,000) [32]. Prevalence in mainland Scotland is very high as well: 229/100,000 [33]. Canada claims the highest national prevalence at 290/100,000 [34]. The prevalence in U.S. has been reported with varying rates: 110 to 192.1/100,000, from the Eastern and Western census, respectively [35]. The majority of global MS epidemiologic studies address prevalence whilst international incidence studies are scarce. Nevertheless, the MS world map exhibits frequent and dynamic changes as more epidemiologic data accumulates from the different regions of the globe.

3. Ubiquitous Application of MS Diagnostic Criteria

The criteria for diagnosing MS have evolved along with advances in knowledge of the disease. The process of diagnosing MS following an initial clinical event, or clinically isolated syndrome (CIS) suggestive of an inflammatory/demyelinating lesion, or lesions, in the CNS, has become more sophisticated, while concomitantly, the international panel authorizing the criteria strive for simplicity and general accessibility of the proposed guidelines. The 2017 McDonald Criteria [36] was designed to serve as a more accessible tool for practitioners and researchers for reaching a faster and more definite MS diagnosis. The criteria aim to increase sensitivity without affecting specificity, reducing the possibility of misdiagnosis, and adding novel aspects in its structure, like the inclusion of symptomatic and asymptomatic lesions, as well as cortical signals detected by MRI, to comply with the concepts of lesions disseminated in space (DIS). Another original addition introduced by the 2017 McDonald international panel is utilizing the presence of unique cerebrospinal fluid (CSF) oligoclonal bands substituting for dissemination in time (DIT) in cases lacking MRI asymptomatic post-gadolinium T1 enhancing images. Assessment of optic pathology, although important, is not included within the current stipulations of the 2017 McDonald Criteria.

Factors affecting realistic applicability of the criteria in all areas of the world are related to limited access to diagnostic technology or to economic constraints. The MSIF reports an increasing trend in the number of MRI machines in emerging countries, almost doubling in a five-year period. Still, 87% of low-income countries [37] do not use the McDonald Criteria reporting criteria, instead utilizing the outdated Poser criteria (1983) [38] which does not require MR imaging for the clinical diagnosis of MS. Another aspect determining effective universal applicability of the criteria is the fact that the most sensitive and recommended methodology for CSF oligoclonal bands analysis, isoelectric focusing immunoblotting [36], is not readily available through local clinical laboratories in countries with developing economies. This technique requires special equipment and expertise to perform the analysis. The older techniques, i.e., agarose gel electrophoresis, are less sensitive and carry substantial risk of providing false-positive results. Many neurological communities in regions facing this dilemma have opted to omit CSF analysis in the diagnostic workup of suspected MS.

The McDonald Criteria panel recognizes that the proposed elements for diagnosis have been acquired from large populations of Western European genetic origins presenting with typical CIS (the initial MS clinical event). The panel emphasizes the need to validate the criteria, either prospectively or retrospectively, in diverse populations, namely in patients from Asia, Latin America, the Middle East, Africa, and other relatively less studied geographical locations. Recent discussions at the Foro Centroamericano y del Caribe para Esclerosis Múltiple (FOCEM) [39] addressed the difficulties in fulfilling the diagnostic criteria in some areas of the world. FOCEM is constituted of neurologists from the six Central American nations, Venezuela, and 26 Caribbean island countries. Most neurological services in these countries have access to MRI, and mostly to 1.5 Tesla equipment; however, practically none of these diagnosticians possess reliable CSF analysis technology to locally perform complimentary analyses. The risk of underdiagnosing in areas of the world where these limitations exist is a realistic concern [40].

It is expected that future availability of economic serological biomarkers will considerably alleviate the diagnostic restrictions existing for MS in some areas of the world.

4. Global MS Care Disparities

MS therapies have flourished in the last three decades whilst becoming more complicated and onerous. The advent of what are recognized as high-efficacy medications applies mostly to DMT for relapsing MS (RMS), with thus far only one MAB approved for primary progressive MS (PPMS). These medications have a greater pharmacological effect than the original first-line, platform, injectable therapies (interferons and glatiramer acetate). International licensing agencies, satisfying an unmet therapeutic need, have approved ocrelizumab, a CD20 cytolytic MAB targeting B lymphocytes, for treatment of PPMS. Several clinical trials are being carried out addressing progressive forms including secondary progressive MS (SPMS). However, making these pharmacological agents accessible to all MS populations is a formidable challenge and realistic socioeconomic preoccupation. Except for the private health enterprise sector of the U.S., most countries of the world rely almost entirely on their official health systems to provide access to MS therapies. For most of the 101 countries that provided data to the MSIF, therapies were partially or fully funded by the government. In the countries affiliated to the MSIF, health services funded by taxation through social security or mandated health insurance covered 76% of the cost of DMT. Global availability of MS medications is notably dissimilar between high-, upper middle-, lower middle- and low-income countries, as described in the Atlas of MS (World Health Organization/MSIF) [41]. The higher the national income, the more availability of medications—not just platform injectable medications, but oral agents and intravenous MAB, as well. Most countries with the lowest national incomes may have access to only one or two first-line DMT. For instance, in Cuba, the only DMT available is the brand Interferon beta 1-a, 44 mcg (Rebif®) [42]; in the Republic of Salvador, the national social security system offers only two medications, both innovators, including a low-dose (Avonex®, 30 mcg) and a high-dose interferon beta 1-a (Rebif®, 44 mcg) [43]. Availability of DMT to MS patients in the world is reviewed in detail at the Atlas of MS 2013, with data provided by the World Bank and the World Health Organization [44]. Availability of medications for all people with MS is not a reality for at least 90 countries of the world. The MSIF document indicates that affordability was ranked as the most common cause of lack of access to therapy in 46% of countries, which rises to 86% in 21 low- and lower-middle-income countries.

The socioeconomic impact of MS in developing countries is a considerable public health concern. These same areas usually display a low prevalence of MS; hence, the disease is not generally appreciated by their health systems. In economically emergent countries in Latin America, for instance, only 9.5% to 42.3% of the MS population have access to a DMT [45]. On the other hand, almost 90% of the economic burden exerted by MS on the country of Colombia is spent just to cover the cost of DMT [46], this cost being dependent on the grade of disability: For a patient with Expanded Disability Score Status (EDSS) 3.0-5.5, the annual cost of MS medications is 25,713 USD, while for a patient with EDSS ≥7.0 in Argentina, it is estimated at 50,712 USD. In general, the cost of DMT is less expensive in European countries and elsewhere, in comparison to the United States where, for example, an interferon for Relapsing Remitting MS (RRMS) may cost as much as 5150 USD/month, and oral fingolimod

5372 USD/month. Other tangible and intangible costs, including medical expenses, rehabilitation procedures, other multidisciplinary care required by MS, loss of work productivity, and the emotional and physical impact on the care givers, add exponentially to the price of MS. The cost increases as disability advances [47]. In many countries where access to DMT is limited, escalation to drugs with higher efficacy is not feasible; hence, the ideal goal of obtaining the therapeutic goal of 'no evidence of disease activity' (NEDA) is consequently and fundamentally challenged. Potential strategies to address these concerns would involve increasing public awareness and knowledge, which eventually should also impact health officials' education and attitudes. Transparency in the process of MS medication acquisition by national health systems would be more efficient and cost-containing by involving neurologists with MS knowledge and independently appointed public commissioners with input from patients support groups in this complex undertaking.

5. Impact of Follow-On Therapeutic Molecules and Biosimilar Medications

The appearance of "generic" medications for MS in international public and private health markets, and prescription formularies of social security programs around the world, has been increasing in development. International regulatory agencies, including the U.S. Food and Drug Administration (FDA) and the European Medicines Agency (EMA), have approved follow-on CBND replacing the innovator Copaxone®. This decision was based on bioequivalence shown by molecular and pharmacological similarity, without requiring clinical studies. Neither the FDA nor EMA have determined approval pathways for follow-on biomedicines such interferons and MAB. In both cases, appropriate phase III clinical data, and even "head-to-head" trials performed on the proposed follow-on medication set against the innovator drug as a substitute, should be required by international licensing agencies. The lack of essential clinical and pharmacological data from biosimilar medications is reflected in the fact in that most international MS associations do not include or consider them as yet in their therapeutic guidelines: These include the American Academy of Neurology, the European Academy of Neurology, the Spanish Society of Neurology, the Catalonia Society of Neurology, Consensus from Peru, Central America and Caribbean countries, among others. Some of the follow-on products manufactured in North Korea, India, Iran, Mexico, Argentina, and Uruguay (outside the sphere of the FDA and EMA), lack data on efficacy and safety of their own, in fact utilizing results obtained from the phase III pivotal trials performed by the innovator (original) products. Follow-on medications have been approved by many international licensing agencies outside the U.S. and the European Union, and are basically unchallenged due to lack of local appropriate technology and education on the subject of the responsible health departments, including the ability to evaluate the biological and immunologic behaviors of the proposed product. Substantial molecular differences have been reported [48] between follow-on and innovator interferon drugs. Analytical studies performed on the interferon 1-a innovators Avonex® (30 mcg) and Rebif® (44 mcg), both produced in the U.S., and the follow-on products Juntab® (Mexico) and CinnoVex® (Iran), both 30 mcg preparations, and the 44 mcg presentations Clausen® (Uruguay) and Blastoferon® (Argentina), these latter examples revealing considerable heterogeneity in immunochemical analyses and in "reporter gene assays" among the follow-on products but not in the brand medications. These studies also demonstrated significant pharmacological and biological potency differences between the innovators and the follow-on products [49]. Studies have consistently shown that lack of clinical data, confounded with absence of demonstration of bioequivalence and interchangeability of biosimilars, do not provide at present time evidence for their efficacy and safety. The economic impacts on individual and public health offered by the follow-on products have not been reflected in significant savings for the health systems [50]. Several international initiatives have developed, like the one promoted by the Latin American Committee for Treatment and Research in MS (LACTRIMS) [51], that encourage practitioners, MS study groups, and MS patient associations (most affiliated to the MSIF) from the region (20 countries) to coordinate with local health officials providing information and education on the licensing process, and even participating as independent advisors, striving for the proposed non-innovative follow-on medications to provide adequate clinical efficacy and safety data.

6. Conclusions

Except for rare exceptions, MS has in fact become a global disease affecting virtually every ethnic and racial group. The widespread epidemiologic presence of the disease has carried tremendous socioeconomic challenges due to the limitation of access and barriers to MS management, notably in countries still undergoing economic development. Considering that comorbidities (obesity, hyperlipidemia, migraine, rheumatological conditions) have been reported to increase the risk of relapse in MS [52], emphasis in management of these comorbidities, including a healthy diet and exercise, should be part of the management paradigm across the globe. Ensuring improved diagnosis, access to treatment, information, and available support resources require coordinated efforts from local and regional neurological MS study groups, societal MS organizations, and patient support groups. The 2017 McDonald panel recognizes this need and encourages MS diagnostic validation in non-Western European ethnicity populations (since 2000, the diverse revisions have applied practically to only Caucasian populations), and to geographic areas where the disease has a low prevalence. Revisions to the MS criteria are conducted every 5–7 years, once new or more advanced diagnostic technology and documented clinical data justify updating the diverse criteria of the proposal. It is expected the next revision will include contributions from the international committees for treatment and research in MS from all areas of the world. Tangible and indirect expenses compound the associated costs of necessary but complex multidisciplinary MS care. In this commentary, these aspects are reviewed from an international perspective while providing awareness and potential paths to alleviate these actual concerns, including addressing the concern of insufficient data on follow-on therapeutic molecules.

Author Contributions: V.M.R. designed and wrote the paper.

References

1. Rossi, S.; Studer, V.; Motta, C.; Polidoro, S.; Perugini, J.; Macchiarulo, G.; Giovannetti, A.M.; Pareja-Gutierrez, L.; Calò, A.; Colonna, I.; et al. Neuroinflammation drives anxiety and depression in relapsing-remitting multiple sclerosis. *Neurology* **2017**, *89*, 1338–1347. [CrossRef] [PubMed]
2. Isoupras, A.; Lordan, R.; Zabetakis, I. Inflammation, not Cholesterol, Is a Cause of Chronic Disease. *Nutrients* **2018**, *10*, 604. [CrossRef] [PubMed]
3. Ontaneda, D.; Thompson, A.J.; Cohen, J.A. Progressive multiple sclerosis: Prospects for disease therapy, repair, and restoration of function. *Lancet* **2017**, *389*, 1357–1366. [CrossRef]
4. Corboy, J.R.; Weinshenker, B.G.; Wingerchuk, D.M. Comment on 2018 American Academy of Neurology guidelines on disease-modifying therapies in MS. *Neurology* **2018**, *90*, 1106–1112. [CrossRef] [PubMed]
5. Rivera, V.M. Multiple Sclerosis in Latin America: Reality and challenge. *Neuroepidemiology* **2009**, *32*, 293–295. [CrossRef] [PubMed]
6. Pearson, J.F.; Alla, S.; Clarke, G.; Taylor, B.V.; Miller, D.H.; Richardson, A.; Mason, D.F. Multiple Sclerosis in New Zealand Māori. *Mult. Scler.* **2014**, *20*, 1892–1895. [CrossRef] [PubMed]
7. Heydarpour, P.; Koshkish, S.; Abtahi, S.; Moradi-Lakeh, M.; Sahraian, M.A. Multiple Sclerosis Epidemiology in Middle East and North Africa: A Systematic review and Meta-Analysis. *Neuroepidemiology* **2015**, *44*, 232–244. [CrossRef] [PubMed]
8. Stachowiak, J. Rising Multiple Sclerosis Rates in Middle East. Available online: https://www.msconnection.org/Blog/October-2015-rising-multiple-sclerosis-rates-in-Middle-East (accessed on 6 September 2018).
9. Callegaro, D.; de Lolio, C.A.; Radvany, J.; Tilbery, C.P.; Mendonça, R.A.; Melo, A.C. Prevalence of Multiple Sclerosis in the city of Sao Paulo, Brazil, in 1990. *Neuroepidemiology* **1992**, *11*, 11–14. [CrossRef] [PubMed]
10. Gonzalez, O.; Sotelo, J. Is the Frequency of Multiple Sclerosis Increasing in Mexico? *J. Neurol. Neurosurg. Psychiatry* **1995**, *59*, 528–530. [CrossRef] [PubMed]

11. Charcot, J.M. *Lectures on the Diseases of the Nervous System. Delivered at la Salpêtrière*; New Sydenham Society: London, UK, 1881; Volume II.

12. Wood, H.C., Jr. *Multiple Sclerosis: The History of a Disease*; Demos Medical Publishing: New York, NY, USA, 2005; pp. 224–250.

13. Alter, M.; Olivares, L. Multiple sclerosis in Mexico: An epidemiologic study. *Arch. Neurol.* **1970**, *23*, 451–454. [CrossRef] [PubMed]

14. Cristiano, E.; Rojas, J.; Romano, M.; Frider, N.; Machnicki, G.; Giunta, D.; Calegaro, D.; Corona, T.; Flores, J.; Gracia, F.; et al. The epidemiology of multiple sclerosis in Latin America and the Caribbean: A systematic review. *Mult. Scler.* **2013**, *19*, 844–854. [CrossRef] [PubMed]

15. De la Maza Flores, M.; Arambide Garcia, G. Prevalence of multiple sclerosis in the Municipality of San Pedro Garza García, Nuevo León (Mexico). *Avances* **2006**, *1*, 8–10.

16. Nazr, Z.; Elemadifar, M.; Khalili, B. Epidemiology of Multiple Sclerosis in the Middle East. A systematic review and meta-analysis. *Mult. Scler. Relat. Disord.* **2014**, *3*, 744. [CrossRef]

17. Gracia, F.; Castillo, L.C.; Benzadón, A.; Larreategui, M.; Villareal, F.; Triana, E.; Arango, A.C.; Lee, D.; Pascale, J.M.; Gomez, E.; et al. Prevalence and Incidence of multiple sclerosis in Panama (2000–2005). *Neuroepidemiology* **2009**, *32*, 287–293. [CrossRef] [PubMed]

18. Ordoñez, G.; Romero, S.; Orozco, L.; Pineda, B.; Jiménez-Morales, S.; Nieto, A.; García-Ortiz, H.; Sotelo, J. Genomewide admixture study in Mexican Mestizos with multiple sclerosis. *Clin. Neurol. Neurosurg.* **2015**, *130*, 55–60. [CrossRef] [PubMed]

19. Rivera, V.M. Multiple Sclerosis in Latin Americans: Genetic Aspects. *Curr. Neurol. Neurosci. Rep.* **2017**, *17*, 57–63. [CrossRef] [PubMed]

20. Flores, J.; González, S.; Morales, X.; Yescas, P.; Ochoa, A.; Corona, T. Absence of multiple sclerosis and demyelinating diseases among Lacandonians, a Pure Amerindian Ethnic Group in Mexico. *Mult. Scler. Int.* **2012**. [CrossRef] [PubMed]

21. Liu, X.; Cui, Y.; Han, J. Estimating epidemiological data of Multiple Sclerosis in hospitalized data in Shandong, Province, China. *Orphanet J. Rare Dis.* **2016**, *11*, 73. [CrossRef] [PubMed]

22. Kira, J. Multiple Sclerosis in the Japanese population. *Lancet Neurol.* **2003**, *2*, 117–127. [CrossRef]

23. Kim, N.H.; Kim, H.J.; Cheong, H.K.; Kim, B.J.; Lee, K.H.; Kim, E.-H.; Kim, E.A.; Kim, S.; Park, M.S.; Yoon, W.T.; et al. Prevalnece of multiple sclerosis in Korea. *Neurology* **2018**, *75*, 1432–1438. [CrossRef] [PubMed]

24. Boiko, A.N. Multiple sclerosis prevalence in Russia and other countries of the former USSR. In *Multiple Sclerosis In Europe: An Epidemiological Update*; Firmhaber, W., Lauer, K., Eds.; Leuchtturm: Darmstadt, Germany, 1994; pp. 219–230.

25. Malkova, N.A.; Shperling, L.P.; Riabukhina, O.V.; Merkulova, E.A. Multiple sclerosis in Eastern Siberia: A 20-year prospective study in Novosibirsk city. *Zh. Nevrol. Psikhiatr. Im. S S Korsakova* **2006**, *3*, 11–16.

26. Boyko, A.; Smirnova, N.; Petrov, S.; Gusev, E. Epidemiology of Multiple Sclerosis in Russia, a historical review. *Mult. Scler. Demyelinating Dis.* **2016**, *1*, 13. [CrossRef]

27. Mohammed, E.M.A. Multiple Sclerosis is prominent in the Gulf states: Review. *Pathogenesis* **2016**, *3*, 19–38. [CrossRef]

28. Inshasi, J.; Thakre, M. Prevalence of multiple sclerosis in Dubai, United Arab Emirates. *Int. J. Neurosci.* **2011**, *121*, 393–398. [CrossRef] [PubMed]

29. Eskandarieh, S.; Heydarpour, P.; Elhami, S.-R.; Sahralan, M.A. Prevalence and Incidence of Multiple Sclerosis in Tehran, Iran. *Iran J. Public Health* **2017**, *45*, 699–704.

30. Najim Al-Din, A.S. Multiple Sclerosis in Kuwait: Clinical and epidemiological study. *J. Neurol. Neurosurg. Psychiatry* **1986**, *49*, 928–931. [CrossRef]

31. Deleu, D.; Mir, D.; Al Tabouki, A.; Mesraoua, R.; Mesraoua, B.; Akhtar, N.; Al Hail, H.; D'souza, A.; Melikyan, G.; Imam, Y.Z.; et al. Prevalence, demographics and clinical characteristics of multiple sclerosis in Qatar. *Mult. Scler.* **2013**, *19*, 816–819. [CrossRef] [PubMed]

32. Visser, E.M.; Wilde, K.; Wilson, J.F.; Yong, K.K.; Counsell, C.E. A new prevalence study of Multiple Sclerosis in Orkney, Shetland and Aberdeen City. *J. Neurol. Neurosurg. Psychiatry* **2012**, *83*, 719–724. [CrossRef] [PubMed]

33. Prevalence and Incidence of Multiple Sclerosis in Scotland. Available online: https://www.mstrust.org.uk (accessed on 6 September 2018).

34. Multiple Sclerosis Canada. Available online: https://mssociety.ca (accessed on 6 September 2018).

35. Dilokthornsakul, O.; Valuck, R.J.; Nair, K.V.; Corboy, J.R.; Allen, R.R.; Campbell, J.D. Multiple sclerosis in the United States commercially insured population. *Neurology* **2016**, *86*, 1014–1021. [CrossRef] [PubMed]

36. Thompson, A.J.; Banwell, B.L.; Barkhof, F.; William, M.C.; Timothy, C.; Giancarlo, C.; Jorge, C.; Franz, F.; Massimo, F.; Mark, S.F.; et al. Diagnosis of multiple sclerosis: 2017 revisions of the McDonald criteria. *Lancet Neurol.* **2018**, *17*, 162–173. [CrossRef]

37. Poser, C.M.; Paty, D.W.; Scheinberg, L.; McDonald, W.I.; Davis, F.A.; Ebers, G.C.; Johnson, K.P.; Sibley, W.A.; Silberberg, D.H.; et al. New diagnostic criteria for multiple sclerosis: Guidelines for research protocols. *Ann. Neurol.* **1983**, *13*, 227–231. [CrossRef] [PubMed]

38. Fortini, A.S.; Sanders, E.L.; Weinshenker, B.G.; Katzmann, J.A. Cerebrospinal Fluid Oligoclonal Bands in the Diagnosis of Multiple Sclerosis. *Am. J. Clin. Pathol.* **2003**, *120*, 672–675. [CrossRef] [PubMed]

39. Available online: http://www.focem.org (accessed on 3 October 2018).

40. Gracia, F.; Armién, B.; Rivera, V. Collaborative Multiple Sclerosis Group of Central America and Spanish Caribbean Region. Multiple Sclerosis in Central American and Spanish Caribbean Region: Should it be Recognized as a Public Health Problem? *J. Epid. Prev. Med.* **2017**, *3*, 134.

41. Browne, P.; Chandraratna, D.; Angood, C.; Tremlett, H.; Baker, C.; Taylor, B.V.; Thompson, A.J. Atlas of Multiple Sclerosis 2013: A growing global problem with widespread inequity. *Neurology* **2014**, *83*, 1022–1024. [CrossRef] [PubMed]

42. Diaz de la Fé, A. Treatment of Multiple Sclerosis in Cuba. Centro Internacional de Rehabilitación Neurológica (CIREN): Havana, Cuba. Available online: www.ciren.cu (accessed on 4 May 2017).

43. Rivera, V.M.; Medina, M.T.; Duron, R.M. Multiple Sclerosis Care in Latin America. *Neurology* **2014**, *82*, 1660–1661. [CrossRef] [PubMed]

44. Available online: www.msif.org/wp-content/upload/2014/09/Atlas-of-MS (accessed on 3 October 2018).

45. Rivera, V.M.; Macias, M.A. Access and barriers to MS care in Latin America. *Mult. Scler. J. Exp. Transl. Clin.* **2017**, *3*. [CrossRef] [PubMed]

46. Jimenez-Pérez, C.E.; Zarco-Montero, L.A.; Castañeda-Cardona, C.; Otálora Esteban, M.; Martínez, A.; Rosselli, D. Current state of Multiple Sclerosis in Colombia. *Acta Neurol. Colomb.* **2015**, *31*, 385–390.

47. Rojas, J.L.; Patrucco, L.; Cristiano, E. Current and emerging treatments for relapsing multiple sclerosis in Argentinean patients: A review. *Deg. Neurol. Neuromusc. Dis.* **2014**, *4*, 103–109.

48. Cuevas, C.; Deisenhammer, F.; You, X.; Scolnik, M.; Buffels, R.; Sperling, B.; Flores Ramirez, F.; Macias Islas, M.; Sauri-Suárez, S. Low immunogenicity but reduced bioavailability of an interferon beta-1a biosimilar compared with its biological parent: Results of MATRIX, a cross-sectional multicenter phase 4 study. *Biosimilars* **2015**, *5*, 1–7.

49. Meager, A.; Dolman, C.; Dilger, P.; Bird, C.; Giovannoni, G.; Schellekens, H.; Thorpe, R.; Wadhwa, M. An Assessment of Biological Potency and Molecular Characteristics of Different Innovator and Noninnovator Interferon-Beta Products. *J. Interferon Cytokine Res.* **2011**, *31*, 383–392. [CrossRef] [PubMed]

50. Macias-Islas, M.A.; Soria-Cedillo, I.; Vazquez-Quintana, M.; Rivera, V.M.; Baca-Muro, V.I.; Lemus-Carmona, E.A.; Chiquete, E. Cost of care according to disease-modifying therapies in Mexicans with multiple sclerosis. *Acta Neurol. Belg.* **2013**, *113*, 415–420. [CrossRef] [PubMed]

51. Steinberg, J.; Fragoso, Y.; Garcia Bonitto, J.R.; Guerra, C.; Rodriguez, V.; Correa, P.; Macias, M.; Novarro, N.; Vizcarra, D.; Orozco, G.; et al. Practical aspects and recommendations concerning the approval and use of biosimilar drugs for the treatment of multiple sclerosis in Latin America. In Proceedings of the X Latin American Committee for Treatments and Research in MS, Asuncion, Paraguay, 22–24 November 2018. Abstract 0098.

52. Kowalek, K.; McKay, K.A.; Patten, S.B.; Fisk, J.D.; Evans, C.; Tremlett, H.; Marrie, R.A.; CIHR Team in Epidemiology and Impact of Comorbidity on Multiple Sclerosis (ECoMS). Comorbidity increases the risk of relapse in multiple sclerosis. *Neurology* **2017**, *89*, 2455–2461. [CrossRef] [PubMed]

11

The Use of Electrochemical Voltammetric Techniques and High-Pressure Liquid Chromatography to Evaluate Conjugation Efficiency of Multiple Sclerosis Peptide-Carrier Conjugates

Efstathios Deskoulidis [1], Sousana Petrouli [1], Vasso Apostolopoulos [2], John Matsoukas [2,3,4,]* and Emmanuel Topoglidis [1,*]

[1]   Materials Science Department, University of Patras, 26504 Patras, Greece; stathis.deskou@gmail.com (E.D.); sousanapetr@gmail.com (S.P.)
[2]   Institute for Health and Sport, Victoria University, Melbourne, VIC 3030, Australia; vasso.apostolopoulos@mail.com
[3]   Newdrug, Patras Science Park, 26500 Patras, Greece
[4]   Department of Physiology and Pharmacology, Cumming School of Medicine, University of Calgary, Alberta, AB T2N 4N1, Canada
*   Correspondence: imats1953@gmail.com (J.M.); etop@upatras.gr (E.T.)

Abstract: Recent studies have shown the ability of electrochemical methods to sense and determine, even at very low concentrations, the presence and quantity of molecules or analytes including pharmaceutical samples. Furthermore, analytical methods, such as high-pressure liquid chromatography (HPLC), can also detect the presence and quantity of peptides at very low concentrations, in a simple, fast, and efficient way, which allows the monitoring of conjugation reactions and its completion. Graphite/SiO$_2$ film electrodes and HPLC methods were previously shown by our group to be efficient to detect drug molecules, such as losartan. We now use these methods to detect the conjugation efficiency of a peptide from the immunogenic region of myelin oligodendrocyte to a carrier, mannan. The HPLC method furthermore confirms the stability of the peptide with time in a simple one pot procedure. Our study provides a general method to monitor, sense and detect the presence of peptides by effectively confirming the conjugation efficiency. Such methods can be used when designing conjugates as potential immunotherapeutics in the treatment of diseases, including multiple sclerosis.

Keywords: mannan; peptide; conjugation; MOG$_{35-55}$; Graphite/SiO$_2$ electrode; voltammetry; HPLC; multiple sclerosis; immunotherapy; vaccine

1. Introduction

Voltammetric techniques, including differential pulse voltammetry (DPV) and cyclic voltammetry (CV), as well as high-performance liquid chromatography (HPLC), were applied to identify and detect a peptide to its conjugated carrier. This study describes for the first time an alternative, fast, low cost and reliable method for the adequate and reliable determination of an active pharmaceutical ingredient (API) in the biocompatible matrix. The performance of the voltammetric techniques is strongly dependent on the performance of the working electrode used. Film electrodes, such as the graphite/SiO$_2$ used in this study, are being used in electrochemistry, as it has a number of advantages over the standard metallic and glass carbon electrodes. These include ease of manufacture requiring lower temperatures, low cost, the high surface area that could be rapidly renovated, simple handling, and their increased conductivity in a wide range of potentials. In addition, these techniques exhibit a wide range of anodic and cathodic peaks and great electrocatalytic activity and stability. All these features are crucial for the correct choice of a working electrode, especially when direct electrochemistry is conducted [1]. We recently demonstrated that these film electrodes modified or not, could be used for electrochemical drug sensing, for validation in food chemistry, and for the immobilization of heme proteins for studying protein/electrode interaction [2–4]. The electrochemical analytical methods were recently applied effectively in the detection of anti-hypertensive drug losartan [3] and have applied this method to detect peptides in peptide-carrier conjugates. The peptide used was the multiple sclerosis (MS) immunogenic peptide from myelin oligodendrocyte (MOG_{35-55}).

Numerous methods have been established for the analytical determination of drugs at low concentrations, using state of the art systems, such as HPLC, high-performance thin-layer chromatography and capillary electrophoresis/capillary electrochromatography [3]. Although these methods provide very accurate and reliable data, they are costly, time consuming, and involve the use of expensive equipment and consumables. In addition, sample pre-treatment is usually necessary. In this sense, electrochemical methods have emerged as low cost, reliable alternatives for the characterization of peptides and drugs. Different electrochemical techniques, involving voltammetry or potentiometry, have been implemented for drug analysis, as they offer ease of preparation and operation, high sensitivity, fast response time, high quantification and detection limits, reasonable selectivity, wide linear range, and are cost effective [3]. In this regard, we applied voltammetry techniques to monitor the conjugation of a peptide to its carrier, for the first time as a proof of concept study.

MS is regarded an autoimmune disease where immune cells (such as, Th1, Th17, macrophages, B cells) and their constituents (pro-inflammatory cytokines) are involved in the pathophysiology of the disease, with destruction of myelin sheath and loss of neurological function [5–10]. In an attempt to develop immunotherapeutics against MS using immunogenic/agonist peptides is to either alter the peptide to make it an antagonist [11–16], make it cyclic [17–19], or conjugate it to an appropriate carrier, which would deliver the peptide in such a manner to either induce tolerance, or alter the profile of T cells from pro-inflammatory (Th1) to anti-inflammatory (Th2) [13–15]. One approach which our team has developed, is to use mannan, a poly-mannose carrier conjugated to MS peptides [20–24]. This approach was developed over 25 years ago by the group of Apostolopoulos et al., to be effective in targeting peptides and proteins to dendritic cells in a number of different cancer vaccine models, some of which were translated to human clinical trials [25–32]. As such, mannan was used as a carrier and conjugated to immunodominant MS peptides including MBP_{83-99}, $PLP_{139-141}$, and MOG_{35-55} or their analogues, and were shown in animal models to tolerize T cells or switch Th1 cells to Th2 cells, depending on the peptide analogue used and showed stimulation of Th2 cells in peripheral blood mononuclear cells from patients with MS [17,21,33–35]. The conjugation of mannan, in its oxidized form (OM), to MOG_{35-55} peptide (MOG_{35-55} was used as an example in this study) via a (Lys-Gly)$_5$ linker [$(KG)_5$] was used and evaluated (OM-$(KG)_5$-MOG_{35-55} conjugate) using voltammetric techniques [1–4,36–38]. The conjugation between OM and peptide (MOG_{35-55}) occurs via formation of Schiff bases between the free amines of the linker $(KG)_5$ and aldehydes of OM. The synthesis and efficacy of these conjugates have been described in numerous studies [23,24,39,40]. However, the extent of conjugation and the redox condition of the participating sugars, such as mannan, are most times assessed by high cost, complicated and lengthy analytical methods, such as capillary electrophoresis and polyacrylamide gel electrophoresis [23,24,39,40].

Among the approaches used in recent years for the immunomodulation of MS, the conjugation of mannan with myelin peptides has shown much promise, including that of OM-$(KG)_5$-MOG_{35-55}, which induces tolerance in mice, providing a promising conjugate for further studies. The electrochemical and HPLC analysis for identification of peptides or their mutants in mannan based conjugates requires specialized techniques, which differ significantly from those methods used for small molecules. In this study, novel analytical methods were developed and applied, that clearly, sense, detect, and confirm the conjugation of OM with MOG_{35-55}. Further, this study makes it possible to accurately evaluate the stability of the peptide component in the conjugate using HPLC [41,42].

2. Materials and Methods

2.1. Materials

Sodium metasilicate (Na_2SiO_3) (SiO_2, 50–53%), NaH_2PO_4, mannan isolated from yeast cells (*Saccharomyces cerevisiae*), potassium ferricyanide, ferrocyanide, and potassium chloride were obtained from Sigma Aldrich Chemie GmbH (Taufkirchen, Germany). MOG_{35-55} and MOG_{37-55} peptides were supplied by NewDrug S.A., Patras Science Park, Greece and purchased from China peptides Inc. The peptide analogue $(Lys-Gly)_5$-MOG_{35-55}, referred as $(KG)_5$-MOG_{35-55}, was synthesized using standard peptide chemistry techniques and previously published by our group. Briefly, Fmoc/tBu methodology was used which included 2-chlorotrityl chloride resin (CLTR-Cl) and N^a-Fmoc (9-fluorenylmethyloxycarboxyl) side chain protected amino acids [43,44]. The purity of the peptides were shown to be >97% by analytical HPLC. Graphite powder (synthetic, APS 7–11 μm, 99%) was obtained from Alfa Aesar. Soda lime glass slides (75 mm × 25 mm × 1.1 mm), with 15 Ohm/sqr Indium Tin Oxide (ITO) coating were obtained from PsiOTec, UK. All chemicals were of analytical grade and used without the need for further purification. All solutions were prepared in deionized water with resistance R = 18 MΩ cm.

2.2. Graphite/SiO₂ Film Electrodes Preparation

The graphite/SiO_2 film electrodes were prepared as described [2,3]. Briefly, silicate liquid polymer (50% Na_2SiO_3; pH 12–13) was gently mixed with 20% graphite powder at 23 °C, until the mixture became homogeneous and acquired a "sticky" texture. The mixture underwent ultrasonication for 2 min for the graphite powder to be fully soluble, and 100 μL of the silicate/graphite suspension were applied on the surface of a conductive ITO glass slide using the "Doctor Blade" technique. Prior to the deposition of the silicate/graphite suspension, the ITO glass slides were cleaned in a detergent solution using an ultrasonic bath for 15 min, and then rinsed with 18 MΩ distilled water and ethanol. Each glass slide was masked with 3M Magic Scotch tape (thickness 62.5 μm; type 810), in order to control the width and the thickness of the mixture spread area. For each graphite/SiO_2 film deposition, one layer of tape was used which provided a size 1 × 1 cm^2 and film thickness of ~66 μm. The films were allowed to dry for 30 min in a class 4000 room, prior to placing them in a preheated oven (330 °C) for 100 min. If required, the liquid suspension could be stored in an insulated flask at 25 °C for later usage. The resulting ITO substrates with the deposited graphite/SiO_2 films were cut in 10 mm × 25 mm pieces before use.

2.3. Characterization of Graphite/SiO₂ Film Electrodes

Field emission scanning electron microscopy (FE-SEM) using an FEI inspect microscope (25 kV) was used to determine morphology and thickness of the Graphite/SiO_2 film. The films were prepared by AU sputtering to increase the conductivity of the samples. Energy dispersive spectroscopy EDS was also used for the elemental analysis of the Graphite/SiO_2/ITO films.

2.4. Preparation of (KG)₅-MOG₃₅₋₅₅ Peptide

MOG_{35-55} agonist peptide was synthesized in our labs, >97% purity, with $(KG)_5$ extended at the N-terminus of the peptide. Peptide was prepared using our methods, either by coupling, catalyzed by microwave radiation in a CEM Liberty microwave system or by using the conventional step by step procedure by solid phase peptide methods (as described in [45]). $(KG)_5$-MOG_{35-55} peptide was also purchased by China Peptides Inc. In house synthesized peptides and purchased peptides were confirmed by HPLC and Mass Spectroscopy for purity and identity.

2.5. Preparation of Oxidized Mannan

Mannan (14 mg) was dissolved in 1 mL phosphate buffer (0.1 M sodium phosphate, pH 6.0), and was oxidized using 0.1 M sodium periodate and incubated at 4 °C for 1 h, after which 10 μL ethanediol was added for 30 min at 4 °C. Oxidized mannan (OM) was passed through a PD-10 column (Sigma Aldrich Chemie) pre-equilibrated in sodium bicarbonate buffer (sodium carbonate: Sodium bicarbonate, pH 9.0). Two ml of OM fraction (7 mg/mL) was collected and kept in the dark.

2.6. Conjugation of Oxidized Mannan to Peptide

To the OM fraction (2 mL; 7 mg/mL, sodium bicarbonate pH 9.0 buffer), 1 mg of $(KG)_5$-MOG_{35-55} peptide was added and allowed to react overnight in the dark at 23 °C. A list of peptides and conjugates are summarized in Table 1.

Table 1. Peptides and conjugates used in this study.

Acronym	Specification
MOG_{35-55}	Myelin oligodendrocyte glycoprotein immunogenic epitope, region 35–55
MOG_{37-55}	Myelin oligodendrocyte glycoprotein immunogenic epitope, region 37–55
$(KG)_5$-MOG_{35-55}	Peptide analogue MOG_{35-55} with $(KG)_5$ at the N-terminus
OM-$(KG)_5$-MOG_{35-55}	Oxidized mannan conjugated to $(KG)_5$-MOG_{35-55}

KG, lysine glycine; MOG, myelin oligodendrocyte glycoprotein; OM, oxidized mannan.

2.7. Monitoring of Conjugation by HPLC

We used a Waters 2695 HPLC (Alliance) system with a photodiode array detector equipped with a Lichrosorb RP-18 reversed phase analytical column (C18 35 μm, 4.6 × 50 mm PIN 186003034). Analysis was achieved with stepped linear gradient of solvent A (0.08% TFA in H_2O) and in solvent B (0.08% TFA in 100% acetonitrile) for 30 min with a flow rate 3 mL/min. The conjugation of OM with $(KG)_5$-MOG_{35-55} peptide was evaluated by HPLC. The $(KG)_5$-MOG_{35-55} HPLC peak disappeared within six hours indicating completion of conjugation to OM.

2.8. Electrochemical/Electrocatalytic Measurements

Electrochemical measurements were conducted using an Autolab PGStat-101 potentiostat (Metrohm, Utrecht, The Netherlands). The electrochemical cell comprised of a 10 mL, three-electrode stirring glass cell with a Teflon cap, a platinum mesh flag as the counter electrode, a $Ag/AgCl/KCl_{sat}$ reference electrode and a Graphite/SiO_2 film on ITO conducting glass as the working electrode. The electrolyte contained a solution of NaH_2PO_4 (10 mM; pH 7.0), which was deoxygenated with argon prior to any measurements and an argon atmosphere was kept throughout the measurements. The DPV measurements took place in a potential range between −1 to +0.05 V. The optimized parameters of DPV correspond to a step potential at 5 mV, amplitude of 50 mV, modulation time of 25 ms with scan rate 100 mV s^{-1} and a frequency of 50 Hz. All potentials are reported against Ag/AgCl and all experiments were carried out at 23 °C.

3. Results and Discussion

3.1. FE-SEM Characterization

The general thickness and surface morphology of the graphite/SiO_2 films were demonstrated by FE-SEM. The top-view of the FE-SEM image (Figure 1a) shows that the surface of the graphite/SiO_2 film is rough and non-uniform with many wrinkles. It exhibits increased porosity and a high effective surface area. Figure 1b presents the cross section of a graphite/SiO_2 film electrode, with an estimated film thickness of ~65 μm as set by the adhesive tape used; the EDS for a graphite/SiO_2 film carried out during the FE-SEM analysis is shown in the Supplementary Materials (SM, Figure S1). The characteristic peaks of Na, O, and Si, due to the use of silicate glue (Na_2SiO_3), are presented in high intensity, thus, the peak of C is presented in lower intensity. Hence, the results validate the reduced concentration of carbon in the mixture used for the fabrication of the graphite/SiO_2 films.

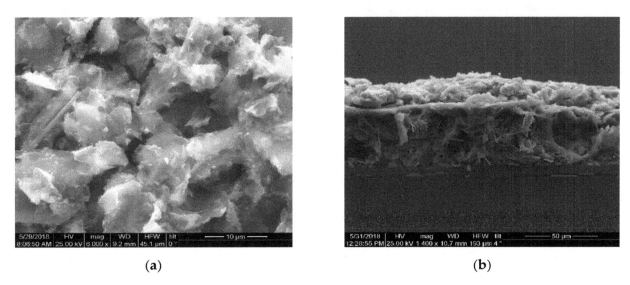

(a)　　　　　　　　　　　　　　　　　(b)

Figure 1. SEM images of the graphite/SiO_2 working electrode from (**a**) top view and (**b**) a cross section.

3.2. UV Characterazation of (KG)₅-MOG₃₅₋₅₅ Peptide with Increasing Amounts of OM

It is known that most peptides exhibit strong absorbance at around 280 nm, due to aromatic amino acids (tyrosine and tryptophan) or disulfide bonds in the peptide sequences [46,47]. Figure 2 shows the UV-vis spectra of (KG)₅-MOG₃₅₋₅₅ with increasing amounts of OM. The increase of absorbance at 280 nm confirms the conjugation of MOG₃₅₋₅₅ peptide to OM. The intensity of the absorption peak at 280 increases until all of the free peptide in solution is conjugated to the OM. It should be noted that the conjugate of (KG)₅-MOG₃₅₋₅₅ with OM took place in solution and not on the surface of the graphite/SiO_2 film electrode as due to its non-transparency it is impossible to monitor the conjugation process on its surface. All the UV-visible absorption spectra of the peptide was recorded using a Shimadzu UV-1800 spectrophotometer.

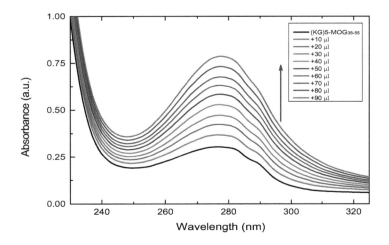

Figure 2. UV-Vis spectral changes of (KG)₅-MOG₃₅₋₅₅ in solution with increasing amounts of OM (10–90 µL).

3.3. Electrochemical Analysis Showing Conjugation of (KG)$_5$-MOG$_{35-55}$ to OM

Electrochemical characteristics of the graphite/SiO$_2$ film electrode were investigated by CV. Figure 3a shows the electrochemical behavior of a bare graphite/SiO$_2$ film electrode in a solution of 0.1 M KCl and 5 mM of [Fe(CN)$_6$]$^{3-/4-}$ through CV in the potential range of +1 to −1 V at different scan rates. Figure 3b shows the currents (anodic and cathodic) from the plots of I vs. square root of scan rate ($v^{1/2}$). Straight lines form for both the anodic and cathodic currents, confirming that a diffusional process has occurred in the reaction of ferrocyanide/ferricyanide. In addition, these results confirm that fast electron transfer occurs on the Graphite/SiO$_2$ film electrode due to its increased conductivity and surface area. In order to calculate the electroactive surface area of the film electrode, the Randles-Sevcik equation was used [36]:

$$i_p = \left(2.69 \times 10^5\right) \times A \times D^{1/2} \times n^{3/2} \times C \times v^{1/2} \tag{1}$$

where i_p corresponds to the maximum current (in Amperes), n is the number of electrons transferred ($n = 1$), D is the diffusion coefficient (cm^2 s^{-1}) of [Fe(CN)$_6$]$^{3-/4-}$ solution (7.6×10^{-6} cm^2 s^{-1}) [37], A is the electrode area (cm^2), C is the concentration (molcm^{-3}) and v is the scan rate (mV s^{-1}) and thus the electroactive surface area of the graphite/SiO$_2$ was estimated to be 0.0039 cm^2.

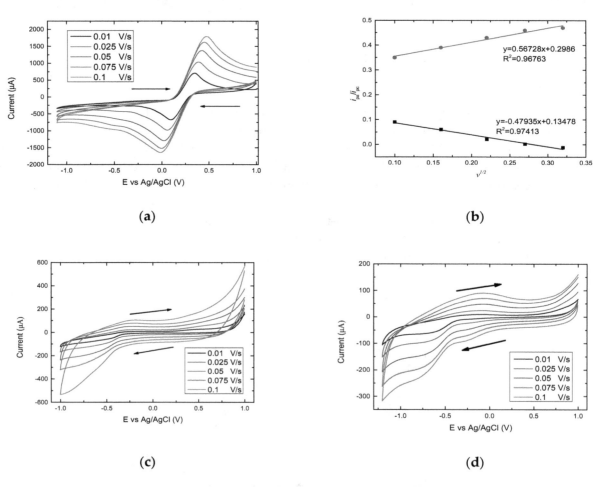

(a)

(b)

(c)

(d)

Figure 3. Cyclic voltammograms (CVs) of (**a**) a bare graphite/SiO$_2$ film electrode in 0.1 M KCl solution containing 5 mM of [Fe(CN)6]$^{3-/4-}$ at different scan rates. (**b**) Plot of anodic and cathodic peak current (Ipa/Ipc) vs. square root of scan rate ($v^{1/2}$). (**c**) A bare graphite/SiO$_2$ film electrode in 10 mM NaH$_2$PO$_4$, pH 7.0 at different scan rates and (**d**) the OM-(KG)$_5$-MOG$_{35-55}$ conjugate on graphite/SiO$_2$ in 10 mM NaH$_2$PO$_4$, pH 7.0 at different scan rates under an Argon atmosphere.

The electrochemical behavior of the graphite/SiO$_2$ film electrode was then investigated in the presence and absence of the MS myelin epitope peptide vaccine (OM-(KG)5-MOG$_{35-55}$). Figure 3c shows the effect of scan rate of a bare graphite/SiO$_2$ electrode, before the detection of the OM-(KG)5-MOG$_{35-55}$, at a scan rate range of 0.01 to 0.1 V s^{-1}. All electrochemical experiments were performed in a peptide free, anaerobic 10 mM NaH$_2$PO$_4$ (pH 7.0). The bare graphite/SiO$_2$ film electrode shows the characteristic charging/de-charging currents, and no cathodic or anodic peaks are observed even at the slowest scan rate (0.01 V s^{-1}). One of the advantages of using graphite paste electrodes is the increased conductivity, which allows a broader study of redox reactions occurring at very high or low biases (ranging from +1 V to −1 V). Further, the slower scan rate applied, the smaller the resulting current is obtained. Figure 3b, on the other hand, showing the CVs of OM-(KG)$_5$-MOG$_{35-55}$ on the graphite/SiO$_2$ film electrode, exhibits not only the characteristic charging/discharging currents assigned to electron injection into sub-band gap/conduction band states of the graphite/SiO$_2$ electrode, but also two reduction peaks around −0.22 V and −0.67 V and a broad re-oxidation peak at −0.1 V.

The redox peak currents were shown to be proportional to the scan rate, characteristic of quasi-reversible behavior. The rate of reaction between the graphite/SiO$_2$ electrode and the conjugate, OM-(KG)$_5$-MOG$_{35-55}$ was not fast enough to maintain equal concentrations of oxidized and reduced species at the surface of the electrode. In addition, the CV responses were shown to be stable, with the waveforms being unperturbed after being scanned several times, whilst no other consumption of the complex occurred nor other undesirable reactions in the phosphate buffer took place.

In Figure 3d, the two cathodic peaks at −0.27 V and −0.7 V and the wide anodic peak approximately at −0.1 V observed are due to the presence of the OM-(KG)$_5$-MOG$_{35-55}$. The two cathodic peaks correspond to the linker molecule (KG)$_5$ used to conjugate the MOG$_{35-55}$ peptide to OM, that contains 5 lysines and 5 glycines to its structure. Thus, the cathodic peaks attributed to the presence of lysines. On the other hand, the wide oxidation peak occurred probably due to superfluity of the free (KG)$_5$-MOG$_{35-55}$ peptide that was not able to conjugate to OM and created the final complex of the OM-(KG)$_5$-MOG$_{35-55}$ conjugate.

The CVs of the constituents of the OM-(KG)$_5$-MOG$_{35-55}$ conjugate are shown in Figure 4. According to Figure 4a, as mentioned earlier, the bare graphite/SiO$_2$ film electrode exhibited no reduction or oxidation peaks which is consistent with the currents being limited by the graphite conductivity at the voltage biases reported herein. On the other hand, the CV of the film electrode in the presence of mannan in 0.1 M buffer exhibited an oxidation peak at approximately 0.5 V, and the CV of the film electrode in the presence of 0.002 mg/mL OM displayed a slight cathodic peak at −0.56 V and the characteristic anodic peak at −0.1 V. At the same time, the electrochemical behavior of peptides MOG$_{35-55}$ and MOG$_{37-55}$ were examined. The main difference between these two peptides is that the MOG$_{35-55}$ peptide contained and additional linker with 5 lysines (KG)$_5$, whilst the MOG$_{37-55}$ peptide included a linker, which only contained 1 lysine. This was confirmed in Figure 4b, which displays the CVs of the Graphite/SiO$_2$ film electrode in the presence of each peptide. The two cathodic and anodic peaks observed are due to the presence of the lysine residues, however, the CV scan of the MOG$_{35-55}$ peptide exhibits a higher current and a wider electrochemical window compared to the CV scan of MOG$_{37-55}$ peptide, as the latter contained only 1 lysine residue.

DPV is a more sensitive approach compared to CV and hence, has been extensively used as a more sensitive method for the detection of molecules in low concentration [38]. In Figure 5, the DPVs are recorded for the bare film electrode, as well as for each part that constitutes the final structure of OM-(KG)$_5$-MOG$_{35-55}$ conjugate on the Graphite/SiO$_2$ working electrode. As can be seen in Figure 5a, the bare graphite/SiO$_2$ is free of any redox peaks. However, in Figure 5b, there are two peaks which correspond to (KG)$_5$-MOG$_{35-55}$ peptide, approximately at −0.65 V and −0.27 V, respectively. Figure 5c shows the DPV of mannan (in 0.1 M phosphate buffer) on the surface of the film electrode, displaying a clear sharper peak at around −0.26 V. The last step in order to evaluate the conjugation of peptide (KG)$_5$-MOG$_{35-55}$ with OM via DPV measurements is depicted in Figure 5d with a clear and distinct peak at −0.28 V and a shoulder peak at −0.62 V, which are actually due to the presence of OM-(KG)$_5$-MOG$_{35-55}$

on the graphite/SiO$_2$ film electrode (after the addition of 0.002 mg/mL of OM). This is a proof of concept study, and we intend to further study the quantification of this and other conjugates, focusing on the limit od detection (LOD) of these conjugates using voltammetric techniques.

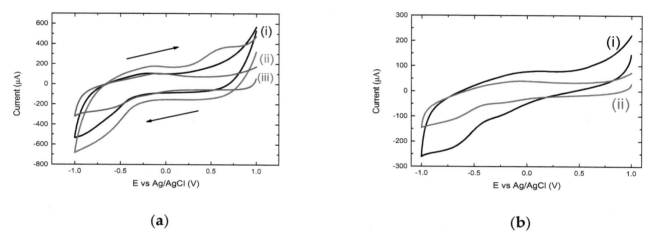

(a)   **(b)**

Figure 4. (**a**) CV scans at a scan rate of 0.1 Vs^{-1} of (i) a bare graphite/SiO$_2$ film electrode, (ii) mannan and (iii) OM-(KG)$_5$-MOG$_{35-55}$ conjugate. (**b**) Depicts the comparison between the CV's of (i) MOG$_{35-55}$ and (ii) MOG$_{37-55}$, both on graphite/SiO$_2$ in 10 mM NaH$_2$PO4, pH 7.0 at scan rate of 0.075 Vs^{-1}.

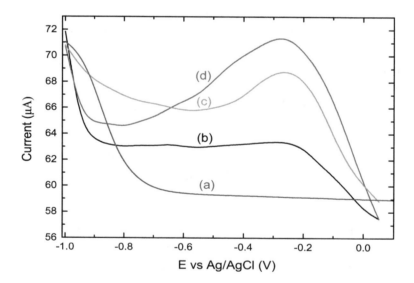

Figure 5. Differential pulse voltammetry (DPVs) comparison of (a) a bare graphite/SiO$_2$ film electrode, (b) (KG)$_5$-MOG$_{35-55}$, (c) mannan, and (d) OM-(KG)$_5$-MOG$_{35-55}$ conjugate on graphite/SiO$_2$ electrode in 10 mM NaH$_2$PO$_4$, pH 7.0.

3.4. Complete Conjugation between (KG)$_5$-MOG$_{35-55}$ Peptide to OM is Monitored by HPLC

Contrarily to the conjugation of MOG$_{35-55}$ peptide with mannan, which did not occur, the reaction of (KG)$_5$-MOG$_{35-55}$ with mannan (oxidized or not) resulted in gradual conjugation of (KG)$_5$-MOG$_{35-55}$ peptide within 6 h depicted in the gradual loss of the HPLC peak during this period (Figure 6). The amino groups of lysine residues within (KG)$_5$ forms a Schiff base reaction with the aldehyde groups of OM (resulting after the oxidation of mannan). The (KG)$_5$-MOG$_{35-55}$ peptide peak at 9.62 gradually disappears within this period, showing complete conjugation of (KG)$_5$-MOG$_{35-55}$ peptide to OM. Figure 6b shows the completion of conjugation within six hours.

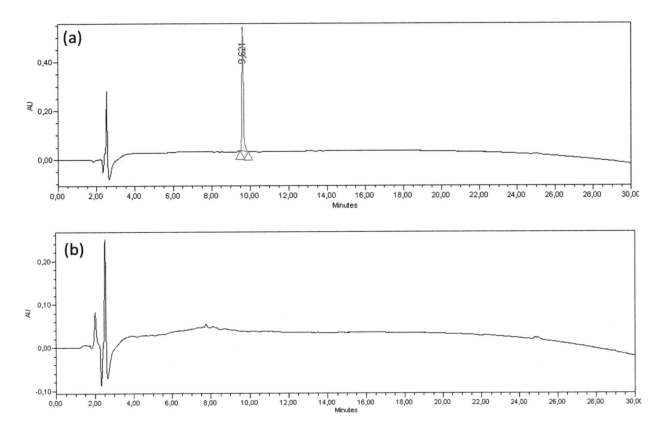

Figure 6. (**a**) High-performance liquid chromatography (HPLC) analysis of $(KG)_5$-$MOG_{35\text{-}55}$–214 nm at the beginning of the conjugation reaction and (**b**) HPLC analysis of OM-$(KG)_5$-$MOG_{35\text{-}55}$ solution after 6 h.

3.5. The Importance of the Linker $(KG)_5$ for Conjugation of Peptides to OM

The conjugation of $MOG_{35\text{-}55}$ peptide to OM was achieved through $(KG)_5$ linker, as previously described [23]. As demonstrated, this approach provides simple and efficient conjugation by the Schiff base reaction, where aldehyde groups of OM reacts with the amino groups of the lysine side chains of the $(KG)_5$-$MOG_{35\text{-}55}$, peptide. In previous similar studies using the linker KG of varying lengths, $(KG)_{n=1\text{-}5}$, we noted that the length of the linker plays a crucial role in the ability of peptides to be efficiently conjugated to the OM scaffold [48].

3.6. Mannan-Peptide Conjugate

In the OM-$(KG)_5$-$MOG_{35\text{-}55}$ conjugate, unreacted aldehyde groups are necessary to immunoregulate the peptide to dendritic cells. This is a result of ethylene glycol addition to blockade further oxidation, and in line with previous studies on MUC1-mannan conjugates in cancer research, which required aldehyde groups in order to activate dendritic cells [39]. The matrix also contains intact mannose units, not oxidized, necessary to bind to the mannose receptor of the dendritic cells and their activation via toll-like receptor 4 [49–52]. In particular, the procedure we followed to produce the mannan-peptide conjugate allows: (i) the presence of antigen peptide $MOG_{35\text{-}55}$ connected with aldehyde groups of the OM through immune bonds (Schiff base) with the amino groups of the lysine side chain in the $(KG)_5$-$MOG_{35\text{-}55}$ peptide. The peptide-OM conjugate is delivered to dendritic cells via the mannan scaffold for regulation of the immune system; (ii) the presence of unreacted aldehyde groups are necessary to modulate dendritic cells; and (iii) the presence intact mannose units, not oxidized, necessary to bind to the mannose receptor of the dendritic cells.

3.7. Chemistry of the Mannose Cleavage

The cis-diols can form a cyclic complex upon oxidation with strong oxidizing agents as periodate. This allows the cleavage of the bond between the two carbons bearing the two hydroxyl groups, leading to the formation of aldehyde groups. Mannose is a carbohydrate, which holds two hydroxyl groups at positions 2,3 of the ring in a cis- position. This allows the oxidizing agent sodium periodate to form a cyclic complex, which finally leads to cleavage of the carbon-carbon bond bearing the cis-hydroxyl groups. This complex cannot be formed if the hydroxyl groups at the adjacent carbon atoms are in a trans position and subsequently this carbon-carbon bond cannot be cleaved. The formation of the cyclic mannose-periodate complex is leading finally to the cleavage of the ring and the formation of the two aldehyde groups. These groups react with the amino groups of the five lysines of the $(KG)_5$-MOG_{35-55} to form double bond imines (Schiff base reaction) thus, the MOG_{35-55} peptide attached to the mannan scaffold. Figure 7 shows the mechanism of cis diol cleavage.

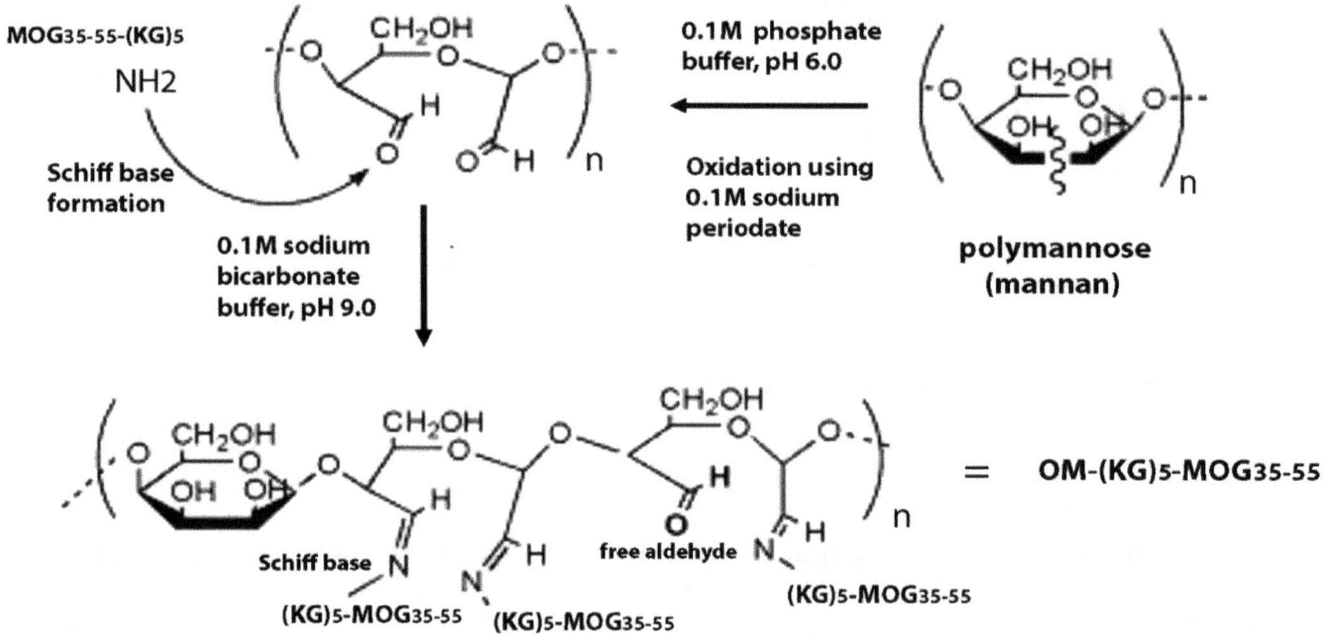

Figure 7. The mechanism of cis diol cleavage. Synthetic scheme of conjugation reaction of peptide with oxidized mannan [35].

4. Conclusions

We developed and confirm an analytical electrochemical method for monitoring the conjugation reaction of peptides to the carrier mannan; $(KG)_5$-MOG_{35-55} was used as the peptide example in this study. Peptide-OM conjugates can serve as potential vaccine candidates as has previously been shown by the group for cancer models and more recently in MS models. Electrochemical voltammetric techniques and HPLC experiments were used to confirm the conjugation of $(KG)_5$-MOG_{35-55} to the aldehyde groups of OM. It is shown that voltammetric technique and HPLC can be used to monitor the conjugation efficiency of peptide-carrier conjugates.

Author Contributions: E.T. conceived and designed exclusively the electrochemical experiments. J.M. and V.A. conceived and designed the biochemical parts, the HPLC measurements and the chemistry of the mannose cleavage; E.D., S.P., E.T. and J.M. performed the experiments; E.T., J.M., E.D. and V.A. analyzed the data; E.T., J.M. and V.A. contributed to reagents/materials/analysis tools; E.D., E.T. and J.M. wrote their respective specialty parts of this paper; V.A. revised and edited the paper. All authors have read and agreed to the published version of the manuscript

Acknowledgments: The authors would like to thank Elias Sakellis from NCSR Demokritos for the SEM images and EDS analysis. V.A. would like to thank the Institute for Health and Sport, Victoria University, for supporting her current efforts into MS research. J.M. would like to thank the General Secretariat for Research and Technology (GSRT) for supporting his MS research.

References

1.   Nosrati, R.; Olad, A.; Maryami, F. The use of graphite/TiO$_2$ nanocomposite additive for preparation of polyacrylic based visible-light induced antibacterial and self-cleaning coating. *Res. Chem. Intermed.* **2018**, *44*, 6219–6237. [CrossRef]

2.   Nikolaou, P.; Deskoulidis, E.; Topoglidis, E.; Kakoulidou, A.T.; Tsopelas, F. Application of chemometrics for detection and modeling of adulteration of fresh cow milk with reconstituted skim milk powder using voltammetric fingerpriting on a graphite/SiO$_2$ hybrid electrode. *Talanta* **2020**, *206*, 120223. [CrossRef] [PubMed]

3.   Nikolaou, P.; Vareli, I.; Deskoulidis, E.; Matsoukas, J.; Vassilakopoulou, A.; Koutselas, I.; Topoglidis, E. Graphite/SiO$_2$ film electrode modified with hybrid organic-inorganic perovskites: Synthesis, optical, electrochemical properties and application in electrochemical sensing of losartan. *J. Solid State Chem.* **2019**, *273*, 17–24. [CrossRef]

4.   Topoglidis, E.; Kolozoff, P.-A.; Tiflidis, C.; Papavasiliou, J.; Sakellis, E. Adsorption and electrochemical behavior of Cyt-c on carbon nanotubes/TiO$_2$ nanocomposite films fabricated at various annealing temperatures. *Colloid Polym. Sci.* **2018**, *296*, 1353–1364. [CrossRef]

5.   Dargahi, N.; Katsara, M.; Tselios, T.; Androutsou, M.E.; De Courten, M.; Matsoukas, J.; Apostolopoulos, V. Multiple sclerosis: Immunopathology and treatment update. *Brain Sci.* **2017**, *7*. [CrossRef]

6.   Katsara, M.; Apostolopoulos, V. Editorial: Multiple Sclerosis: Pathogenesis and Therapeutics. *Med. Chem.* **2018**, *14*, 104–105. [CrossRef]

7.   Katsara, M.; Matsoukas, J.; Deraos, G.; Apostolopoulos, V. Towards immunotherapeutic drugs and vaccines against multiple sclerosis. *Acta Biochim. Biophys. Sin.* **2008**, *40*, 636–642. [CrossRef]

8.   Katsara, M.; Tselios, T.; Deraos, S.; Deraos, G.; Matsoukas, M.T.; Lazoura, E.; Matsoukas, J.; Apostolopoulos, V. Round and round we go: Cyclic peptides in disease. *Curr. Med. Chem.* **2006**, *13*, 2221–2232. [CrossRef]

9.   Steinman, L. Multiple sclerosis: A coordinated immunological attack against myelin in the central nervous system. *Cell* **1996**, *85*, 299–302. [CrossRef]

10. Steinman, L. Multiple sclerosis: A two-stage disease. *Nat. Immunol.* **2001**, *2*, 762–764. [CrossRef]

11. Candia, M.; Kratzer, B.; Pickl, W.F. On Peptides and Altered Peptide Ligands: From Origin, Mode of Action and Design to Clinical Application (Immunotherapy). *Int. Arch. Allergy Immunol.* **2016**, *170*, 211–233. [CrossRef] [PubMed]

12. Katsara, M.; Minigo, G.; Plebanski, M.; Apostolopoulos, V. The good, the bad and the ugly: How altered peptide ligands modulate immunity. *Expert Opin. Biol. Ther.* **2008**, *8*, 1873–1884. [CrossRef] [PubMed]

13. Katsara, M.; Yuriev, E.; Ramsland, P.A.; Deraos, G.; Tselios, T.; Matsoukas, J.; Apostolopoulos, V. A double mutation of MBP(83-99) peptide induces IL-4 responses and antagonizes IFN-gamma responses. *J. Neuroimmunol.* **2008**, *200*, 77–89. [CrossRef]

14. Katsara, M.; Yuriev, E.; Ramsland, P.A.; Deraos, G.; Tselios, T.; Matsoukas, J.; Apostolopoulos, V. Mannosylation of mutated MBP83-99 peptides diverts immune responses from Th1 to Th2. *Mol. Immunol.* **2008**, *45*, 3661–3670. [CrossRef]

15. Katsara, M.; Yuriev, E.; Ramsland, P.A.; Tselios, T.; Deraos, G.; Lourbopoulos, A.; Grigoriadis, N.; Matsoukas, J.; Apostolopoulos, V. Altered peptide ligands of myelin basic protein (MBP87-99) conjugated to reduced mannan modulate immune responses in mice. *Immunology* **2009**, *128*, 521–533. [CrossRef]

16. Trager, N.N.M.; Butler, J.T.; Harmon, J.; Mount, J.; Podbielska, M.; Haque, A.; Banik, N.L.; Beeson, C.C. A Novel Aza-MBP Altered Peptide Ligand for the Treatment of Experimental Autoimmune Encephalomyelitis. *Mol. Neurobiol.* **2018**, *55*, 267–275. [CrossRef]

17. Katsara, M.; Deraos, S.; Tselios, T.V.; Pietersz, G.; Matsoukas, J.; Apostolopoulos, V. Immune responses of linear and cyclic PLP139-151 mutant peptides in SJL/J mice: Peptides in their free state versus mannan conjugation. *Immunotherapy* **2014**, *6*, 709–724. [CrossRef]

18. Lourbopoulos, A.; Deraos, G.; Matsoukas, M.T.; Touloumi, O.; Giannakopoulou, A.; Kalbacher, H.; Grigoriadis, N.; Apostolopoulos, V.; Matsoukas, J. Cyclic MOG35-55 ameliorates clinical and neuropathological features of experimental autoimmune encephalomyelitis. *Bioorg. Med. Chem.* **2017**, *25*, 4163–4174. [CrossRef]

19. Lourbopoulos, A.; Matsoukas, M.T.; Katsara, M.; Deraos, G.; Giannakopoulou, A.; Lagoudaki, R.; Grigoriadis, N.; Matsoukas, J.; Apostolopoulos, V. Cyclization of PLP139-151 peptide reduces its encephalitogenic potential in experimental autoimmune encephalomyelitis. *Bioorg. Med. Chem.* **2018**, *26*, 2221–2228. [CrossRef]

20. Apostolopoulos, V.; Rostami, A.; Matsoukas, J. The Long Road of Immunotherapeutics against Multiple Sclerosis. *Brain Sci.* **2020**, *10*. [CrossRef]

21. Day, S.; Tselios, T.; Androutsou, M.E.; Tapeinou, A.; Frilligou, I.; Stojanovska, L.; Matsoukas, J.; Apostolopoulos, V. Mannosylated Linear and Cyclic Single Amino Acid Mutant Peptides Using a Small 10 Amino Acid Linker Constitute Promising Candidates Against Multiple Sclerosis. *Front. Immunol.* **2015**, *6*, 136. [CrossRef] [PubMed]

22. Deraos, G.; Rodi, M.; Kalbacher, H.; Chatzantoni, K.; Karagiannis, F.; Synodinos, L.; Plotas, P.; Papalois, A.; Dimisianos, N.; Papathanasopoulos, P.; et al. Properties of myelin altered peptide ligand cyclo(87-99)(Ala91,Ala96)MBP87-99 render it a promising drug lead for immunotherapy of multiple sclerosis. *Eur. J. Med. Chem.* **2015**, *101*, 13–23. [CrossRef] [PubMed]

23. Tapeinou, A.; Androutsou, M.E.; Kyrtata, K.; Vlamis-Gardikas, A.; Apostolopoulos, V.; Matsoukas, J.; Tselios, T. Conjugation of a peptide to mannan and its confirmation by tricine sodium dodecyl sulfate-polyacrylamide gel electrophoresis. *Anal. Biochem.* **2015**, *485*, 43–45. [CrossRef] [PubMed]

24. Tselios, T.V.; Lamari, F.N.; Karathanasopoulou, I.; Katsara, M.; Apostolopoulos, V.; Pietersz, G.A.; Matsoukas, J.M.; Karamanos, N.K. Synthesis and study of the electrophoretic behavior of mannan conjugates with cyclic peptide analogue of myelin basic protein using lysine-glycine linker. *Anal. Biochem.* **2005**, *347*, 121–128. [CrossRef]

25. Apostolopoulos, V.; Pietersz, G.A.; Tsibanis, A.; Tsikkinis, A.; Drakaki, H.; Loveland, B.E.; Piddlesden, S.J.; Plebanski, M.; Pouniotis, D.S.; Alexis, M.N.; et al. Pilot phase III immunotherapy study in early-stage breast cancer patients using oxidized mannan-MUC1 [ISRCTN71711835]. *Breast Cancer Res.* **2006**, *8*, R27. [CrossRef]

26. Apostolopoulos, V.; Pietersz, G.A.; Tsibanis, A.; Tsikkinis, A.; Stojanovska, L.; McKenzie, I.F.; Vassilaros, S. Dendritic cell immunotherapy: Clinical outcomes. *Clin. Transl. Immunol.* **2014**, *3*, e21. [CrossRef]

27. Karanikas, V.; Hwang, L.A.; Pearson, J.; Ong, C.S.; Apostolopoulos, V.; Vaughan, H.; Xing, P.X.; Jamieson, G.; Pietersz, G.; Tait, B.; et al. Antibody and T cell responses of patients with adenocarcinoma immunized with mannan-MUC1 fusion protein. *J. Clin. Investig.* **1997**, *100*, 2783–2792. [CrossRef]

28. Karanikas, V.; Lodding, J.; Maino, V.C.; McKenzie, I.F. Flow cytometric measurement of intracellular cytokines detects immune responses in MUC1 immunotherapy. *Clin. Cancer Res.* **2000**, *6*, 829–837.

29. Karanikas, V.; Thynne, G.; Mitchell, P.; Ong, C.S.; Gunawardana, D.; Blum, R.; Pearson, J.; Lodding, J.; Pietersz, G.; Broadbent, R.; et al. Mannan Mucin-1 Peptide Immunization: Influence of Cyclophosphamide and the Route of Injection. *J. Immunother* **2001**, *24*, 172–183. [CrossRef]

30. Loveland, B.E.; Zhao, A.; White, S.; Gan, H.; Hamilton, K.; Xing, P.X.; Pietersz, G.A.; Apostolopoulos, V.; Vaughan, H.; Karanikas, V.; et al. Mannan-MUC1-pulsed dendritic cell immunotherapy: A phase I trial in patients with adenocarcinoma. *Clin. Cancer Res.* **2006**, *12*, 869–877. [CrossRef]

31. Mitchell, P.L.; Quinn, M.A.; Grant, P.T.; Allen, D.G.; Jobling, T.W.; White, S.C.; Zhao, A.; Karanikas, V.; Vaughan, H.; Pietersz, G.; et al. A phase 2, single-arm study of an autologous dendritic cell treatment against mucin 1 in patients with advanced epithelial ovarian cancer. *J. Immunother Cancer* **2014**, *2*, 16. [CrossRef]

32. Vassilaros, S.; Tsibanis, A.; Tsikkinis, A.; Pietersz, G.A.; McKenzie, I.F.; Apostolopoulos, V. Up to 15-year clinical follow-up of a pilot Phase III immunotherapy study in stage II breast cancer patients using oxidized mannan-MUC1. *Immunotherapy* **2013**, *5*, 1177–1182. [CrossRef] [PubMed]

33. Deraos, G.; Chatzantoni, K.; Matsoukas, M.T.; Tselios, T.; Deraos, S.; Katsara, M.; Papathanasopoulos, P.; Vynios, D.; Apostolopoulos, V.; Mouzaki, A.; et al. Citrullination of linear and cyclic altered peptide ligands from myelin basic protein (MBP(87-99)) epitope elicits a Th1 polarized response by T cells isolated from multiple sclerosis patients: Implications in triggering disease. *J. Med. Chem.* **2008**, *51*, 7834–7842. [CrossRef] [PubMed]

34. Matsoukas, J.; Apostolopoulos, V.; Kalbacher, H.; Papini, A.M.; Tselios, T.; Chatzantoni, K.; Biagioli, T.; Lolli, F.; Deraos, S.; Papathanassopoulos, P.; et al. Design and synthesis of a novel potent myelin basic protein epitope 87-99 cyclic analogue: Enhanced stability and biological properties of mimics render them a potentially new class of immunomodulators. *J. Med. Chem.* **2005**, *48*, 1470–1480. [CrossRef] [PubMed]

35. Tselios, T.; Apostolopoulos, V.; Daliani, I.; Deraos, S.; Grdadolnik, S.; Mavromoustakos, T.; Melachrinou, M.; Thymianou, S.; Probert, L.; Mouzaki, A.; et al. Antagonistic effects of human cyclic MBP(87-99) altered peptide ligands in experimental allergic encephalomyelitis and human T-cell proliferation. *J. Med. Chem.* **2002**, *45*, 275–283. [CrossRef]

36. Song, M.-J.; Hwang, S.W.; Whang, D. Amperometric hydrogen peroxide biosensor based on a modified gold electrode with silver nanowires. *J. Appl. Electrochem.* **2010**, *40*, 2099–2105. [CrossRef]

37. Konopka, S.J.; McDuffie, B. Diffusion coefficients of ferri-and ferrocyanide ions in aqueous media, using twin-electrode thin-layer electrochemistry. *Anal. Chem.* **1970**, *42*, 1741–1746. [CrossRef]

38. Hussain, G.; Silvester, D.S. Comparison of Voltammetric Techniques for Ammonia Sensing in Ionic Liquids. *Electroanalysis* **2018**, *30*, 75–83. [CrossRef]

39. Apostolopoulos, V.; Pietersz, G.A.; Gordon, S.; Martinez-Pomares, L.; McKenzie, I.F. Aldehyde-mannan antigen complexes target the MHC class I antigen-presentation pathway. *Eur. J. Immunol.* **2000**, *30*, 1714–1723. [CrossRef]

40. Apostolopoulos, V.; Pietersz, G.A.; Loveland, B.E.; Sandrin, M.S.; McKenzie, I.F. Oxidative/reductive conjugation of mannan to antigen selects for T1 or T2 immune responses. *Proc. Natl. Acad. Sci. USA* **1995**, *92*, 10128–10132. [CrossRef]

41. Grunwald, J.; Rejtar, T.; Sawant, R.; Wang, Z.; Torchilin, V.P. TAT peptide and its conjugates: Proteolytic stability. *Bioconjug. Chem.* **2009**, *20*, 1531–1537. [CrossRef]

42. Lemus, R.; Karol, M.H. Conjugation of haptens. *Methods Mol. Med.* **2008**, *138*, 167–182. [CrossRef]

43. Berthet, M.; Martinez, J.; Parrot, I. MgI$_2$ -chemoselective cleavage for removal of amino acid protecting groups: A fresh vision for peptide synthesis. *Biopolymers* **2017**, *108*. [CrossRef]

44. Isidro-Llobet, A.; Alvarez, M.; Albericio, F. Amino acid-protecting groups. *Chem. Rev.* **2009**, *109*, 2455–2504. [CrossRef]

45. Apostolopoulos, V.; Deraos, G.; Matsoukas, M.T.; Day, S.; Stojanovska, L.; Tselios, T.; Androutsou, M.E.; Matsoukas, J. Cyclic citrullinated MBP87-99 peptide stimulates T cell responses: Implications in triggering disease. *Bioorg. Med. Chem.* **2017**, *25*, 528–538. [CrossRef] [PubMed]

46. Pagba, C.V.; McCaslin, T.G.; Veglia, G.; Porcelli, F.; Yohannan, J.; Guo, Z.; McDaniel, M.; Barry, B.A. A tyrosine-tryptophan dyad and radical-based charge transfer in a ribonucleotide reductase-inspired maquette. *Nat. Commun.* **2015**, *6*, 10010. [CrossRef] [PubMed]

47. Zhai, J.; Zhao, L.; Zheng, L.; Gao, F.; Gao, L.; Liu, R.; Wang, Y.; Gao, X. Peptide–Au Cluster Probe: Precisely Detecting Epidermal Growth Factor Receptor of Three Tumor Cell Lines at a Single-Cell Level. *ACS Omega* **2017**, *2*, 276–282. [CrossRef] [PubMed]

48. Tapeinou, A. Design, synthesis and evaluation of analogues of myelin protein immunodominant epitopes implemented in multiple sclerosis. *Eur. J. Med. Chem.* **2017**, *143*, 621–631. [CrossRef] [PubMed]

49. Apostolopoulos, V.; Barnes, N.; Pietersz, G.A.; McKenzie, I.F. Ex vivo targeting of the macrophage mannose receptor generates anti-tumor CTL responses. *Vaccine* **2000**, *18*, 3174–3184. [CrossRef]

50. Apostolopoulos, V.; Pietersz, G.A.; McKenzie, I.F. Cell-mediated immune responses to MUC1 fusion protein coupled to mannan. *Vaccine* **1996**, *14*, 930–938. [CrossRef]

51. Sheng, K.C.; Kalkanidis, M.; Pouniotis, D.S.; Wright, M.D.; Pietersz, G.A.; Apostolopoulos, V. The adjuvanticity of a mannosylated antigen reveals TLR4 functionality essential for subset specialization and functional maturation of mouse dendritic cells. *J. Immunol.* **2008**, *181*, 2455–2464. [CrossRef] [PubMed]

52. Sheng, K.C.; Pouniotis, D.S.; Wright, M.D.; Tang, C.K.; Lazoura, E.; Pietersz, G.A.; Apostolopoulos, V. Mannan derivatives induce phenotypic and functional maturation of mouse dendritic cells. *Immunology* **2006**, *118*, 372–383. [CrossRef] [PubMed]

12

Longitudinal Serum Neurofilament Levels of Multiple Sclerosis Patients Before and After Treatment with First-Line Immunomodulatory Therapies

André Huss [1], Makbule Senel [1], Ahmed Abdelhak [1,2,3], Benjamin Mayer [4], Jan Kassubek [1], Albert C. Ludolph [1], Markus Otto [1] and Hayrettin Tumani [1,5,*]

[1] Department of Neurology, University Hospital of Ulm, Oberer Eselsberg 45, 89081 Ulm, Germany; andre.huss@uni-ulm.de (A.H.); makbule.senel@uni-ulm.de (M.S.); ahmed.abdelhak@ucsf.edu (A.A.); jan.kassubek@uni-ulm.de (J.K.); Albert.Ludolph@rku.de (A.C.L.); markus.otto@uni-ulm.de (M.O.)
[2] Department of Neurology and Stroke, University Hospital of Tübingen, Hoppe-Seyler-Alle 3, 72076 Tübingen, Germany
[3] Hertie institute of clinical of clinical brain research, University of Tübingen, Hoppe-Seyler-Alle 3, 72076 Tübingen, Germany
[4] Institute of Epidemiology and Medical Biometry, Ulm University, Schwabstraße 13, 89075 Ulm, Germany; benjamin.mayer@uni-ulm.de
[5] Speciality Clinic of Neurology Dietenbronn, Dietenbronn 7, 88477 Schwendi, Germany
* Correspondence: hayrettin.tumani@uni-ulm.de

Abstract: Serum neurofilament light chain (NfL) has been shown to correlate with neuroaxonal damage in multiple sclerosis (MS) and various other neurological diseases. While serum NfL is now regularly reported in clinical approval studies, there is a lack of longitudinal data from patients treated with established basic immunotherapies outside of study conditions. In total, 34 patients with early relapsing-remitting MS (RRMS) were included. The follow-up period was 24 months with regular follow-up visits after 3, 6, 9, 12 and 18 months. Therapy with glatiramer acetate was initiated in 20 patients and with interferon-beta in 12 patients. The disease course was monitored by the events of relapses, Expanded Disability Status Scale (EDSS) score and MRI parameters. Overall, serum NfL levels were higher at time points with a current relapse event than at time points without relapse (12.8 pg/mL vs. 9.7 pg/mL, $p = 0.011$). At follow-up, relapse-free patients showed significantly reduced serum NfL levels starting from 9 months compared to baseline ($p < 0.05$) and reduced levels after 12 months compared to baseline ($p = 0.013$) in patients without EDSS progression for 12 months. In this explorative observational study, our data suggest that the longitudinal measurement of serum NfL may be useful in addition to MRI to monitor disease activity and therapy response.

Keywords: multiple sclerosis; serum neurofilament; immunomodulatory therapies; therapy-response marker

1. Introduction

Multiple sclerosis (MS) is a chronic inflammatory disease of the central nervous system (CNS) characterized by demyelination and axonal loss [1]. The current concept of MS pathology is based on infiltrating immune B- and T-cells via the blood–brain barrier, local antibody production and activation of glial cells [2,3]. These processes are thought to lead to primary demyelination followed by neurodegeneration [2]. In recent years, several neurochemical markers have been established for the characterization of pathological molecular processes. One of the most extensively investigated markers for neuroaxonal loss is neurofilament light chain (NfL) [4–6]. NfL is one of four neurofilament subunits and the most abundant one, making it a popular target for neurological diseases [7]. Here, NfL showed superior sensitivity for MS than the phosphorylated subunit of neurofilament [8].

Initially investigated using standard immunoassays, NfL in the cerebrospinal fluid (CSF) from MS patients was found to correlate with disease course and activity [9,10]. In the early phase of the disease, it has a prognostic value [5,11,12] and can be used as a treatment response marker [13]. However, NfL is not specific for MS, is rather a general marker for neurodegenerative processes [14,15] and changes with the normal aging brain [16], which needs to be considered when looking at NfL changes over time.

As detection methods were developed over the years, highly sensitive immunoassays became available and allowed the analysis of brain-derived proteins, not only in the CSF, but in serum as well [17]. Beyond showing a good correlation with CSF values, serum NfL has already thoroughly been investigated in MS [18], i.e., it has been shown to correlate with clinical and radiological disease activity (relapses, new/enlarged T2 lesions and gadolinium-enhancing lesions in magnetic resonance imaging (MRI)) [19–22]. The most important advantage of serum analyses is the possibility of serial sampling and consecutive analysis of biomarkers. Thus, NfL is regularly used in clinical trials to monitor therapy efficacy, and it is on the footsteps of being used as a secondary outcome parameter in clinical trials [23].

In most studies, group effects of treatments on neurofilaments are investigated, which already indicate the applicability of serum NfL as a therapy response marker [22,24] and as a prognostic marker for long-term clinical outcomes in MS [25]. However, longitudinal data of intraindividual NfL levels over disease course under immunomodulatory therapies in well-characterized MS patients are widely missing and only described rarely [26,27].

In this study, we analyzed consecutive samples of MS patients in the early phase of the disease, before and after the initiation of disease-modifying treatment with either glatiramer acetate or interferon-beta over a follow-up period of 24 months. Serum NfL levels at each visit were correlated to clinical outcome parameters (relapse and Expanded Disability Status Scale (EDSS)), serum cytokine profile, cognitive functions and MRI parameters of disease activity and progression.

The aim of this study was (a) to show the effect of immunomodulatory therapies on serum NfL levels in MS patients over disease course, (b) to evaluate the relationship between NfL and MRI parameters reflecting disease progression, such as T2 lesion load, (c) to evaluate possible correlation with cognitive functions and (d) to compare serum NfL levels with the serum cytokine profile.

2. Experimental Section

2.1. Patients

In total, 34 patients who attended the Department of Neurology at the University Hospital Ulm between 2002 and 2004 before initiation of disease-modifying treatment (DMT) were included in the study. Initially, the MS diagnosis was made on the diagnostic criteria valid at time of study inclusion (McDonald 2001), but were adjusted for the most recent updates of the McDonald criteria (McDonald 2017). After study inclusion, 20 patients started treatment with glatiramer acetate, 12 patients were treated with interferon-beta (Avonex, Betaferon and Rebif) and 2 patients rejected DMT. All patients were then followed-up for 24 months with visits every 3 months in the first year and every 6 months in the second year. At all visits, clinical assessments including relapse evaluation, EDSS, Paced Auditory Serial Addition Test (PASAT), and serum sampling were performed. Relapses were defined as focal neurological disturbance lasting more than 24 h, without an alternate explanation. Furthermore, 17 patients received magnetic resonance imaging (MRI) scans at baseline, 12 months and 24 months. Detailed patients' characteristics are shown in Table 1 and the study schedule is shown in Table 2. Relapses were treated with high-dose corticosteroids (50–1000 mg) over 3–5 days after exclusion of contraindications. Age did not differ between patients with and without at least one relapse during follow-up and did not correlate with serum NfL levels at baseline.

Table 1. Patients' characteristics.

Characteristics	Median Values with IQR, $n = 34$
Age	33 (29–40)
EDSS baseline	1.5 (1.0–2.0)
Serum NfL baseline (pg/mL)	10.2 (8.4–14.7)
Relapse within 12 months (n)	14
Relapse within 24 months (n)	16
Treatment after baseline	
Glatiramer acetate	20
Interferon-beta	12
No disease-modifying therapy	2

EDSS = Expanded Disability Status Scale; NfL = Neurofilament light chain; IQR = Interquartile range.

Table 2. Study schedule and number of available data.

	Baseline	3 Months	6 Months	9 Months	12 Months	18 Months	24 Months
Clinical assessment	34	32	32	32	33	34	34
EDSS	31	30	27	30	32	32	32
Serum NfL	34	29	29	32	33	31	24
MRI (T2 lesion load)	17				17		17
Serum cytokine profile	29	29	29	29	29	29	29
PASAT	32	32	31	30	32	30	31

EDSS, Expanded Disability Status Scale; PASAT, Paced Auditory Serial Addition Test; NfL, neurofilament light chain; MRI, magnetic resonance imaging.

2.2. NfL Measurements

Serum samples were stored in the local biobank according to recommended biobanking protocols at −80 °C [28]. Serum NfL was measured using the Simoa technology (Quanterix Corporation, Lexington, MA, USA). Samples were diluted, as recommended by the manufacturer, and concentrations were calculated using the corresponding standard curve.

2.3. Cytokines Measurements

Cytokine profiles including IFN-γ, osteopontin (OPN), IL-2, IL-4 and IL-10 were determined in serum at study onset and at every visit during follow-up using the electrochemiluminescence detection multiplex technology of Meso Scale Discovery (MSD, Gaithersburg, MD, USA) according to the manufacturer's instructions as previously reported [29].

2.4. MRI Scans

MRI scans of the brain and spinal cord were performed on a 1.5 Tesla clinical MRI scanner (Symphony Siemens, Erlangen, Germany) and the total number of hyperintense lesions in T2-weighted scans at the different time points were visually quantified by an experienced rater.

2.5. Cognitive Functions

Cognitive functions were assessed at every time point by the Paced Auditory Serial Addition Test (PASAT). Here, information processing speed and flexibility, as well as calculation ability are tested, which also means that this is not a global measure of cognitive dysfunction, but rather targets specific cognitive executive functions frequently affected in MS.

2.6. Statistical Methods

All statistical tests were performed using the GraphPad Prism 8 software (GraphPad Software Inc., La Jolla, CA, USA). Shapiro–Wilk test was used to examine the distribution of the data. Mann–Whitney U test was used to compare medians in skewed distributed parameters for unpaired samples and Wilcoxon matched-pairs signed-rank test for paired samples. Correlation analyses were performed with Spearman's rank correlation and corrected for multiple testing by the Bonferroni method. A p-value ≤ 0.05 was considered as statistically significant.

2.7. Ethical Statement

The study was reviewed by the appropriate ethics committee of the University of Ulm (approval number 79/2001, approval date 14.11.2001) and was performed in accordance with the ethical standards of the current version of the Declaration of Helsinki. Written informed consent was obtained from all patients participating in this study.

3. Results

3.1. Serum NfL at Time Points With and Without Active Relapse

We categorized serum NfL levels of all time points accordingly whether an active relapse was present or not. Additionally, the change of serum NfL values at a time point with an active relapse in comparison with the previous time point was determined. Here, the absolute change of serum NfL values (pg/mL) and the percentage change was calculated (tx-tx-1). Significantly higher serum NfL levels were observed for time points with an active relapse compared with time points with no relapse (Figure 1A, $p < 0.05$). This was also true for the percentage change (Figure 1C, $p < 0.05$), but not for the absolute change of serum NfL (Figure 1B, $p = 0.15$).

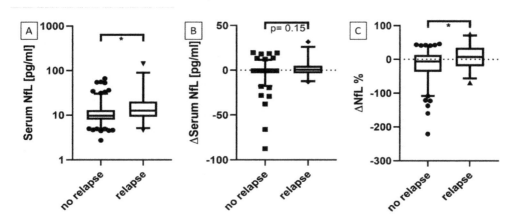

Figure 1. Serum NfL and time points with or without an active relapse. (**A**) Comparison of serum NfL levels during time points with and without an active relapse. (**B**) Comparison of the change of serum NfL between a time point with an active relapse and the previous time point. (**C**) Comparison of the percentage change of serum NfL between a time point with an active relapse and the previous time point. * $p < 0.05$.

3.2. Serum NfL Levels During Follow-Up Period of 24 Months

3.2.1. Patients with Relapses vs. No Relapse

In patients with a relapse-free disease course of 12 months and 24 months, serum NfL decreased significantly between baseline and time points 12 months and 18 months and time points 9, 12, 18 and

24 months, respectively (Figure 2A,B, blue triangles facing down, $p < 0.05$). There were no significant differences for baseline and follow-up visits of serum NfL levels in patients with at least one relapse within 12 or 24 months (Figure 2A,B). Furthermore, serum NfL levels in patients with a relapse within 12 months were significantly higher than in patients without a relapse within 12 months at time points 9 and 12 months (Figure 2A, $p < 0.05$).

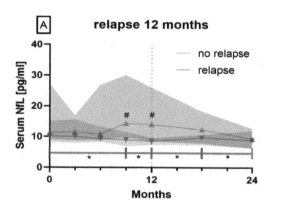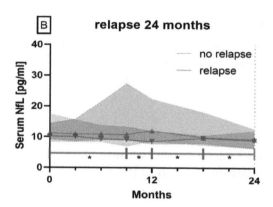

Figure 2. Serum NfL levels over 12 and 24 months in patients with (red triangle facing up) and without relapse (blue triangle facing down) for (**A**) 12 or (**B**) 24 months. Symbols show median values, colored range indicates 95% confidence interval (CI), * $p < 0.05$ for intragroup differences, # $p < 0.05$ for intergroup differences.

3.2.2. Patients with EDSS Progression vs. Stable or Improved EDSS

In patients showing EDSS progression within 12 months and patients with a stable or improved EDSS for 24 months, no differences concerning their NfL levels were observed. However, in patients with a stable or improving EDSS within 12 months, serum NfL levels decreased significantly between baseline and time points 12 and 18 months (Figure 3A, $p < 0.05$). Considering 24 months of observation, patients with EDSS progression showed serum NfL levels that differed significantly from baseline serum NfL levels after 3 and 18 months (Figure 3B, $p < 0.05$).

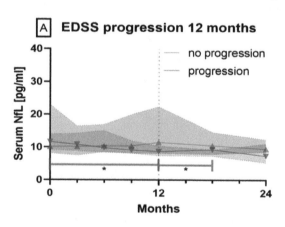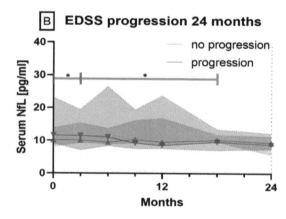

Figure 3. Serum NfL levels over 12 and 24 months in patients with (red triangle up) and without EDSS progression (blue triangle down) within (**A**) 12 or (**B**) 24 months. Symbols show median values, colored range indicates 95% CI, * $p < 0.05$.

3.3. Correlation of Serum NfL with

3.3.1. Age

There was no significant correlation of serum NfL and age in our cohort ($r < 0.3, p > 0.05$). However, age effects on serum NfL have been described [9,16]. As we mainly compared longitudinal sNfL values from the same individual over a limited period (24 months), no correction for age was made.

3.3.2. Serum Cytokine Profile in All Patients

We performed correlation analyses for serum NfL and serum IFN-γ, OPN, IL-2, IL-4 and IL-10 and for all time points. There was no significant correlation between serum NfL and the cytokine profile ($r < 0.3$, $p > 0.05$).

3.4. PASAT

To see whether serum NfL is associated with cognitive decline in MS patients, we performed a correlation analysis of serum NfL and PASAT at all time points (Figure 4). After correcting for multiple testing, a significant correlation between PASAT at month 24 and serum NfL at time points 3 and 18 remained (Spearman $r = 0.64$ and 0.57 and adjusted p-value = 0.005 and 0.029, respectively).

	Pasat t24	Pasat t18	Pasat t12	Pasat t9	Pasat t6	Pasat t3	Pasat t0
Serum NfL t0	0.40	0.28	0.28	0.04	0.22	0.20	0.22
Serum NfL t3	0.64	0.53	0.50	0.23	0.47	0.23	0.33
Serum NfL t6	0.51	0.46	0.34	0.28	0.48	0.24	0.30
Serum NfL t9	0.40	0.35	0.27	0.22	0.28	0.37	0.13
Serum NfL t12	0.27	0.25	0.28	0.11	0.21	0.32	0.09
Serum NfL t18	0.57	0.36	0.33	0.45	0.36	0.42	0.29
Serum NfL t24	0.16	0.12	0.13	0.16	0.15	0.16	0.20

Figure 4. Correlation matrix of Spearman correlation analysis for serum NfL and PASAT. Numbers in the cells are showing the respective Spearman correlation coefficient.

3.5. EDSS in Patients with Active Disease within 24 Months

To see whether serum NfL is associated with the disability in MS patients, we performed a correlation analysis of serum NfL and EDSS at all time points (Figure 5).

	EDSSt24	EDSSt18	EDSSt12	EDSSt9	EDSSt6	EDSSt3	EDSSt0
Serum NfL t0		-0.04	-0.11	-0.12	-0.09	0.04	-0.24
Serum NfL t3	0.23	-0.18	-0.11	-0.17	0.05	-0.12	-0.26
Serum NfL t6	-0.37	-0.32	-0.39	-0.33	-0.34	-0.35	-0.44
Serum NfL t9	-0.11	-0.14	0.01	-0.07	0.03	-0.28	-0.31
Serum NfL t12	-0.01	0.02	0.18	0.02	0.02	-0.07	-0.35
Serum NfL t18	0.18	-0.20	-0.05	0.10	0.09	-0.21	-0.16
Serum NfL t24	0.10	0.04	0.11	-0.05	0.08		0.03

Figure 5. Correlation matrix of Spearman correlation analysis for serum NfL and EDSS. Numbers in the cells are showing the respective Spearman correlation coefficient.

We did not observe significant correlations for serum NfL and EDSS at any time point in the group with active disease (at least one relapse) within 24 months.

3.6. Individual Serum NfL Courses in Patients Treated with Glatiramer Acetate

The serum NfL courses of all patients treated with glatiramer acetate with available MRI scans (T2 lesions) are illustrated. Additionally, for every available time point, the EDSS and occurred relapses are shown (Figure 6).

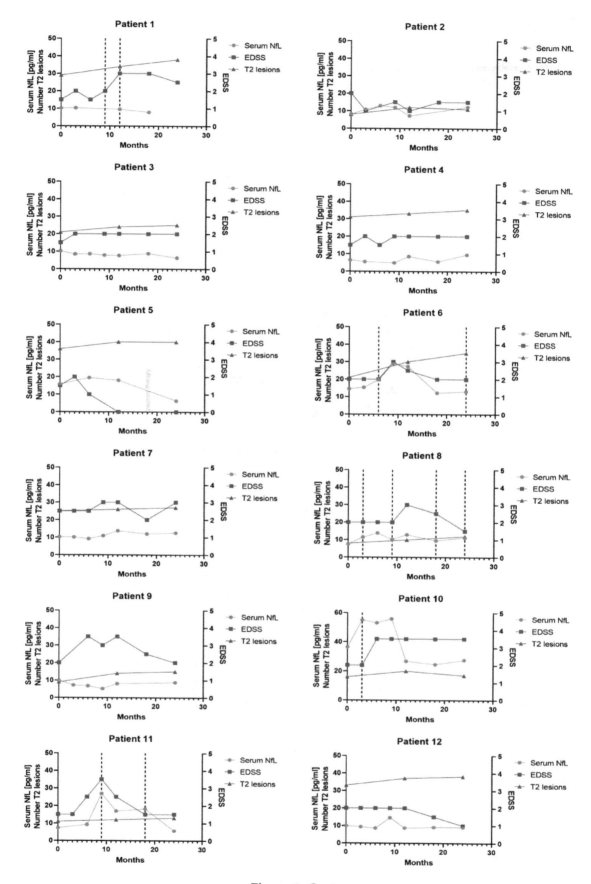

Figure 6. *Cont.*

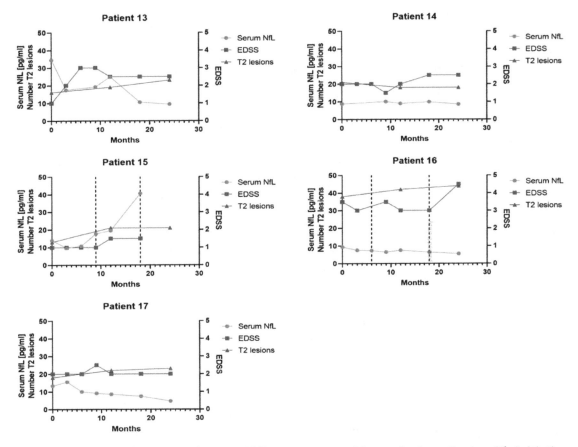

Figure 6. Illustration of individual serum NfL courses over 24 months in patients with initiation of disease-modifying treatment with glatiramer acetate after baseline. Green circles, red squares and blue triangles show serum NfL values (left y-axis), EDSS (right y-axis) and the number of T2 lesions (left y-axis), respectively. Vertical dashed lines show events of clinical activity in the form of a relapse at this time point.

4. Discussion

Neurodegeneration and axonal loss are major hallmarks of MS [2]. NfL has been extensively investigated as a biomarker for those molecular processes [6,9,11]. Initially NfL was exclusively analyzed in CSF, but with improved analytical sensitivity, serum analyses became possible as well [17]. Serum NfL shows a good correlation with CSF level and thereby offers a window to monitor axonal loss in MS patients consecutively [18,22]. Therefore, numerous studies including serum NfL in MS are available and it is used frequently in clinical trials [9,11,23,30]. However, longitudinal serum NfL assessments are scarce [26,27], especially in individual MS patients before and after initiation of first-line therapies. For this purpose, we aimed at characterizing the influence of those therapies on serum NfL levels.

Our data suggested that serum NfL may be suitable as a marker for therapy responsiveness based on the following findings: (a) sNfL levels stayed at a consistent low level or even dropped significantly in relapse-free patients over time and (b) sNfL levels after 9 and 12 months were significantly lower in patients without relapse within 12 months compared with patients suffering from a relapse during this time period.

However, we want to point out that most MS patients in the early phase of the disease, which is the case for most of our patients, show serum NfL levels that are within a normal age-adjusted range [16].

Furthermore, our data showed that serum NfL levels were associated with relapses as they were higher in time points with a present relapse compared with non-relapse time points.

The individual serum NfL courses showed that effects that were seen on a group basis did not always hold for every individual. Although serum NfL levels increased during the event of a relapse and decreased after high-dose corticosteroid therapy in most patients, there were exceptions (e.g., patient 16). More consistently, in our cohort, we observed that serum NfL levels stayed at a constant low level in therapy-responsive patients, which might be helpful in therapy monitoring of patients treated with first-line therapies. Our data suggested that this effect can be seen after 9 months. Whereas a sampling interval of 3 or even 6 months seems appropriate in patients without disease activity, other studies of highly active and more severely affected patients suggest a sampling interval and serum NfL testing every month [26]. We did not observe a positive correlation between serum NfL and EDSS for all time points, which is not surprising as this was also not seen in other studies [31] or only described in larger cohorts and with patients more severely affected by the disease and accordingly with higher EDSS [22,32]. The same was true for the correlation of serum NfL and PASAT as cognitive functions are only mildly affected in the early phase of the disease [33]. Even though, in a previous study, we observed an association of a more active disease course with higher levels of pro-inflammatory cytokines and lower levels of anti-inflammatory cytokines in a subpopulation of our study cohort [29], there was no correlation of serum NfL with any of the observed cytokines in the present study.

We also want to discuss the shortcomings of this study. As this was a retrospective analysis of serum NfL in a prospectively collected cohort, pre-analytical effects on serum NfL outcomes must be considered as samples were stored for more than 10 years. However, the observed values were in the same range as those of comparable patients [30,34,35] and of particular interest as no other therapies were available at this time and thereby we were able to monitor long-term outcomes of serum NfL in this specific study population. We can also not completely rule out spontaneous processes or regression that influences serum NfL (sNfL) levels, as we did not include untreated, stable MS patients. As this was an explorative study, these findings need to be confirmed in independent studies and it is desirable to have more detailed MRI data (e.g., number of gadolinium-enhanced lesions, atrophy, etc.) and complete data sets for every patient in those future studies because, for example, T1-hypointense lesions explain the severity of clinical disability better than T2-hyperintense white matter lesions and gadolinium-enhancing lesions correlate better with active disease status. Missing correlation with EDSS was similar to previous findings [31]. However, we were also unable to detect any correlations with the analyzed cytokines. This might be due to the small sample size or that inflammatory processes were either not present in patients or not displayed in the serum of those patients.

Monitoring of subclinical disease activity using MRI is an established procedure in the care of MS patients. Due to the method's invasiveness, this is not possible for CSF examination, although CSF parameters are appropriate to reflect intrathecal inflammatory processes. Serum NfL appears to be a promising marker for monitoring subclinical disease activity, as demonstrated in this cohort with longitudinal data collection under the same therapy over 24 months. However, this effect may not be seen in every patient as shown in our single-patient illustrations. In a heterogeneous disease like MS, a single biomarker is not sufficient to completely monitor and evaluate therapy efficacy. For this reason, all available information, clinical and paraclinical, should be gathered and taken into account for clinical decision making.

In summary, our study presents the first results on the effect of first-line therapies on serum NfL levels in mildly affected MS patients over 24 months. Here, serum NfL seems especially helpful in detecting therapy-responsive patients, but we also want to address the need for identifying factors that might influence serum NfL values. Among others, this includes processes involved in the transport of NfL from the CSF into serum as well as NfL clearance. The more we know about non-disease-related mechanisms that affect serum NfL, the better we can model serum NfL courses and identify real changes that are caused by pathological processes.

Author Contributions: Conceptualization, H.T.; data curation, A.H.; analysis, A.H. and B.M.; funding acquisition, H.T.; investigation, A.H.; methodology, J.K. and M.O.; project administration, A.C.L. and H.T.; resources, M.O.;

supervision, A.C.L. and H.T.; validation, M.S. and A.A.; visualization, A.H.; writing—original draft, A.H.; writing—review and editing, M.S., A.A., J.K., A.C.L., M.O. and H.T. All authors have read and agreed to the published version of the manuscript.

Acknowledgments: We kindly thank all patients for their participation in this study and all members of our local biobank, CSF and research lab for their excellent work. We would like to thank Paula Klassen for the linguistic and grammatical revision of the manuscript.

References

1. Compston, A.; Coles, A. Multiple sclerosis. *Lancet* **2002**, *359*, 1221–1231. [CrossRef]

2. Compston, A.; Coles, A. Multiple Sclerosis. *Lancet* **2008**, *372*, 1502–1517. [CrossRef]

3. Kamm, C.P.; Uitdehaag, B.M.; Polman, C.H. Multiple sclerosis: Current knowledge and future outlook. *Eur. Neurol.* **2014**, *72*, 132–141. [CrossRef] [PubMed]

4. Petzold, A.; Keir, G.; Green, A.J.E.; Giovannoni, G.; Thompson, E.J. A specific ELISA for measuring neurofilament heavy chain phosphoforms. *J. Immunol. Methods* **2003**, *278*, 179–190. [CrossRef]

5. Teunissen, C.E.; Khalil, M. Neurofilaments as biomarkers in multiple sclerosis. *Mult. Scler. J.* **2012**, *18*, 552–556. [CrossRef] [PubMed]

6. Yuan, A.; Rao, M.; Veeranna; Nixon, R.A. Neurofilaments and neurofilament proteins in health and disease. *Cold Spring Harb. Perspect. Biol.* **2017**, *9*, a018309. [CrossRef]

7. Gaetani, L.; Blennow, K.; Calabresi, P.; Di Filippo, M.; Parnetti, L.; Zetterberg, H. Neurofilament light chain as a biomarker in neurological disorders. *J. Neurol. Neurosurg. Psychiatry* **2019**, *90*, 870–881. [CrossRef]

8. Kuhle, J.; Plattner, K.; Bestwick, J.P.; Lindberg, R.L.; Ramagopalan, S.V.; Norgren, N.; Nissim, A.; Malaspina, A.; Leppert, D.; Giovannoni, G.; et al. A comparative study of CSF neurofilament light and heavy chain protein in MS. *Mult. Scler. J.* **2013**, *19*, 1597–1603. [CrossRef]

9. Khalil, M.; Teunissen, C.E.; Otto, M.; Piehl, F.; Sormani, M.P.; Gattringer, T.; Barro, C.; Kappos, L.; Comabella, M.; Fazekas, F.; et al. Neurofilaments as biomarkers in neurological disorders. *Nat. Rev. Neurol.* **2018**, *14*, 577–589. [CrossRef]

10. Khalil, M.; Salzer, J. CSF neurofilament light. *Neurology* **2016**, *87*, 1068–1069. [CrossRef]

11. Brettschneider, J.; Petzold, A.; Junker, A.; Tumani, H. Axonal damage markers in the cerebrospinal fluid of patients with clinically isolated syndrome improve predicting conversion to definite multiple sclerosis. *Mult. Scler. J.* **2006**, *12*, 143–148. [CrossRef] [PubMed]

12. Arrambide, G.; Espejo, C.; Eixarch, H.; Villar, L.M.; Alvarez-Cermeño, J.C.; Picón, C.; Kuhle, J.; Disanto, G.; Kappos, L.; Sastre-Garriga, J.; et al. Neurofilament light chain level is a weak risk factor for the development of MS. *Neurology* **2016**, *87*, 1076–1084. [CrossRef] [PubMed]

13. Gunnarsson, M.; Malmeström, C.; Axelsson, M.; Sundström, P.; Dahle, C.; Vrethem, M.; Olsson, T.P.; Piehl, F.; Norgren, N.; Rosengren, L.E.; et al. Axonal damage in relapsing multiple sclerosis is markedly reduced by natalizumab. *Ann. Neurol.* **2010**, *69*, 83–89. [CrossRef]

14. Bridel, C.; Van Wieringen, W.N.; Zetterberg, H.; Tijms, B.M.; Teunissen, C.E.; Alvarez-Cermeño, J.C.; Andreasson, U.; Axelsson, M.; Bäckström, D.C.; Bartos, A.; et al. Diagnostic value of cerebrospinal fluid neurofilament light protein in neurology. *JAMA Neurol.* **2019**, *76*, 1035–1048. [CrossRef] [PubMed]

15. Delaby, C.; Alcolea, D.; Carmona-Iragui, M.; Illán-Gala, I.; Morenas-Rodríguez, E.; Barroeta, I.; Altuna, M.; Estellés, T.; Santos-Santos, M.; Turon-Sans, J.; et al. Differential levels of Neurofilament Light protein in cerebrospinal fluid in patients with a wide range of neurodegenerative disorders. *Sci. Rep.* **2020**, *10*, 1–8. [CrossRef] [PubMed]

16. Khalil, M.; Pirpamer, L.; Hofer, E.; Voortman, M.M.; Barro, C.; Leppert, D.; Benkert, P.; Ropele, S.; Enzinger, C.; Fazekas, F.; et al. Serum neurofilament light levels in normal aging and their association with morphologic brain changes. *Nat. Commun.* **2020**, *11*, 812. [CrossRef]

17. Rissin, D.M.; Kan, C.W.; Campbell, T.G.; Howes, S.C.; Fournier, D.R.; Song, L.; Piech, T.; Patel, P.P.; Chang, L.; Rivnak, A.J.; et al. Single-molecule enzyme-linked immunosorbent assay detects serum proteins at subfemtomolar concentrations. *Nat. Biotechnol.* **2010**, *28*, 595–599. [CrossRef]

18. Kuhle, J.; Barro, C.; Andreasson, U.; Derfuss, T.; Lindberg, R.; Sandelius, Å.; Liman, V.; Norgren, N.; Blennow, K.; Zetterberg, H. Comparison of three analytical platforms for quantification of the neurofilament light chain in blood samples: ELISA, electrochemiluminescence immunoassay and Simoa. *Clin. Chem. Lab. Med.* **2016**, *54*, 1655–1661. [CrossRef]

19. Kuhle, J.; Barro, C.; Disanto, G.; Mathias, A.; Soneson, C.; Bonnier, G.; Yaldizli, Ö.; Regeniter, A.; Derfuss, T.; Canales, M.; et al. Serum neurofilament light chain in early relapsing remitting MS is increased and correlates with CSF levels and with MRI measures of disease severity. *Mult. Scler. J.* **2016**, *22*, 1550–1559. [CrossRef]

20. Kuhle, J.; Nourbakhsh, B.; Grant, D.; Morant, S.; Barro, C.; Yaldizli, Ö.; Pelletier, D.; Giovannoni, G.; Waubant, E.; Gnanapavan, S. Serum neurofilament is associated with progression of brain atrophy and disability in early MS. *Neurology* **2017**, *88*, 826–831. [CrossRef]

21. Siller, N.; Kuhle, J.; Muthuraman, M.; Barro, C.; Uphaus, T.; Groppa, S.; Kappos, L.; Zipp, F.; Bittner, S. Serum neurofilament light chain is a biomarker of acute and chronic neuronal damage in early multiple sclerosis. *Mult. Scler. J.* **2018**, *25*, 678–686. [CrossRef] [PubMed]

22. Disanto, G.; Barro, C.; Benkert, P.; Naegelin, Y.; Schädelin, S.; Giardiello, A.; Zecca, C.; Blennow, K.; Zetterberg, H.; Leppert, D.; et al. Serum Neurofilament light: A biomarker of neuronal damage in multiple sclerosis. *Ann. Neurol.* **2017**, *81*, 857–870. [CrossRef]

23. Sormani, M.P.; Haering, D.A.; Kropshofer, H.; Leppert, D.; Kundu, U.; Barro, C.; Kappos, L.; Tomic, D.; Kuhle, J. Blood neurofilament light as a potential endpoint in Phase 2 studies in MS. *Ann. Clin. Transl. Neurol.* **2019**, *6*, 1081–1089. [CrossRef]

24. Sejbæk, T.; Nielsen, H.H.; Penner, N.; Plavina, T.; Mendoza, J.P.; Martin, N.A.; Elkjaer, M.L.; Ravnborg, M.H.; Illes, Z. Dimethyl fumarate decreases neurofilament light chain in CSF and blood of treatment naïve relapsing MS patients. *J. Neurol. Neurosurg. Psychiatry* **2019**, *90*, 1324–1330. [CrossRef]

25. Thebault, S.; Abdoli, M.; Fereshtehnejad, S.-M.; Tessier, D.; Tabard-Cossa, V.; Freedman, M.S. Serum neurofilament light chain predicts long term clinical outcomes in multiple sclerosis. *Sci. Rep.* **2020**, *10*, 10381. [CrossRef] [PubMed]

26. Akgün, K.; Kretschmann, N.; Haase, R.; Proschmann, U.; Kitzler, H.H.; Reichmann, H.; Ziemssen, T. Profiling individual clinical responses by high-frequency serum neurofilament assessment in MS. *Neurol. Neuroimmunol. Neuroinflamm.* **2019**, *6*, e555. [CrossRef] [PubMed]

27. Hyun, J.-W.; Kim, Y.; Kim, G.; Kim, S.-H.; Kim, H.J. Longitudinal analysis of serum neurofilament light chain: A potential therapeutic monitoring biomarker for multiple sclerosis. *Mult. Scler. J.* **2019**, *26*, 659–667. [CrossRef]

28. Teunissen, C.E.; Petzold, A.; Bennett, J.L.; Berven, F.S.; Brundin, L.; Comabella, M.; Franciotta, D.; Frederiksen, J.L.; Fleming, J.O.; Furlan, R.; et al. A consensus protocol for the standardization of cerebrospinal fluid collection and biobanking. *Neurology* **2009**, *73*, 1914–1922. [CrossRef]

29. Tumani, H.; Kassubek, J.; Hijazi, M.; Lehmensiek, V.; Unrath, A.; Süssmuth, S.; Lauda, F.; Kapfer, T.; Fang, L.; Senel, M.; et al. Patterns of TH1/TH2 cytokines predict clinical response in multiple sclerosis patients treated with glatiramer acetate. *Eur. Neurol.* **2011**, *65*, 164–169. [CrossRef]

30. Novakova, L.; Zetterberg, H.; Sundström, P.; Axelsson, M.; Khademi, M.; Gunnarsson, M.; Malmeström, C.; Svenningsson, A.; Olsson, T.; Piehl, F.; et al. Monitoring disease activity in multiple sclerosis using serum neurofilament light protein. *Neurology* **2017**, *89*, 2230–2237. [CrossRef]

31. Abdelhak, A.; Huss, A.; Kassubek, J.; Tumani, H.; Otto, M. Serum GFAP as a biomarker for disease severity in multiple sclerosis. *Sci. Rep.* **2018**, *8*, 14798. [CrossRef]

32. Högel, H.; Rissanen, E.; Barro, C.; Matilainen, M.; Nylund, M.; Kuhle, J.; Airas, L. Serum glial fibrillary acidic protein correlates with multiple sclerosis disease severity. *Mult. Scler. J.* **2018**, *26*, 210–219. [CrossRef] [PubMed]

33. Johnen, A.; Bürkner, P.-C.; Landmeyer, N.C.; Ambrosius, B.; Calabrese, P.; Motte, J.; Hessler, N.; Antony, G.; König, I.R.; Klotz, L.; et al. Can we predict cognitive decline after initial diagnosis of multiple sclerosis? Results from the German National early MS cohort (KKNMS). *J. Neurol.* **2018**, *266*, 386–397. [CrossRef] [PubMed]

34. Håkansson, I.; Tisell, A.; Cassel, P.; Blennow, K.; Zetterberg, H.; Lundberg, P.; Dahle, C.; Vrethem, M.; Ernerudh, J. Neurofilament levels, disease activity and brain volume during follow-up in multiple sclerosis. *J. Neuroinflamm.* **2018**, *15*, 209. [CrossRef] [PubMed]

13

PBMC of Multiple Sclerosis Patients Show Deregulation of OPA1 Processing Associated with Increased ROS and PHB2 Protein Levels

Domenico De Rasmo [1,*], Anna Ferretta [2], Silvia Russo [2], Maddalena Ruggieri [2], Piergiorgio Lasorella [2], Damiano Paolicelli [2], Maria Trojano [2] and Anna Signorile [2,*]

[1] CNR-Institute of Biomembranes, Bioenergetics and Molecular Biotechnologies, 70126 Bari, Italy
[2] Department of Basic Medical Sciences, Neurosciences and Sense Organs, University of Bari "Aldo Moro", 70124 Bari, Italy; anna.ferretta@uniba.it (A.F.); silvia.russo92@gmail.com (S.R.); maddalena.ruggieri@uniba.it (M.R.); p.lasorella@studenti.uniba.it (P.L.); damiano.paolicelli@uniba.it (D.P.); maria.trojano@uniba.it (M.T.)
*   Correspondence: d.derasmo@ibiom.cnr.it (D.D.R.); anna.signorile@uniba.it (A.S.);

Abstract: Multiple sclerosis (MS) is an autoimmune disease in which activated lymphocytes affect the central nervous system. Increase of reactive oxygen species (ROS), impairment of mitochondria-mediated apoptosis and mitochondrial alterations have been reported in peripheral lymphocytes of MS patients. Mitochondria-mediated apoptosis is regulated by several mechanisms and proteins. Among others, optic atrophy 1 (OPA1) protein plays a key role in the regulating mitochondrial dynamics, cristae architecture and release of pro-apoptotic factors. Very interesting, mutations in OPA1 gene, have been associated with multiple sclerosis-like disorder. We have analyzed OPA1 and some factors involved in its regulation. Fifteen patients with MS and fifteen healthy control subjects (HC) were enrolled into the study and peripheral blood mononuclear cells (PBMCs) were isolated. H_2O_2 level was measured spectrofluorimetrically, OPA1, PHB2, SIRT3, and OMA1 were analyzed by western blotting. Statistical analysis was performed using Student's t-test. The results showed that PBMC of MS patients were characterized by a deregulation of OPA1 processing associated with increased H_2O_2 production, inactivation of OMA1 and increase of PHB2 protein level. The presented data suggest that the alteration of PHB2, OMA1, and OPA1 processing could be involved in resistance towards apoptosis. These molecular parameters could also be useful to assess disease activity.

Keywords: multiple sclerosis; PBMCs; mitochondria; ROS; OPA1; PHB2; OMA1

1. Introduction

Multiple sclerosis (MS) is a complex neurodegenerative disease that involves immune and central nervous system (CNS) [1,2]. MS is expressed in different clinical forms including primary progressive (PP), secondary progressive (SP), progressive relapsing (RP) and relapsing-remitting (RR), which is the most prevalent form [3]. The pathogenesis of MS involves the loss of blood–brain barrier integrity with the consequent invasion of lymphocytes into the CNS resulting in tissue damage [4].

Despite the knowledge of genetics, cell biology and immunology, obtained in the last years, the ultimate etiology or specific elements that trigger MS remain unknown. The etiopathogenesis and pathophysiology of MS involves different factors, among others mitochondrial dysfunction and oxidative stress (OS) play a key role and have a further modulatory effect on many aspects of the disease. OS plays an important role in activation of immune cells, especially T cells [5–7], and recently it has been reported that peripheral blood mononuclear cells (PBMCs) of MS patients show impaired redox status associated with mitochondrial alterations [5]. A number of mechanisms participate in the maintenance of the immune homeostasis avoiding the development of autoimmune diseases. The apoptosis is an important anti-autoimmune process that deletes potentially pathogenic autoreactive lymphocytes, limiting the immune response-dependent tissue damage [8,9]. It has been shown that deletion of autoreactive lymphocytes by apoptosis is defective in patients with MS, thereby permitting these cells to perpetuate a continuous cycle of inflammation within the CNS [10,11]. In particular, the impairment of mitochondria-mediated apoptosis in Cd4+ T lymphocytes [12], as well as, a reduction of mitochondrial respiration are reported in MS patients [13]. Mitochondria have a main role in both cell death and life and they are a major source of reactive oxygen species (ROS) production. At the same time, mitochondria are responsive to OS and are critical in modulating apoptosis in response themselves to a variety of stress signals.

Several mitochondria parameters such as mitochondrial respiratory chain activity, ROS production, dynamics (fusion and fission), and mitochondria cristae architecture are involved in mitochondria-mediated apoptosis [14–16]. Among mitochondrial proteins involved in apoptosis mechanism, optic atrophy 1 (OPA1) is a mitochondrial dynamin like GTPase that has attracted great attention for its role in the regulating mitochondrial fusion and fission, the stability of the mitochondrial respiratory chain complexes, pro-apoptotic cytochrome c release and the maintenance of mitochondrial cristae architecture [17]. Very interesting, it is reported that mutations in OPA1 gene, resulting in autosomal dominant optic atrophy (ADOA), are associated with multiple sclerosis-like disorder in patients [18].

OPA1 undergoes constitutive processing leading to the conversion of the un-cleaved long OPA1 (L-OPA1) in a cleaved short OPA1 (S-OPA1) forms. Various stress conditions, including apoptotic stimulation are associated with the conversion of L-OPA1 into S-OPA1. The processing and activity of OPA1 is regulated by mitochondrial proteases, such as OMA1, cellular energetic condition [19], post-translational modification, such as acetylation status [20,21], and oxidative stress [20,22]. OMA1-mediated processing of OPA1 is a cellular stress response, in fact, although OMA1 is constitutively active, it display strongly enhanced activity in response to OS [23]. Furthermore, OPA1 stability is controlled by prohibitin 2 (PHB2) [24] a chaperon like protein, localizes in nucleus, plasma membrane, and mitochondria. Evidences indicate that mitochondrial PHB2 is over expressed under conditions of oxidative stress [25]. Interesting, PHB2 has been found up-regulated in lymphocytes of MS patients [26]. OPA1 processing is also modulated by its acetylation status mediated by SIRT3 enzyme, a mitochondrial deacetylase that also plays an important role in apoptosis [20]. In this work we have analyzed the protein level, and proteolytic processing of OPA1 and its stress-associated regulators, OMA1, SIRT3, and PHB2 in PBMCs of MS patients.

2. Experimental Section

2.1. Patients

Fifteen patients with MS according to McDonald criteria [27] and fifteen healthy volunteers control subjects (HC) were enrolled into the study. The patients and HC subjects were selected by the Centre of Multiple Sclerosis at Department of Basic Medical Sciences Neurosciences and Sense Organs, University of Bari. All patients had to be without any immunomodulatory treatment at least 6 months prior to study entry. All subjects gave their informed consent for inclusion before they participated in the study. The study was conducted in accordance with the Declaration of Helsinki and the protocol was approved by the Ethics Committee of Azienda Policlinico di Bari (Project identification code 5275). Table 1 reports demographic and clinical characteristics of MS patients and healthy subjects. For all data, no significant difference was observed between males and females as well as between RR and SP forms of MS.

Table 1. Demographic and clinical characteristics of patients with multiple sclerosis (MS) and healthy control subjects (HC) enrolled into the study. (SP: secondary progressive, RR: relapsing-remitting, EDSS: Expanded Disability Status Scale, SEM: standard error of mean.

	MS	HC
Subject (number)	15	15
Age (year)	45 ± 2.46 SEM	44.92 ± 3.92 SEM
Gender	12 Females 3 Males	6 Females 9 Males
MS form	11 RR 4 SP	
Disease duration(year)	14.4 ± 1.70 SEM	
EDSS	4.2 ± 0.34 SEM	

2.2. Sample Preparation

Peripheral blood mononuclear cells (PBMCs) were isolated from K3-EDTA blood by centrifugation on a Ficoll-Hypaque density gradient (density: 1.077 g/mL; Amersham Pharmacia Biotech, Buckinghamshire, UK), washed twice and resuspended in PBS. Total protein concentration was determined by Bio Rad protein assay.

2.3. Electrophoretic Procedures and Western Blotting

Protein of PBMCs were resuspended in RIPA lysis buffer, separated by 7.5% SDS-polyacrylamide gel electrophoresis (PAGE) and transferred into a nitrocellulose membrane. The membrane was blocked with 5% fatty acid free dry milk in 500 mM NaCl, 0.05% Tween 20, 20 mM Tris, pH 7.4 (TTBS) for 3 h at 4 °C and probed over night with antibodies against OPA1 (whole molecule of OPA1 protein was used as the immunogen) (Thermo scientific, Pierce Antibodies, Lausanne, Switzerland), PHB2 (Invitrogen, Paisley, UK), OMA1, SIRT3 (Cell Signalling, Danvers, MA, USA) and β-actin (Sigma-Aldrich, St. Louis, MO, USA). After being washed in TTBS, the membranes were incubated for 60 min with anti-rabbit or anti-mouse IgG peroxidase-conjugated. Immunodetection was then performed, after further TTBS washes, with the enhanced chemiluminescence (ECL) (Euroclone, Paignton, UK). Densitometric analysis, expressed as arbitrary densitometric units (ADU), electrophoretic profile and relative front (Rf) determinations were performed by Image Lab Touch 2.4 software (BioRad, Milan, Italy). Rf indicates the relative movement of the band from the top.

2.4. H_2O_2 Assay

H_2O_2 level was determined by the cell permeant probe 2'-7'-dichlorodihydrofluorescin diacetate (DCFDA). PBMCs were incubated with 10 μM DCFDA in the dark at 37 °C for 20 min, pelleted at 600× g for 5 min, washed and resuspended in the assay buffer (100 mM potassium phosphate, pH 7.4, 2 mM $MgCl_2$). An aliquot was used for protein determination. The H_2O_2 dependent oxidation of the fluorescent probe (507 nm excitation and 530 nm emission wavelengths) was measured by a Jasco FP6200 spectrofluorimeter (Jasco SRL, Cremella, Italy).

2.5. Data Analysis

All presented data are means ± standard error of mean (SEM). Statistical difference was determined by Student' t-test. p-value of 0.05 was considered as statistically significant (*** $p < 0.001$; ** $p < 0.01$; * $p < 0.05$).

Correlation plots for controls and MS have been performing with Excel Microsoft software using Pearson's correlation analysis. P-values less than 0.05 were considered statistically significant.

3. Results

Fifteen HC and fifteen MS subjects (see Table 1) were enrolled in the study. The patients group included 12 females and 3 males and 11 RR forms and 4 SP forms of MS (see Table 1). The PBMC cellular lysate was used to investigate on the OPA1 protein level and processing by Western blotting analysis using a specific antibody (Figure 1).

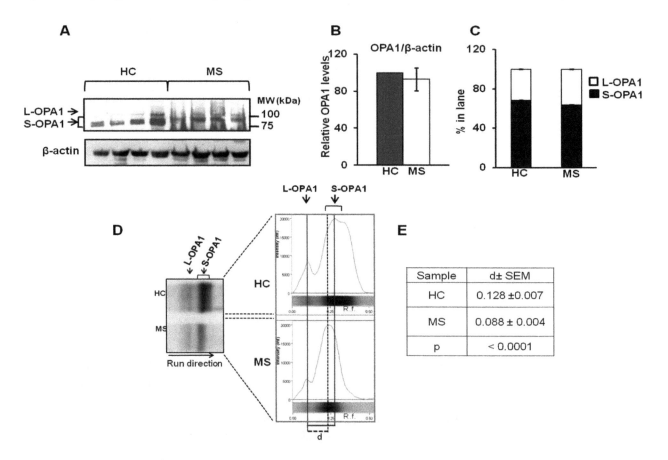

Figure 1. Optic atrophy 1 (OPA1) protein level and processing in peripheral blood mononuclear cells (PBMCs) from HC and MS patients. (**A**) Representative images of western blotting analysis. The PBMC proteins from HC and MS were loaded on 7.5% SDS-PAGE. After separation, the proteins were transferred on nitrocellulose membranes and immunoblotted with the antibody against OPA1. Protein loading was assessed with β-actin antibody. (**B**) The total protein level of OPA1 (L+S forms) was evaluated by densitometric analysis. The arbitrary densitometric units (ADU) of OPA1 were normalized to ADU of β-actin and the mean of HC set to 100%. The histograms represent the percentage values MS patients with respect to HC. The values are means ± SEM of different samples. (**C**) The histograms represent the percentage of ADU of long (L) and short (S), forms of OPA1 in each lane. The values are means ± SEM of samples. (**D**) Left panel, representative image of electrophoretic mobility of immune-revealed bands of OPA1 in PBMCs from HC and MS. Right panel, the images of the western blotting were analyzed by Image Lab Touch 2.4 software (BioRAD) for determination of electrophoretic profile of each lane and calculation of relative front (Rf) of L-OPA1 and S-OPA1 bands (see Table S1). Rf indicates the relative movement of the band from the top of the gel. "d" represents the difference between Rf of S-OPA1 and Rf of L-OPA1 in each lane. (**E**) The table reports the means values of "d" ± SEM of different samples. ($p < 0.001$, Student's t-test).

The antibody against OPA1 protein, immuno-revealed in both HC and MS groups a long form (L) and short forms (S) of OPA1 (Figure 1A). Densitometric analysis of immuno-revealed bands of OPA1 (L+S) showed the same level of total OPA1protein in MS group with respect to HC (Figure 1B). No difference was observed in percentage of L and S form of OPA1 between HC and SM samples

(Figure 1C). Interestingly, the image analysis of western blotting revealed two bands of S-OPA1 in HC and one band of S-OPA1with a different electrophoretic mobility with respect to HC samples in MS (Figure 1A,D). Analysis by Image Lab Touch 2.4 software confirmed the presence of two S-OPA1 bands in HC and one S-OPA1 band in MS as shown by curve peaks (Figure 1D). Moreover, the determination of Rf of L-OPA1 and S-OPA1 bands revealed a significant decrease in Rf of S-OPA1 in MS sample with respect to HC (see Table S1). No differences were observed in Rf of L-OPA1 between HC and MS samples (Table S1). Calculation of difference between Rf of S-OPA1 band and L-OPA1 band in each lane ("d"), revealed a significant decrease of "d" in MS samples with respect to HC (Figure 1D,E). This suggested that processing of OPA1, in MS samples, generated a S-OPA1 form at a higher molecular weight with respect to HC.

Processing of OPA1 is regulated by different proteins and cellular conditions such as oxidative stress. Measurement of H_2O_2 level, detected by the redox-sensitive fluorescent probe DCFDA, showed increased ROS production in the PBMCs of MS patients compared to HC (Figure 2).

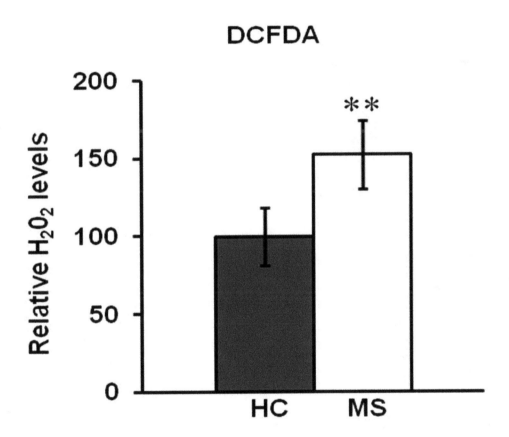

Figure 2. H_2O_2 production in PBMC of HC and MS patients. H_2O_2 level was detected spectrofluorimetrically by dichlorodihydrofluorescin (DCFDA) probe. The mean of HC was set to 100% and the mean value of MS expressed as percentage of intensity of fluorescence respect to HC. The histograms represent the means of values ± SEM. (** $p < 0.01$; Student's t-test).

This result prompted to investigate on stress regulated protein OMA1, PHB2 and SIRT3 that are involved in OPA1 processing and stabilization [20,22,25]. Activation of OMA1 protease is accompanied by its autocatalytic degradation that results in the complete turnover of protein [22]. Western blotting analysis of OMA1 did not show the activation of this protease in PBMCs from MS samples as revealed by the increased ratio between inactive and active forms (Figure 3A,B). We next examined PHB2 level by western blot analysis with specific antibody. An increased PHB2 protein level was observed in MS patients (Figure 3C,D) compared to HC samples, while no difference was observed for SIRT3 protein level (Figure 3C,D).

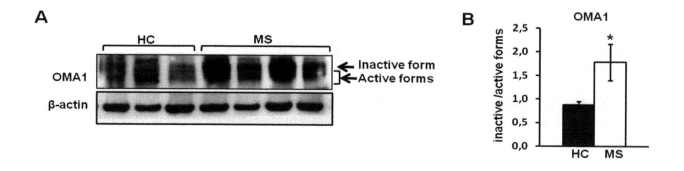

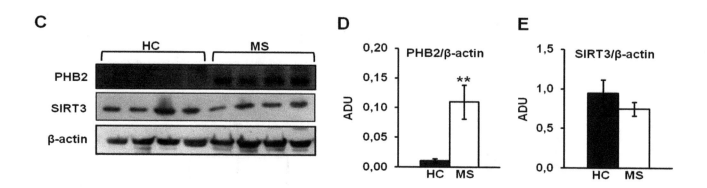

Figure 3. OMA1, SIRT3, and PHB2 in PBMCs of HC and MS patients. (**A,C**) Representative images of Western blotting analysis. Proteins from PBMC from HC and MS were loaded on 7.5% SDS-PAGE. After separation, the proteins were transferred on nitrocellulose membranes and immunoblotted with the antibodies against OMA1, SIRT3, and PHB2. Protein loading was assessed with β-actin antibody. The immunoblotting against β-actin in panel C is the same shown in the Figure 1A, belonging to the same experiment series (**B,D**). (**B**) The histograms represent the means of ratio values ± SEM between the ADU of inactive and active forms of OMA1 in HC and MS subjects. (**D,E**) The ADU of PHB2 and SIRT3 were normalized to ADU of β-actin. The histograms represent the means of values of ADU ± SEM of samples. (* $p < 0.05$, ** $p < 0.01$; Student's t-test).

To explore whether the alterations in the analyzed molecular parameters can cross correlate with each other, a correlation analysis was performed for HC and MS groups. The results in HC indicated a remarkable positive correlation of SIRT3 changes with changes of L- and S-OPA1 balance. This correlation was lost in MS group. In addition, in MS group, a significant positive correlation was observed between H_2O_2 level and PHB2 (Figure 4B), and negative correlations between H_2O_2 and L- and S-OPA1 balance (Figure 4C) and between PHB2 and L- and S-OPA1 balance (Figure 4D).

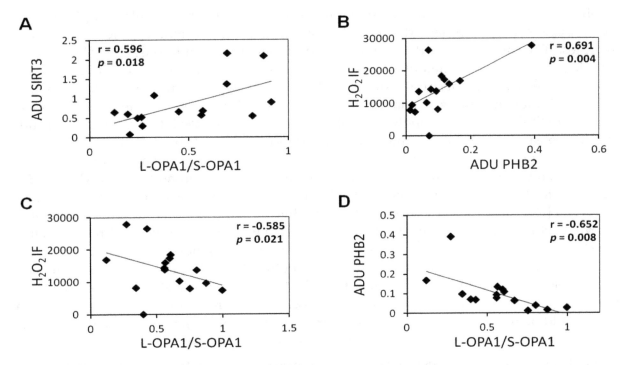

Figure 4. Correlation plots. Empty squares indicates HC group, full squares indicates MS group (**A**)Scatter plot and linear regression of data of relationship between SIRT3 protein level, expressed in ADU, and L-OPA1/S-OPA1 balance in HC group (correlation coefficient, r = 0.596; P, 0.021). (**B**) Scatter plot and linear regression of data of relationship between H_2O_2, expressed in intensity of fluorescence (IF), and PHB2 protein level, expressed in ADU in MS group (correlation coefficient, r = −0.691; P, 0.004). (**C**) Scatter plot and linear regression of data of relationship between H_2O_2 and L-OPA1/S-OPA1 balance in MS group (correlation coefficient r = −0.585, P,0.021). (**D**) Scatter plot and linear regression of data of relationship between PHB2 protein expression and cleaved long OPA1 (L-OPA1)/cleaved short OPA1 (S-OPA1) balance in MS group (correlation coefficient, r = −0.652; P = 0.008). Degree of freedom 13.

4. Discussion

The pathogenesis of MS involves autoreactive T lymphocytes that have the capacity to invade the CNS causing demyelization and axonal damage [4]. The deletion of autoreactive lymphocytes is normally mediated by apoptosis, however, an escape from mitochondria-mediated apoptosis has been reported in lymphocytes of MS patients [12]. Mitochondria from MS lymphocytes also show a decrease of mitochondrial respiration [13] associated with a specific decrease of complex I and complex IV activities [28], and, of note, mitochondria have been found to range in shape and size and showed thickened cristae [29]. Mitochondrial dependent apoptosis is also depending on mitochondrial respiration, shape and structure. A growing body of evidence suggests that OPA1 participates through several mechanisms in defining mitochondrial shape and structure of cristae [14] and modulating mitochondrial respiration [17]. This modulates cell susceptibility towards apoptotic stimuli [14]. Augmented level of OPA1, formation of OPA1 oligomers and a correct balance of L and S forms are considered anti-apoptotic factors [17]. In light of this and the data reporting that OPA1 mutations are associated with multiple sclerosis-like symptoms [18], in this work, we analyzed OPA1 and its modulators in PBMCs of MS patients compared to HC. Fifteen healthy controls and fifteen subjects affected by MS were enrolled in the study. The patients group included 12 females and 3 males and 11 RR forms and 4 SP forms of MS (see Table 1). No significant difference was observed between males and females subjects as well as between RR and SP forms.

Our results showed the same level of OPA1 total protein (L+S) in HC and SM samples and no differences were observed in the balance between L and S forms of OPA1 in PBMC of HC and MS patients. Interesting the analysis of the electrophoretic migration of immune-revealed bands of OPA1 in lymphocytes of MS samples showed only one S-form at a higher molecular weight in MS with respect to the two S forms observed in HC, thus suggesting a characteristic processing of OPA1 in MS samples. The functions of OPA1 are regulated, under stress conditions, by OMA1-dependent proteolytic cleavage. As expected PBMCs of MS patients show increased level of ROS that, anyway, not results in the activation of stress-induced OMA1 [22], as shown by the accumulation of inactive form of OMA1, thus suggesting an adaptation to exposure at chronic OS. Of note, it was reported that suppression of OMA1 activity strongly prevented cytochrome *c* release into the cytosol [30] and cells lacking the protease OMA1 showed an increased resistance to external apoptotic stimuli [31,32]. OPA1, beyond the proteolytic control, is also under the control of alternative splicing. Eight different OPA1 isoforms, generated by alternative splicing of four exons near the amino terminus (Figure S1), are characterized for the presence, or absence, of at least three different proteolytic cleavage sites, named S1, S2, and S3 [33]. The S1 site is cleaved by OMA1 while S2 and S3 by Ymel1 protease. The presence of isoform 3, which contains S3 and S1 cleavage sites (see Figure S1), together with the inactivation of OMA1 protease (see also [32]), could explain the shift of electrophoretic mobility observed in MS patients. Although YME1L and OMA1 constitutively control OPA1, the proteolytic processing of OPA1 is more complex, in fact, other proteases can act on OPA1 under particular stress condition or metabolic demands [33,34], thus, the involvement of other mitochondrial proteases cannot be ruled out. In this contest, should be noted that, in MS, several proteases are involved [35,36] and that mitochondrial proteases are often involved in the pathogenesis of neurological diseases [37].

It has been reported that SIRT3 has an important role in a variety of oxidative stress-mediated cellular responses [38], in the regulation of bioenergetic function and antioxidant defense of mitochondria under OS conditions [39]. OS regulated SIRT3 protein level that, in turn, is involved in mitochondrial apoptosis by modulating OPA1 acetylation/processing [20]. In particular, sustained level of SIRT3 protein favors the apoptosis resistance, while a decrease promotes cell death [20]. We have also investigated on SIRT3 protein level; however, despite the increased ROS production in MS, no difference has been observed in MS lymphocytes compared to HC samples. Although the SIRT3 protein level was unchanged, this could be interpreted as a loss of response of lymphocytes of MS patients to OS. The data on SIRT3 and OMA1 suggest a deregulation of normally stress response mechanisms of these proteins in PBMCs of MS patients.

Furthermore, OPA1 processing and stability is also controlled by PHB2 protein. In mitochondrial inner membrane, PHB2 protein forms with PHB1 a large membrane-bound complex [40,41]. This complex is required for OPA1 stability [42], indeed the deletion of PHB2 leads to the impaired cellular proliferation, aberrant mitochondrial cristae morphogenesis, and apoptosis [24,42], while an over-expression of PHB2 is reported to protect cells from apoptosis [43]. We show, according with others [26] and as response to OS [25], a strong increase of PHB2 protein level in MS samples, thus representing another element of resistance to apoptosis. It worth mentioning that an elevated autophagic flux has been reported in autoreactive T cells, both in patients and in the mouse model of experimental autoimmune encephalomyelitis [44]. It has been found that PHB2 participates in the mitophagy process (selective autophagy) by functioning as mitochondrial receptor in autophagosome formation [45].

Interestingly, using Pearson's correlation analysis, we found a positive correlation in HC group between SIRT3 changes and changes of L- and S-OPA1 balance. This is in agreement with the findings showing that the SIRT3-dependent deacetylation of L-OPA1 inhibits its proteolytic processing to form S-OPA1 [20]. This correlation was lost in the MS group, while changes of L- and S-OPA1 balance, PHB2 protein level and H_2O_2 correlated each other. In facts, under condition of oxidative stress, an increased cleavage of L-OPA1 to produce S-OPA1 has been observed [20] as well as an increase of PHB2 expression [25]. The over expression of PHB2 has been found to protect the cell from oxidative stress-dependent apoptosis [43].

5. Conclusions

Our data showed that, in PBMCs of MS patients, oxidative stress is associated with increased level of PHB2 and stabilization of OMA1. We propose that the alteration of PHB2, OMA1, and OPA1 is involved in the apoptosis resistance. We hypothesize involvement of specific proteolytic processing of OPA1 in lymphocytes of MS patients. Other investigations will be needed to define the mechanisms at the bases of this deregulations and the possible proteases involved in the characteristic processing of OPA1 in MS samples. The specific OPA1 electrophoretic profile and an increased level of PHB2 in MS patients could also be taken in account to assess disease activity. Understanding of the molecular mechanisms underlying these deregulations could shed light on new therapeutic interventions.

Author Contributions: Conceptualization, A.S. and D.D.R.; methodology, A.S. and D.D.R.; software, A.S. and D.D.R.; validation, A.S. and D.D.R.; formal analysis, A.S. and D.D.R.; resources, M.R., P.L., D.P., M.T.; data curation, A.S., D.D.R., A.F., S.R., M.R., D.P.; writing—original draft preparation, A.S. and D.D.R.; writing—review and editing, A.S., D.D.R., M.T., A.F., S.R., M.R., D.P.; supervision, A.S. and D.D.R.; project administration, A.S. and D.D.R.; funding acquisition, A.S. All authors have read and agreed to the published version of the manuscript.

References

1. Tobore, T.O. Towards a comprehensive etiopathogenetic and pathophysiological theory of multiple sclerosis. *Int. J. Neurosci.* **2020**, *130*, 279–300. [CrossRef]

2. Lassmann, H.; Brück, W.; Lucchinetti, C.F. The immunopathology of multiple sclerosis: An overview. *Brain Pathol.* **2007**, *17*, 210–218. [CrossRef]

3. Loma, I.; Heyman, R. Multiple sclerosis: Pathogenesis and treatment. *Curr. Neuropharmacol.* **2011**, *9*, 409–416. [CrossRef]

4. Sospedra, M.; Martin, R. Immunology of multiple sclerosis. *Annu. Rev. Immunol.* **2005**, *23*, 683–747. [CrossRef]

5. Gonzalo, H.; Nogueras, L.; Gil-Sánchez, A.; Hervás, J.V.; Valcheva, P.; González-Mingot, C.; Martin-Gari, M.; Canudes, M.; Peralta, S.; Solana, M.J.; et al. Impairment of Mitochondrial Redox Status in Peripheral Lymphocytes of Multiple Sclerosis Patients. *Front. Neurosci.* **2019**, *13*, 938. [CrossRef]

6. Gilgun-Sherki, Y.; Melamed, E.; Offen, D. The role of oxidative stress in the pathogenesis of multiple sclerosis: The need for effective antioxidant therapy. *J. Neurol.* **2004**, *251*, 261–268.

7. Ohl, K.; Tenbrock, K.; Kipp, M. Oxidative stress in multiple sclerosis: Central and peripheral mode of action. *Exp. Neurol.* **2016**, *277*, 58–67. [CrossRef] [PubMed]

8. Comabella, M.; Khoury, S.J. Immunopathogenesis of multiple sclerosis. *Clin. Immunol.* **2012**, *142*, 2–8. [CrossRef] [PubMed]

9. McFarland, H.F.; Martin, R. Multiple sclerosis: A complicated picture of autoimmunity. *Nat. Immunol.* **2007**, *8*, 913–919. [CrossRef] [PubMed]

10. Segal, B.M.; Cross, A.H. Fas(t) track to apoptosis in MS: TNF receptors may suppress or potentiate CNS demyelination. *Neurology* **2000**, *55*, 906–907. [CrossRef] [PubMed]

11. Ruggieri, M.; Avolio, C.; Scacco, S.; Pica, C.; Lia, A.; Zimatore, G.B.; Papa, S.; Livrea, P.; Trojano, M. Glatiramer acetate induces pro-apoptotic mechanisms involving Bcl-2, Bax and Cyt-c in peripheral lymphocytes from multiple sclerosis patients. *J. Neurol.* **2006**, *253*, 231–236. [CrossRef]

12. Julià, E.; Edo, M.C.; Horga, A.; Montalban, X.; Comabella, M. Differential susceptibility to apoptosis of CD4+T cells expressing CCR5 and CXCR3 in patients with MS. *Clin. Immunol.* **2009**, *133*, 364–374. [CrossRef]

13. La Rocca, C.; Carbone, F.; De Rosa, V.; Colamatteo, A.; Galgani, M.; Perna, F.; Lanzillo, R.; Brescia Morra, V.; Orefice, G.; Cerillo, I.; et al. Immunometabolic profiling of T cells from patients with relapsing-remitting multiple sclerosis reveals an impairment in glycolysis and mitochondrial respiration. *Metabolism* **2017**, *77*, 39–46. [CrossRef]

14. Benard, G.; Rossignol, R. Ultrastructure of the mitochondrion and its bearing on function and bioenergetics. *Antioxid. Redox Signal.* **2008**, *10*, 1313–1342. [CrossRef]

15. Kalkavan, H.; Green, D.R. MOMP, cell suicide as a BCL-2 family business. *Cell Death Differ.* **2018**, *25*, 46–55. [CrossRef]

16. Wai, T.; Langer, T. Mitochondrial Dynamics and Metabolic Regulation. *Trends Endocrinol. Metab.* **2016**, *27*, 105–117. [CrossRef]

17. Pernas, L.; Scorrano, L. Mito-Morphosis: Mitochondrial Fusion, Fission, and Cristae Remodeling as Key Mediators of Cellular Function. *Annu. Rev. Physiol.* **2016**, *78*, 505–531. [CrossRef]

18. Yu-Wai-Man, P.; Spyropoulos, A.; Duncan, H.J.; Guadagno, J.V.; Chinnery, P.F. A multiple sclerosis-like disorder in patients with OPA1 mutations. *Ann. Clin. Trans. Neurol.* **2016**, *3*, 723–729. [CrossRef]

19. Patten, D.A.; Wong, J.; Khacho, M.; Soubannier, V.; Mailloux, R.J.; Pilon-Larose, K.; MacLaurin, J.G.; Park, D.S.; McBride, H.M.; Trinkle-Mulcahy, L.; et al. OPA1-dependent cristae modulation is essential for cellular adaptation to metabolic demand. *EMBO J.* **2014**, *33*, 2676–2691. [CrossRef]

20. Signorile, A.; Santeramo, A.; Tamma, G.; Pellegrino, T.; D'Oria, S.; Lattanzio, P.; De Rasmo, D. Mitochondrial cAMP prevents apoptosis modulating Sirt3 protein level and OPA1 processing in cardiac myoblast cells. Biochim. Biophys. *Acta Mol. Cell. Res.* **2017**, *1864*, 355–366. [CrossRef]

21. MacVicar, T.; Langer, T. OPA1 processing in cell death and disease—The long and short of it. *J. Cell Sci.* **2016**, *129*, 2297–2306. [CrossRef]

22. Baker, M.J.; Lampe, P.A.; Stojanovski, D.; Korwitz, A.; Anand, R.; Tatsuta, T.; Langer, T. Stress-induced OMA1 activation and autocatalytic turnover regulate OPA1-dependent mitochondrial dynamics. *EMBO J.* **2014**, *33*, 578–593. [CrossRef]

23. Rainbolt, T.K.; Lebeau, J.; Puchades, C.; Wiseman, R.L. Reciprocal Degradation of YME1L and OMA1 Adapts Mitochondrial Proteolytic Activity during Stress. *Cell Rep.* **2016**, *14*, 2041–2049. [CrossRef]

24. Merkwirth, C.; Dargazanli, S.; Tatsuta, T.; Geimer, S.; Löwer, B.; Wunderlich, F.T.; von Kleist-Retzow, J.C.; Waisman, A.; Westermann, B.; Langer, T. Prohibitins control cell proliferation and apoptosis by regulating OPA1-dependent cristae morphogenesis in mitochondria. *Genes Dev.* **2008**, *22*, 476–488. [CrossRef]

25. Ross, J.A.; Robles-Escajeda, E.; Oaxaca, D.M.; Padilla, D.L.; Kirken, R.A. The prohibitin protein complex promotes mitochondrial stabilization and cell survival in hematologic malignancies. *Oncotarget* **2017**, *8*, 65445–65456. [CrossRef]

26. Kumar, M.K.S.; Nair, S.; Mony, U.; Kalingavarman, S.; Venkat, R.; Sivanarayanan, T.B.; Unni, A.K.K.; Rajeshkannan, R.; Anandakuttan, A.; Radhakrishnan, S.; et al. Significance of elevated Prohibitin 1 levels in Multiple Sclerosis patients lymphocytes towards the assessment of subclinical disease activity and its role in the central nervous system pathology of disease. *Int. J. Biol. Macromol.* **2018**, *110*, 573–581. [CrossRef]

27. Polman, C.H.; Reingold, S.C.; Banwell, B.; Clanet, M.; Cohen, J.A.; Filippi, M.; Fujihara, K.; Havrdova, E.; Hutchinson, M.; Kappos, L.; et al. Diagnostic criteria for multiple sclerosis: 2010 revisions to the McDonaldcriteria. *Ann. Neurol.* **2011**, *69*, 292–302. [CrossRef]

28. De Riccardis, L.; Rizzello, A.; Ferramosca, A.; Urso, E.; De Robertis, F.; Danieli, A.; Giudetti, A.M.; Trianni, G.; Zara, V.; Maffia, M. Bioenergetics profile of CD4+T cells in relapsing remittingmultiple sclerosissubjects. *J. Biotechnol.* **2015**, *202*, 31–39. [CrossRef]

29. Djaldetti, R.; Achiron, A.; Ziv, I.; Djaldetti, M. Lymphocyte ultrastructure in patients with multiple sclerosis. *Biomed. Pharmacother.* **1995**, *49*, 300–303. [CrossRef]

30. Jiang, X.; Jiang, H.; Shen, Z.; Wang, X. Activation of mitochondrial protease OMA1 by Bax and Bak promotes cytochrome c release during apoptosis. *Proc. Natl. Acad. Sci. USA* **2014**, *111*, 14782–14787. [CrossRef]

31. Anand, R.; Wai, T.; Baker, M.J.; Kladt, N.; Schauss, A.C.; Rugarli, E.; Langer, T. The i-AAA protease YME1L and OMA1 cleave OPA1 to balance mitochondrial fusion and fission. *J. Cell Biol.* **2014**, *204*, 919–929. [CrossRef]

32. Quirós, P.M.; Ramsay, A.J.; Sala, D.; Fernández-Vizarra, E.; Rodríguez, F.; Peinado, J.R.; Fernández-García, M.S.; Vega, J.A.; Enríquez, J.A.; Zorzano, A.; et al. Loss of mitochondrial proteaseOMA1alters processing of the GTPase OPA1 and causes obesity and defective thermogenesis in mice. *EMBO J.* **2012**, *31*, 2117–2133. [CrossRef]

33. Van der Bliek, A.M.; Shen, Q.; Kawajiri, S. Mechanisms of mitochondrial fission and fusion. *Cold Spring Harb. Perspect. Biol.* **2013**, *5*, a011072. [CrossRef]

34. Sood, A.; Jeyaraju, D.V.; Prudent, J.; Caron, A.; Lemieux, P.; McBride, H.M.; Laplante, M.; Tóth, K.; Pellegrini, L. A Mitofusin-2-dependent inactivating cleavage of Opa1 links changes in mitochondria cristae and ER contacts in the postprandial liver. *Proc. Natl. Acad. Sci. USA* **2014**, *111*, 16017–16022. [CrossRef]

35. Scarisbrick, I.A. The multiple sclerosis degradome: Enzymatic cascades in development and progression of central nervous system inflammatory disease. In *Advances in Multiple Sclerosis and Experimental Demyelinating Diseases*; Springer: Berlin/Heidelberg, Germany, 2008; Volume 318, pp. 133–175.

36. Muri, L.; Leppert, D.; Grandgirard, D.; Leib, S.L. MMPs and ADAMs in neurological infectious diseases and multiple sclerosis. *Cell. Mol. Life Sci.* **2019**, *76*, 3097–3116. [CrossRef]

37. Kozin, M.S.; Kulakova, O.G.; Favorova, O.O. Involvement of Mitochondria in Neurodegeneration in Multiple Sclerosis. *Biochemistry* **2018**, *83*, 813–830. [CrossRef]

38. Singh, C.K.; Chhabra, G.; Ndiaye, M.A.; Garcia-Peterson, L.M.; Mack, N.J.; Ahmad, N. The Role of Sirtuins in Antioxidant and Redox Signaling. *Antioxid. Redox Signal.* **2018**, *28*, 643–661. [CrossRef]

39. Wu, Y.T.; Wu, S.B.; Wei, Y.H. Roles of sirtuins in the regulation of antioxidant defense and bioenergetic function of mitochondria under oxidative stress. *Free Radic. Res.* **2014**, *48*, 1070–1084. [CrossRef]

40. Nijtmans, L.G.; Artal, S.M.; Grivell, L.A.; Coates, P.J. The mitochondrial PHB complex: Roles in mitochondrial respiratory complex assembly, ageing and degenerative disease. *Cell. Mol. Life Sci.* **2002**, *59*, 143–155. [CrossRef]

41. Signorile, A.; Sgaramella, G.; Bellomo, F.; De Rasmo, D. Prohibitins: A Critical Role in Mitochondrial Functions and Implication in Diseases. *Cells* **2019**, *8*, E71. [CrossRef]

42. Merkwirth, C.; Langer, T. Prohibitin function within mitochondria: Essential roles for cell proliferation and cristae morphogenesis. *Biochim. Biophys. Acta* **2009**, *1793*, 27–32. [CrossRef]

43. Muraguchi, T.; Kawawa, A.; Kubota, S. Prohibitin protects against hypoxia-induced H9c2 cardiomyocyte cell death. *Biomed. Res.* **2010**, *31*, 113–122. [CrossRef]

44. Alirezaei, M.; Fox, H.S.; Flynn, C.T.; Moore, C.S.; Hebb, A.L.; Frausto, R.F.; Bhan, V.; Kiosses, W.B.; Whitton, J.L.; Robertson, G.S.; et al. Elevated ATG5 expression in autoimmune demyelination and multiple sclerosis. *Autophagy* **2009**, *5*, 152–158. [CrossRef]

45. Wei, Y.; Chiang, W.C.; Sumpter, R., Jr.; Mishra, P.; Levine, B. Prohibitin 2 Is an Inner Mitochondrial Membrane Mitophagy Receptor. *Cell* **2017**, *168*, 224–238. [CrossRef]

14

Microbiome in Multiple Sclerosis: Where are we, What we Know and do not Know

Marina Kleopatra Boziki [1], Evangelia Kesidou [1], Paschalis Theotokis [1],
Alexios-Fotios A. Mentis [2,3], Eleni Karafoulidou [1], Mikhail Melnikov [4,5], Anastasia Sviridova [4,5],
Vladimir Rogovski [6], Alexey Boyko [4,5,*] and Nikolaos Grigoriadis [1,*]

[1] 2nd Neurological University Department, Aristotle University of Thessaloniki, AHEPA General Hospital,
54634 Thessaloniki, Greece; bozikim@auth.gr (M.K.B.); bioevangelia@yahoo.gr (E.K.);
ptheotokis@gmail.com (P.T.); elenikarafoulidou95@hotmail.com (E.K.)

[2] Public Health Laboratories, Hellenic Pasteur Institute, Athens 11521, Greece; mentisaf@gmail.com

[3] Laboratory of Microbiology, University Hospital of Larissa, School of Medicine, University of Thessaly,
41110 Larissa, Greece

[4] Department of Neurology, Neurosurgery and Medical Genetics, Pirogov Russian National Research Medical
University, Moscow 117997, Russia; medikms@yandex.ru (M.M.); anastasiya-ana@yandex.ru (A.S.)

[5] Department of Neuroimmunology, Federal Center of Cerebrovascular Pathology and Stroke,
Moscow 117342, Russia

[6] Department of Molecular Pharmacology and Radiobiology, Pirogov Russian National Research Medical
University, Moscow 117997, Russia; qwer555@mail.ru

* Correspondence: boykoan13@gmail.com (A.B.); ngrigoriadis@auth.gr (N.G.);

Abstract: An increase of multiple sclerosis (MS) incidence has been reported during the last decade, and this may be connected to environmental factors. This review article aims to encapsulate the current advances targeting the study of the gut–brain axis, which mediates the communication between the central nervous system and the gut microbiome. Clinical data arising from many research studies, which have assessed the effects of administered disease-modifying treatments in MS patients to the gut microbiome, are also recapitulated.

Keywords: gut microbiome; gut–brain axis; metagenomics; multiple sclerosis; disease-modifying treatments

1. Introduction

The prevalence of multiple sclerosis (MS) has reportedly increased over the last few decades, showing both higher absolute numbers of patients and a real increase in MS incidence [1,2]. Overall, the number of patients afflicted with MS may be increasing due to a prolongation of their life expectancy and of the disease duration. Moreover, the integration of MAGNIMS (magnetic resonance imaging in multiple sclerosis) consensus in the diagnostic criteria for MS and the universal application of these criteria, together with their constant re-evaluation in order to achieve optimal sensitivity and specificity, allow for more accurate and early diagnoses [3,4]. The development of novel disease-modifying treatments (DMTs) that are effective in controlling disease activity and delaying progression (even in cases with highly active disease [5]), as well as the increase in physician's awareness towards complications of the disease (such as spasticity, urinary disturbance, and chronic infections [6]), are also measures that increase life quality, and ultimately survival, for patients with MS. Moreover, the combined efforts of medical societies worldwide towards the development and application of universal registries and patient databases have led to improved case ascertainment that has also contributed to the observed increase of MS frequency [7]. In addition to the aforementioned advances in the health system and the medical services provided, a true increase in the incidence of MS has occurred in several ethnic populations over the last few decades. This is indicated by (i) the minimal number of ethnic populations that still remain free of the disease; (ii) a well-documented increase of the frequency of MS in previously low-incidence populations, such as in Asia, Southern and Eastern Europe; and (iii) the wider age window, i.e., younger than 16 and older than 50 years of age, in which the disease onset occurs [1,8,9]. According to the hygiene hypothesis, advanced civilization and technological progress in the recent past led to an improvement of the hygiene level of the overall life conditions for several ethnic populations and this improvement may be linked to increased MS frequency. In this respect, the observed alterations in MS incidence may be linked to an environmental shift towards a more MS-predisposing status. Another likely scenario is that the relative significance of the environmental factor with respect to MS pathogenesis has increased in the 21st Century.

This review aims to summarize the recent advances that have been achieved in the analysis of gut microbiota, an environmental factor with a well-described impact in autoimmunity, and to provide a critical assessment of the derived knowledge with respect to the role of gut microbiota in MS pathogenesis. Moreover, we attempt to form key questions in order to position the derived knowledge into a valuable context with respect to personalized medicine and patient-tailored therapeutic approaches.

2. The Environmental Factor in Autoimmune Disease

A complex interplay between genetic and environmental factors is necessary for the development of autoimmunity. In MS, genetically predisposing factors have been recognized, with specific polymorphisms of the major histocompatibility complex (MHC), namely the human leukocyte antigen (HLA) system, to be the factors accounting for the majority of cases [10]. For instance, beta chain of HLA (HLA-DRB1) and DQ beta 1 chain of HLA (HLA-DQB1)polymorphisms have been implicated in MS predisposition in Caucasians. In addition, more than 130 single nucleotide polymorphisms (SNPs) implicated in various responses of the innate and adaptive immune system, as well as in cell survival and/or pathways of cellular death, have been recognized. However, even by considering the cumulative effect of these polymorphisms, the effect of the genetic factor itself does not account for more than 30% of MS cases [10]. Environmental factors have long been implicated in MS pathogenesis, and they include lifestyle conditions, such as smoking and the level of physical exercise, as well as the type of overall diet (e.g., Western, Eastern, or Mediterranean) and/or specific dietary parameters, such as vitamin D and salt intake [11,12]. Recently, it became evident that dietary and lifestyle conditions may exert a profound impact on the gastrointestinal tract (GI) and, more specifically, the intestine. This is an organ that appears to pose a significant role in regulating several responses of the signaling systems of the human organism, namely the endocrine, the immune, and, more remotely, the central nervous system (CNS) [13,14].

More importantly, the genetic factor itself is the main factor that is present upon the prenatal and immediate postnatal stage that determines predisposition towards disease at a level that remains relatively constant throughout life. Nonetheless, its outcome is subject to the effect of several environmental factors that are, overall, actively present throughout life. Each factor acts for an individual period of time and possibly affects a specific stage of disease pathogenesis, namely the predisposition, onset, and/or course of the disease [15]. According to the classical paradigm of genetics–environment interplay, gene polymorphisms are constant for a given individual and exert an effect upon their phenotype that remains constant throughout life. Environmental factors, on the other hand, continue to exert a biological effect that may be cumulative for the time period that the factor is present, or they may act as triggers that induce the onset of disease. An environmental factor may, therefore (i) act before the biological onset of the disease, thus contributing towards predisposition; (ii) act upon disease onset (trigger); or (iii) be present during the disease course, according to the LEARn (Latent Early Life-Associated Regulation) model, an epigenetic model of disease development described by Lahiri et al. Similarly, the GERSMS (Genetic and Environmental Risk Score) has been proposed as a means to quantify a combined estimate of an individual's genetic burden and environmental exposures [16]. Special notice has been taken with respect to (i) the Western diet (ii) other lifestyle conditions, such as smoking, lack of physical excersise etc.; (iii) specific virus infections, such as the Epstein-Barr virus; (iv) the wide use of antibiotics; and (iv) the high sanitary level, as factors that promote pro-inflammatory responses; Several of these factors are present early (age <15 years old) in life [17].

3. Gut Microbiota and the Role of Intestinal Dysbiosis

The human GI tract is colonized by approximately 1014 different populations of microorganisms. Overall, gut microbiota are nowadays regarded as a separate organ in the human body, weighing approximately 2 kg and carrying information that is at least 100 times larger than the number of human genes for an individual [18]. Under steady-state conditions, these microorganisms are symbiotic, in the sense that they contribute to the homeostasis of the human organism. More specifically, gut microbiota (i) contribute to the maintenance of the motility and permeability of the gut; (ii) prevent colonization by pathogens; (iii) mediate nutrient metabolism; (iv) participate in the production of vitamins, such as vitamin B complex, vitamin K, and folate; and (v) promote intestinal epithelial functions, such as absorption and secretion [18]. Recently, gut microbiota have been shown to shape the immune responses of innate and adaptive immunity, both locally (at the level of the GI mucosa) and systemically, thus affecting remote organs [19]. Data stemming from two large metagenomic databases, i.e., the MetaHIT (Metagenomics of the Human Intestinal Tract) and the Human Microbiome Project, isolated 2172 species in humans that were classified into 12 different phyla, with 93.5% of them belonging to the Proteobacteria, Firmicutes, Actinobacteria, and Bacteroidetes [20]. Large fractions of the phyla Firmicutes and Bacteroidetes reportedly include the genera *Prevotella*, *Bacteroides*, and *Ruminococcus*, and these are followed in size by Actinobacteria [20]. Moreover, the relative composition of the gut microbiota does not appear to be constant throughout different parts of the GI tract. Rather, there appears to be some degree of regional specialization with respect to the exact microbes that colonize each part of the gut [21]. For instance, frequent *Lactobacilli* are present in the duodenum, whereas both *Lactobacilli* and *Streptococci* are abundant in the jejunum. A large diversity has been described for the colon with the caecum and the appendix; these are two areas that also bear larger burden of microorganisms, in terms of absolute numbers [21]. Similarly, the diversity in microbiota across the GI tract leads to differential profiles of the metabolites that are produced as a result of the various microbiota mediating nutrient absorption and metabolism: In the stomach and the duodenum, vitamin A and aryl hydrocarbon receptors (AHR) ligands are primarily produced, whereas in the colon, a gradual shift towards higher short-chain fatty acid (SCFA) production is evident [22]. The structural architecture of the GI tract, as well as the differences in cellular composition and the pH of the adjacent mucosa, account for the alterations in the microbial composition and in the associated metabolites across the GI tract. Disequilibrium in the relative composition of intestinal microbiota has recently been recognized as a common underlying condition in several autoimmune diseases. The alteration of the intestinal microbial community that might lead to either animal or human diseases is termed intestinal or gut dysbiosis. Intestinal microbiota have been proven to shape immune responses and to affect the neural and endocrine systems of the gut. All these pathways exert remote signaling in the human body and thus bear implications for systemic and organ-specific autoimmunity, as in the case of the CNS [19].

4. The Gut Microbiota in MS

4.1. Immunoregulation and the Gut–Brain Axis

The enteric nervous system has long been recognized as a second brain. More recently, the gut–brain axis has been recognized as a bi-directional communication system from the CNS to the gut and vice versa; this communication is mediated by neuronal connections, neuroendocrine signals, general humoral signals, and immune signaling [23]. The CNS regulates gut function by promoting gut motility via a dense innervation system and by orchestrating local immune responses through the high numbers of immune cells that are present in the gut. These humoral signals are delivered by the utilization of common molecular mediators, such as pro-inflammatory cytokines, neuropeptides (like cholecystokinin (CCK) and leptin), and neurotransmitters (like dopamine (DA), serotonin (5-HT), gamma-aminobutyric acid (GABA), acetylcholine (Ach), and glutamate [22]). Conversely, structures in immediate proximity to the microbiota—such as the intestinal epithelial cells and immune cells in gut-associated lymphatic tissue (GALT) and the enteric nervous system (ENS)—mediate the transmission of signaling pathways from the gut towards the CNS. In this respect, gut microbiota may modulate the host via several pathways that originate in parts of the neuroendocrine, neural, and immune systems [23].

For instance, structurally distinct lipopolysaccharide (LPS), a characteristic component of the outer envelope of many microbes, exhibits a differential immunogenic profile in terms of the associated cytokines that are produced as a response by the host [24]. Toll-like receptor (TLR) signaling, a part of the pattern-recognition receptor (PRR) signaling, appears to be a key mediator of the host's immune response towards bacteria, as it is the first-line sensing pathway that recognizes microbial structural patterns.

Moreover, the recognition of bacterial structures by the TLR system prevents microbial translocation towards the deep layers of the gut lumen, as demonstrated in myeloid differentiation primary response 88 (MyD88) -/- mice that lack the expression of epithelial MyD88-dependent TLR [25]. In the bi-directional communication between the microbes and the host, it is therefore evident that the host may also regulate microbial colonization by the early recruitment of sensing and defense mechanisms. For example, cluster of differentiation antigen (CD) 1d (CD1d)+ invariant natural killer T (iNKT) cells and γδ intraepithelial lymphocytes (γδ IELs) are T-cell subsets that respond to microbial antigens. These cells were shown to regulate bacterial colonization in the gut [26]. Local immunoglobulin A (IgA) production by B-cells is also regarded as a factor regulating gut microflora composition and density [27,28]. Conversely, germinal center formation and the production of IgA are shaped by activation of T-follicular helper cells; the latter is induced by microbes and mediated by programmed cell death protein 1 (PD-1) [28].

4.2. Gut Microbiota and Innate Immunity

Overall, microbiota are essential for priming the gastro-intestinal immune system to evoke specific immune responses: With respect to the innate immune system, several subsets of cells that participate antigen presentation respond to microbial stimuli by enhancing cytokine and chemokine production. The mucosa-associated invariant T (MAIT) cells, which express an invariant α T-cell receptor (TCR) chain and the non-classical MHC-I related protein located in mucosal tissues (e.g., intestinal lamina propria), produce diverse pro-inflammatory cytokines, such as interleukin (IL)-17, interferon gamma (IFNγ), granzyme B, or tumor necrosis factor alpha (TNFα) [29]. By expressing various chemokine receptors, MAIT cells exhibit a migratory capacity into remote tissues [29]. Natural killer (NK)-cells increase the expression of co-stimulatory molecules in response to microbial stimuli. NK cells are essential for the priming of other immune cells and the coordination of the overall host immune response by the production of IL-4, IL-13, and IFNγ, as well as the promotion of chemokine (C-X-C motif) ligand 16 (CXCL16) production by epithelial cells [29]. Dendritic cells and macrophages are, as is known, the classical antigen-presenting cells, and they play a key role in first-line host defense and the modulation of adaptive immunity. In so doing, they enhance the production of pro-IL-1β and its processing to bioactive IL-1β by caspase-1, thus discriminating between pathogenic and protective bacteria and dietary components [30].

4.3. Gut Microbiota and Adaptive Immunity

The adaptive immune system also exhibits the capacity for microbe-driven responses. T-helper (Th)-17 cells are prevalent in the intestine, and they are important for the gastro-intestinal host defense, as they secrete cytokines that are involved in the regulation of inflammation (IL-17A, IL-17F, and IL-22).

Specific microbes are capable of eliciting a differential T-effector phenotype (e.g., Th17 and Tregs) in the intestines and lymph nodes of mice that exhibit predisposition towards autoimmunity [31,32]. In germ-free mice or antibiotics-treated mice, the number of Th17 cells is reduced along with attenuated pro-inflammatory responses [33]. Moreover, mice that are resistant to autoimmunity exhibit the preferential sequestration of Th17 cells in the intestine, whereas peripheral blood Th17 repopulation by the administration of anti-(a4b7) integrin monoclonal antibodies rescues the autoimmune disease phenotype [34]. In this respect, the intestine appears to be a key regulating organ of immune system responses [34,35]. T regulatory (Treg) cells are two- to three-folds higher in abundance in the gastro-intestinal tract compared to other tissues. Mice with compromised gut microbiota, such as germ-free mice or antibiotic-treated mice, display a reduced frequency of Treg cells, and these Treg cells exhibit impaired anti-inflammatory cytokine-secretion, especially IL-10. In these mice, re-colonization by gut microbes promotes the function and frequency of Treg cells [32,36]. Moreover, bacterial antigens, such as LPS, are necessary for class-switch recombination in B cells towards IgA production. Additionally, B-cells primed by bacterial antigens have been shown to participate in antigen presentation and IgA selection in the germinal centers of the GALT (e.g., Peyer's patches) [37].

4.4. The Role of Microbial Metabolites

Apart from microbial structural components that may serve as antigens that shape immune responses in the intestine with implications for systemic disease, other molecular mediators also exhibit the capacity to induce pro- or anti-inflammatory reactions. Metabolites of microbial origin are present in the intestine, often as a by-product of nutrient degradation; these molecules may stimulate immune cells towards activated phenotype and cytokine production. SCFAs are metabolites produced by intestinal microbes that mediate a well-known anti-inflammatory effect. SCFAs inhibit histone deacetylases (HDACs) on Treg and microglia, a mechanism mediated by G-protein-coupled receptors (GPRs) [38]. Moreover, SCFAs may stimulate dendritic cells (DCs) towards the production of anti-inflammatory molecules, such as retinoic acid (RA) and transforming growth factor beta (TGFβ). Tryptophan metabolites evidently shape the phenotype of T cell subsets by promoting the production of either pro-inflammatory Th1 cytokines, such as IFN-γ and IL-2, or anti-inflammatory Th2 cytokines, such as IL-4 and IL-10 [38]. Tryptophan metabolites may also promote the Th17 pro-inflammatory phenotype by acting on AHR, a signaling pathway known to also affect astrocyte activation in the CNS as a response to microbial stimuli from the systemic circulation [38].

4.5. The Role of Intestinal Barrier

Clinical and experimental evidence on the role of the intestinal barrier and its structural and functional integrity has recently elucidated aspects of the interplay between intestinal microbes and the host. An impaired intestinal barrier is regarded a common underlying condition in several autoimmune diseases of the gut that exhibit systemic implications, such as inflammatory bowel disease (IBD). In this respect, impaired intestinal barrier integrity exposes the cells of the local and, more importantly, of the systemic immune system to stimuli of microbial origin with a potential to elicit immune responses, as suggested in the context of the leaky gut theory. Intestinal dysbiosis appears to mediate barrier dysfunction, as this microbiome-related process may induce changes in mucus composition, enterocyte apoptosis and tight junction dysfunction through the translocation of associated structural components, as well as bacterial translocation to the lamina propria [39]. These alterations lead to an increased homing of lymphocytes in the lamina propria, the immunological layer of the intestinal barrier, and, in doing such, they contribute in the host's predisposition towards local and systemic autoimmune responses. In the case of MS, such intestinal barrier alterations are linked to the presence of increased LPS and LPS-mediated signaling in the lamina propria, leading to chronic low-grade inflammation and endotoxemia [39]. Concomitant reduction in SCFAs associated to dysbiosis, that is, reduced microbial diversity, a condition frequently described in MS, results in compromised intestinal barrier and thus predisposes towards systemic pro-inflammatory reactions.

In the CNS, microglia and astrocytes respond to pro-inflammatory stimuli from systemic circulation and acquire activated phenotypes, thus further promoting pro-inflammatory milieu in the context of CNS autoimmunity [39]. In this respect, the intestinal barrier has recently emerged as a novel target of pharmacological intervention in MS. This is because the restoration of the intestinal barrier may reduce the exposure of the cellular components of the systemic immune system to microbial derivatives and the associated pro-inflammatory cascade.

4.6. Mechanisms of Immune-Modulation by Intestinal Microbiota—Experimental Evidence

Experimental evidence has dictated that the presence of intestinal microbiota is necessary in order for CNS autoimmunity to develop. In a myelin oligodendrocyte glycoprotein-specific t cell receptor (MOG-TCR) transgenic mouse model of spontaneous disease, experimental autoimmune encephalomyelitis (EAE) does not occur under germ-free (GF) conditions, whereas mice transferred from GF conditions into a conventional environment develop spontaneous EAE after few weeks of transfer [40]. Interestingly, MOG-TCR transgenic mice of a genetic background that is resistant towards autoimmunity, namely the B10.S mice, do not exhibit spontaneous EAE, even under conventional conditions [34]. In these mice, a preferential sequestration of Th17 pro-inflammatory T-cells in the intestine has been observed. The administration of anti-$\alpha 4\beta 7$, a monoclonal antibody (mAb) that blocks intestinal integrin, has been found to be able to repopulate peripheral blood with Th17 T-cells and to rescue the disease phenotype [34]. The intestine thus appears as an organ with the ability to control systemic autoimmune responses with implication towards CNS autoimmunity [41]. In a similar context, the modulation of gut microbiota, as achieved by antibiotic administration, reduces the severity of conventional EAE. In an experimental setting, specific immune responses have been linked with single bacteria, such as in the case of Clostridia and Bacteroides fragilis derived from human feces that have the potential to induce Foxp3+ T regulatory cells, thus ameliorating EAE [42]. The fecal transplantation of MOG-TCR transgenic mice with human feces stemming from twins discordant for MS has only been found to result in the development of spontaneous EAE in mice recipients for feces stemming from twins with MS. In contrast, mice recipients for feces stemming from healthy twins have not been found to develop the disease [43]. GF mice recipients for the human feces of MS patients have also been found to develop severe EAE, coupled with alterations in the peripheral immune profile [44]. More specifically, fecal transplantation with material provided by healthy adults has been found to result in the induction of T regulatory cells in the mesenteric lymph nodes of the recipient mice, thus, overall, exerting an immune-regulatory response [44]. Conversely, the administration of Lactobacilli has been repeatedly shown to protect form EAE by the induction of IL-4, IL-10, TGF-$\beta 1$, and IL-27 [45,46] by mediating an increase in IL-10+ and Foxp3+ T regulatory cells [47–49].

However, findings often observed in EAE fail to be translated to human disease due to the differences that the model exhibits. With the exception of spontaneous models, EAE requires myelin peptide immunization with a strong adjuvant. This is a condition that exerts especially skewed immune responses towards inflammation and results in a monophasic disease of inflammatory origin with little demyelination compared to the human disease [50]. In TCR transgenic mice that exhibit spontaneous disease, more than 90% of the circulating T-cells bear transgenic, autoreactive TCRs [51,52]. This is a condition that also does not accurately depict CNS autoimmunity in humans. In this respect, a detailed profiling of human microbiota appears to be a necessary approach to elucidate human-specific mechanisms. These mechanisms stem from interactions between the gut microbiota and the host, and they show the potential to induce autoimmune responses with relevance to the CNS.

4.7. Mechanisms of Immune-Modulation by Intestinal Microbiota—Clinical Evidence

During the last five years, several clinical studies have provided evidence indicating that in MS, the gut microbiome is altered. In an approach similar to the experimental model, initial studies linked alterations in the relative abundance of Clostridia, in the context of gut dysbiosis with MS. However, the clinical relevance—with respect to whether these alterations contribute towards susceptibility for

MS or, instead, they exert a relative protective effect—remains controversial both for adult [53,54] and pediatric populations [55,56]. In 2016, two case control studies reported distinct patterns of gut microbiota composition by the use of 16S ribosomal ribonucleic acid rRNA metagenomics analysis [57,58] (for further discussion on the potential of metagenomic techniques as applied to MS, see [59,60]). These studies provided evidence of reduced diversity in the gut microbiome of MS patients compared to controls. Interestingly, this reduction was evident for patients with active MS, whereas patients in remission exhibited comparable diversity levels to the healthy population. Further studies verified this association of disease activity status with alterations of the relative abundance of microbes in the gut, with Firmicutes and Bacteroidetes exhibiting higher relative abundances reviewed by Kozhieva et al. [61]. These studies indicated the following: Though it is widely accepted that the gut microbiome in patients with MS is characterized by moderate dysbiosis, a clear and consistent multiple sclerosis microbiome phenotype has not been described. Moreover, given that a myriad of microbes have been implicated in MS, it is unlikely that, in the future, a single microbial organism will be isolated and characterized as an environmental trigger towards disease. This is in striking contrast with the paradigm stemming from mouse EAE. According to the latter, triggering of CNS autoimmunity by microbes provides mechanistic insight with respect to the molecular pathways that lead from the local immune responses in the gut to systemic inflammation and, eventually, to organ-specific autoimmunity towards the CNS [31,32].

Recently, a systematic review [62] of MS case-control studies with respect to gut microbiota composition concluded that, although differences in the diversity of microbiota were not reported by the majority of the included studies, several studies reported consistent patterns with respect to the taxonomic relative abundance. These findings further elucidated pattern alterations in the overall gut microbial composition of patients with MS compared to controls. Further prospective studies are necessary in order to establish a causative relation between these microbial pattern alterations and the disease pathogenesis and/or exacerbation. Notably, the majority of the reviewed studies referred to the Relapsing-remmitting type of MS(RRMS). A recent study addressed the differential gut microbiota profile in patients with primary progressive MS (PPMS), relatively to healthy controls [63]. As in the case of patients with RRMS, patients with PPMS have exhibited differences in a minority of a-diversity indices, whereas pattern differences have been observed at a taxonomic level [63].

In line with the observations described above, diet and dietary supplementation has recently emerged a major factor that affects gut microbiota's relative composition. It has been proposed that a diet that is rich in vegetables, complex carbohydrates (fibers) combined with probiotics, vitamin D supplementation, vitamin A supplementation, and lipoic acid promotes gut eubiosis. This is coupled with a concomitant increase in microbial diversity and microbe-associated anti-inflammatory mediators, such as SCFAs, microbial anti-inflammatory molecules (MAMs), histone deacetylase inhibitors, AHR receptor agonists, and an increase of the Treg/Th17 ratio [64]. Conversely, a Western diet rich in animal fat and trans-fatty acids, with a high sugar and salt intake, promotes gut dysbiosis and results in (i) an increased presence of pro-inflammatory mediators such as TNFa, IL-6, and IL-17; and (ii) increased gut barrier and blood–brain barrier (BBB) permeability with implications for systemic and CNS autoimmunity [64]. More specifically, gut dysbiosis predisposes one to intestinal inflammation, which is characterized by alterations in the immunological barrier layer of the lamina propria towards pro-inflammatory milieu in the GALT and an increase in the presence of endotoxin/LPS in the intestinal mucosa. The further translocation of LPS and other bacterial components, as well as whole bacteria in the deep layers of the intestinal wall and the local secondary lymphoid organs (such as the mesenteric lymph nodes) allows for the generation of circulating activated T-cells in the context of low-grade endotoxemia [39,64]. These systemic alterations (i) compromise the integrity of the BBB, (ii) allow for pro-inflammatory stimuli to cross the BBB towards the CNS, and (iii) affect microglia and astrocyte activation status, thus predisposing one towards neuroinflammation.

Clinical evidence of the possible causal relationship between the gut microbiota profile and the CNS autoimmunity stems from more interventional approaches that actively alter gut microflora composition; such approaches include fecal microbiota transplantation (FMT), an investigational method that has been used successfully to treat cases of severe enterocolitis [65,66] More specifically, prolonged antibiotic administration in certain individuals may cause expansion of *Clostridium difficile* (*C. difficile*) at the expense of symbiotic bacteria, thus serving as an example of intestinal dysbiosis and *C. difficile*-related severe enterocolitis. FMT protocols require that fecal material from a healthy donor, following careful donor screening and appropriate preparation procedures, is transferred to a patient, either via colonoscopy or via an oral route as capsule ingestion [67]. Due to risks linked with transplantation (i.e., possible transmittable disease) and colonoscopy procedures, FMT is reserved for cases that are refractory to the antibiotics that are typically prescribed against enterocolitis due to *C. difficile*. Recently, FMT has been advocated as an attractive therapeutic approach for several diseases that are linked to intestinal dysbiosis, either of the intestine, such as IBD [68,69] or systemic extragastric and CNS disease [70,71] (and reviewed in [72]). Isolated case reports have described the beneficial effects of FMT over MS disease course, and a clinical trial of FMT for patients with MS is currently underway [73].

5. Disease-Modifying Treatment (DMT) and Gut Microbiota

In the management of MS, DMTs serve as prophylactic treatments towards clinical and radiological disease activity, whereas other medications are prescribed for symptom management. The later are more often prescribed in the context of disability accumulation, such as gamma-Aminobutyric acid-type B $GABA_B$ receptor agonists (e.g., baclofen) for limb spasticity and a-adrenergic inhibitors for the control of overactive bladders. Several of these regimens are known to alter the profile of the gut microbiota [39]. Recently, several oral DMTs were shown to inhibit the growth of *Clostridium* in vitro. This feature has been proposed to contribute to the DMTs' overall anti-inflammatory mechanism of action [74,75]. In this study, fingolimod was proven to be bactericidal, whereas teriflunomide and dimethyl fumarate (DMF) exerted a bacteriostatic effect. Clinical data stemming from metagenomics analysis of gut microbiota alterations in patients receiving DMF and glatiramer acetate (GA) further verified that DMTs exert a profound effect on the relative composition of gut microbiota. The above could shed light into potential additional mechanisms of action [76].

5.1. Interferon-β

With respect to IFNβ, several lines of investigation have indicated that it may modify the immunological properties of the intestinal barrier. IFNβ is a member of the type 1 interferon (T1IFN) family, and it is considered a major cytokine that mediates local responses to viral, bacterial, and other antigen stimuli in the intestine (reviewed in [77]). In a mouse model of pneumococcal lung infection, IFNβ treatment led to the upregulation of tight junction proteins in lung epithelial and blood vessel endothelial layers, thus reducing lung–blood barrier permeability and preventing invasive pneumococcal infection [78]. Furthermore, IFNβ, produced by DCs following stimulation by gut commensal microbiota, was recently shown to mediate Treg proliferation in the intestine [79]. A clinical case-control study exploring the effect of IFNβ administration in patients with MS recently reported an increase of *Prevotella*, a known probiotic, in patients with MS treated with IFNβ. This increase was comparable to healthy controls, whereas untreated patients exhibited a reduced relative abundance of probiotics [80].

5.2. Glatiramer Acetate

GA is a myelin-basic protein (MBP) analog and a long-administered first-line DMT treatment for MS. In line with its anti-inflammatory properties, GA is known to ameliorate colonic injury in an experimental model of colitis by inducing a reduction in TNFa and a concomitant increase in Tregs, IL-10, and TGFb-producing cells [81]. Moreover, the role of GA in stabilizing the intestinal barrier and promoting tissue repair, as documented by analysis of syndecan-1 expression, was shown in a model of IBD [82]. In EAE, GA administration ameliorated the disease phenotype coupled with an increase in gut *Prevotella*, and the administration of GA combined with GI colonization with live *Prevotella* led to the further attenuation of disease [83]. GA treatment in patients with MS was shown to exert an effect in the relative abundance of gut microbiota, especially the Lachnospiraceae and Veillonellaceae families [76]. Similarly, another case-control study in patients with RRMS treated with GA reported alterations in the relative composition of the gut microbiome with respect to several *Clostridium* [84].

5.3. Dimethyl Fumarate

DMF is a long-prescribed DMT for psoriasis that was more recently approved as a first-line treatment for MS. In an experimental setting, DMF was shown to promote an increase in the relative abundance of probiotics and to stabilize the intestinal barrier. A concomitant increase in SCFA-producing microbes was shown to further promote the systemic anti-inflammatory effect of the drug [85]. Similarly, DMF administration in Lewis rats was shown to mediate (i) a reduction in the TLR-4 expression by the GALT, (ii) a reduction in IFNγ, and (iii) a concomitant increase in lamina propria's Foxp-3+ expression and the abundance of CD4+CD25+ Tregs in Peyer's patches [86]. A case-control study implementing metagenomics techniques reported an association between DMF treatment and decreased relative abundance of Firmicutes and Clostridia, as well as an increase of Bacteroidetes, relative to untreated patients [76].

5.4. Teriflunomide

Teriflunomide, another oral, first-line DMT approved as a prophylactic treatment for RRMS, has been shown to modify immune responses in the intestine by promoting the local proliferation of CD39+ Tregs. Thus, it exerted anti-inflammatory action that ameliorated CNS inflammation in a mouse model of EAE [87].

5.5. Natalizumab

Natalizumab (NTZ) is an injectable second-line DMT that has been approved for patients with highly active RRMS. NTZ is a monoclonal antibody targeting a4-integrin, a family that includes adhesion molecules expressed in T-cells. Integrins exhibit tissue specificity with a4b1 expressed in the CNS, whereas a4b7 is expressed in the intestine. NTZ is not selective; therefore, by inhibiting T-cell trafficking towards the CNS, it also blocks T-cell circulation in the gut. In addition to its beneficial effect in MS, NTZ has been shown to be effective in ameliorating the symptoms of IBD [88]. The administration of NTZ has been proposed as preferred treatment approach for patients with RRMS and IBD co-morbidity [88]. Furthermore, IBD is a well-described condition characterized by intestinal dysbiosis and local immune dysregulation. In this respect, also in patients with RRMS that do not exhibit signs of IBD, the amelioration of T-cell trafficking in the gut by NTZ may contribute to the drug's anti-inflammatory effect by inhibiting the circulation of activated T-cells in the gut. The gut has recently been proposed as a regulating organ with respect to the peripheral circulation of activated T-cells, with implications for CNS autoimmunity. In mice resistant to EAE that exhibit the preferential sequestration of autoreactive Th17 T-cells in the intestine, the administration of the a4b7 mAb led to the re-population of peripheral blood with Th17 T-cells and rescued the disease phenotype [34]. Interestingly, in this MOG-TCR transgenic mouse model, the selective accumulation of autoreactive T-cells in the intestine acts as a mechanism of immune tolerance that contributes in resistance towards EAE [34]. In the context of MS, it is reasonable to assume that the blocking of T-cell trafficking in the intestine may ameliorate the exposure of the immune system to stimuli of microbial origin. This amelioration could be performed by reducing antigen sampling and, subsequently, T-cell clonal expansion and activation in response to these antigens. As gut dysbiosis, and the associated local immune dysregulation, is frequently reported in patients with RRMS, this concomitant effect may serve as an additional mode of action for NTZ in RRMS.

5.6. Fingolimod

Fingolimod is an oral second-line DMT that is indicated as prophylactic treatment for highly active RRMS. Fingolimod is a sphingosine-1-phosphate (S1P) agonist, acting on four out of five S1P receptors, on various organs and cell types. Fingolimod ligation on S1P receptors leads to the downregulation of the S1P receptor expression; therefore, the drug is considered as a functional antagonist of S1P signaling. On a physiological level, S1P receptor expression is necessary for the lymphocytes, either naïve or activated, to egress from the secondary lymphoid organs, such as the peripheral lymph nodes. Due to this mechanism of action, fingolimod inhibits the egress of lymphocytes from lymph nodes to the peripheral blood stream. Thus, it ameliorates systemic immune responses and CNS-targeted autoimmunity. Similarly, other S1P ligands have been tested for intestinal autoimmune disease, such as IBD, as they exhibit the potential to ameliorate the transmigration of immune cells across the intestine [89]. Fingolimod has been shown to ameliorate experimental colitis [90], and two S1P ligands are currently being tested in terms of safety and efficacy in phase II and phase III clinical trials on colitis [88]. Interestingly, S1P signaling has been shown to regulate innate lymphoid cell (ILC) transmigration from intestinal lamina propria towards systemic circulation and other lymphoid organs, thus regulating infectious and inflammatory responses [91]. In a transgenic mouse model of enteric nervous system pathology resembling Parkinson's disease (PD) due to a-synuclein accumulation, fingolimod resulted in an enhanced gut motility and increased levels of brain-derived neurotrophic factor (BDNF) [92]. Moreover, S1P ligation has been shown to exert a stabilizing effect towards barrier function [93,94] and the BBB [95], with implications for EAE and MS [96–98]. Fingolimod may potentially exert an effect on the gut microbiome's relative composition, as it has been shown to regulate IgA plasmablasts' maturation from the intestinal Peyer's patches, a first-line defense mechanism of the host towards microbe colonization [99,100]. Moreover, fingolimod was shown to exert a direct anti-microbial effect by inhibiting the growth of *Clostridium* and the associated endotoxin production in vitro [74].

5.7. Alemtuzumab

Alemtuzumab is an anti-CD52 monoclonal antibody inducing T-cell and B-cell depletion in peripheral blood. It was originally used for the treatment of chronic B-cell lymphocytic leukemia. Recently, alemtuzumab has been approved for the treatment of highly active RRMS for patients with breakthrough disease that were previously exposed to other first- and/or second-line DMTs [101]. Apart from the obvious effect of alemtuzumab in depleting circulating primarily B- and T-cell lymphocytes, the long-term immunomodulating effect is mediated by alterations that the drug causes in the peripheral immune cell pool following repopulation. Some of these alterations are attributed to the homeostatic proliferation of mature lymphocytes that the drug promotes in peripheral tissues [102]. Due to this effect, the administration of alemtuzumab has been linked with an increased susceptibility towards autoimmune comorbidities, such as autoimmune thyroid disease, membranous glomerulonephritis, autoimmune hepatitis, and immune thrombocytopenic purpura [103]. Colitis due to *Clostridium* was the cause of fatal outcome in one patient with RRMS who received alemtuzumab [104], whereas another patient presented with pancolitis during the first course of alemtuzumab treatment [105]. Susceptibility towards infection was the assumed underlying cause in both cases. With respect to the second case, an immune-mediated mechanism contributing to sepsis has also been proposed [105]. Evidence stemming from a cynomolgus monkey model indicated that the intestinal barrier may be disrupted during alemtuzumab treatment [106]. In macaques monkeys, a single dose of alemtuzumab resulted in (i) intestinal epithelial cell loss, (ii) increased apoptosis in the villi, and (iii) an abnormal Paneth cell morphology [107]. Mouse anti-CD52 mAb also resulted in increased numbers of IELs undergoing apoptosis and disrupted intestinal barrier function in mice [108]. In a cynomolgus monkey model, alemtuzumab administration resulted in profound alterations in the relative composition of gut microbiota, namely Lactobacillales, Enterobacterales, and Clostridiales, as well as the genera *Prevotella* and *Faecalibacterium*. These alterations were primarily linked to alterations in the relative abundance of TCRαβ+ or TCRγδ+ T cells [109]. These data indicate that alemtuzumab administration exerts a profound effect on the intestinal homeostasis with respect to tissue integrity, barrier function, immune properties, and microbiome profile. However, it remains unknown whether these alterations are beneficial in the context of CNS autoimmunity, or, instead, if, in a proportion of patients, the overall beneficiary effect of alemtuzumab in subsiding disease activity is counterbalanced by a detrimental effect in intestinal function.

6. Conclusions: Treat the Microbiome—Treat MS?

The combined efforts of the scientific community in the field of MS have been focused on identifying strategies that may be implemented in order to either modify the peripheral immune responses or, as proposed by the less successful approach to date, to enhance neuroprotection and the endogenous regenerative capacity of the CNS. In addition to the classical paradigm of immune–brain interaction in the context of MS, the intestine has emerged as an additional regulating organ of responses that take place both in the immunological and the nervous (central and peripheral) counterparts. In this respect, the gut commensal microbiota may serve as environmental factors that shape the intestinal milieu. The modification of gut microbiota by either dietary (e.g., probiotic supplementation) or medicinal approaches (e.g., antibiotic administration) may serve as additional therapeutic strategies for MS prophylaxis [110]. More interventional approaches, such as FMT, have also been proposed. Moreover, the relative composition of gut microbiota may also serve as an indicator of reciprocal host–microorganism interactions. Further longitudinal studies that implement the profiling of intestinal microbiota during the pre-clinical phase and over the course of the disease are needed in order to elucidate this assumption. MS is a complex autoimmune disease with clinical variability. As such, the establishment of a causative role for intestinal microbiota towards disease pathogenesis requires combined efforts from the field of metagenomics and other "-omics" approaches [59,60,111] with the capacity for high throughput data production and the application of these data in the context of translational medicine.

With respect to future directions, we consider gut microbiota modulation as a promising intervention for the management of MS. Understanding the pathways that the gut microbiota implicate in order to shape host's immune responses may elucidate therapeutic targets, such as the induction of immune regulatory cell populations via the promotion of an "anti-inflammatory" gut microflora. Similar interventions, possibly in combination with DMTs, may contribute in promoting treatment efficacy and optimal response. As several newly available DMTs confer significant and potentially severe adverse effects, gut microbiota modification has emerged as a promising, and possibly less interventional, additional approach.

Author Contributions: M.K.B. conducted data collection, design, writing, overall preparation of the manuscript and synthesis. E.K. (Evangelia Kesidou), P.T., A.-F.A.M., E.K. (Eleni Karafoulidou), M.M., A.S., V.R. participated in data collection and preparation of the manuscript. A.B. and N.G. were responsible for conception and critical review of the manuscript. All authors have read and agreed to the published version of the manuscript.

References

1. Global Health Metrics. Global, regional, and national incidence, prevalence, and years lived with disability for 328 diseases and injuries for 195 countries, 1990–2016: A systematic analysis for the Global Burden of Disease Study 2016. *Lancet* **2017**, *390*, 1211–1259. [CrossRef]
2. Grytten, N.; Torkildsen, O.; Myhr, K.M. Time trends in the incidence and prevalence of multiple sclerosis in Norway during eight decades. *Acta Neurol. Scand.* **2015**, *132*, 29–36. [CrossRef] [PubMed]
3. Filippi, M.; Rocca, M.A.; Ciccarelli, O.; De Stefano, N.; Evangelou, N.; Kappos, L.; Rovira, A.; Sastre-Garriga, J.; Tintore, M.; Frederiksen, J.L.; et al. MRI criteria for the diagnosis of multiple sclerosis: MAGNIMS consensus guidelines. *Lancet Neurol.* **2016**, *15*, 292–303. [CrossRef]

4. Thompson, A.J.; Banwell, B.L.; Barkhof, F.; Carroll, W.M.; Coetzee, T.; Comi, G.; Correale, J.; Fazekas, F.; Filippi, M.; Freedman, M.S.; et al. Diagnosis of multiple sclerosis: 2017 revisions of the McDonald criteria. *Lancet Neurol.* **2018**, *17*, 162–173. [CrossRef]

5. Tintore, M.; Vidal-Jordana, A.; Sastre-Garriga, J. Treatment of multiple sclerosis—Success from bench to bedside. *Nat. Rev. Neurol.* **2019**, *15*, 53–58. [CrossRef]

6. Henze, T.; Rieckmann, P.; Toyka, K.V. Symptomatic treatment of multiple sclerosis. Multiple Sclerosis Therapy Consensus Group (MSTCG) of the German Multiple Sclerosis Society. *Eur. Neurol.* **2006**, *56*. [CrossRef]

7. Glaser, A.; Stahmann, A.; Meissner, T.; Flachenecker, P.; Horakova, D.; Zaratin, P.; Brichetto, G.; Pugliatti, M.; Rienhoff, O.; Vukusic, S.; et al. Multiple sclerosis registries in Europe—An updated mapping survey. *Mult. Scler. Relat Disord.* **2019**, *27*, 171–178. [CrossRef]

8. McKay, K.A.; Hillert, J.; Manouchehrinia, A. Long-term disability progression of pediatric-onset multiple sclerosis. *Neurology* **2019**, *92*, e2764–e2773. [CrossRef] [PubMed]

9. Guillemin, F.; Baumann, C.; Epstein, J.; Kerschen, P.; Garot, T.; Mathey, G.; Debouverie, M. Older Age at Multiple Sclerosis Onset Is an Independent Factor of Poor Prognosis: A Population-Based Cohort Study. *Neuroepidemiology* **2017**, *48*, 179–187. [CrossRef] [PubMed]

10. Patsopoulos, N.A. Genetics of Multiple Sclerosis: An Overview and New Directions. *Cold Spring Harb. Perspect. Med.* **2018**, *8*. [CrossRef] [PubMed]

11. Belbasis, L.; Bellou, V.; Evangelou, E.; Ioannidis, J.P.; Tzoulaki, I. Environmental risk factors and multiple sclerosis: An umbrella review of systematic reviews and meta-analyses. *Lancet Neurol.* **2015**, *14*, 263–273. [CrossRef]

12. Zheng, C.; He, L.; Liu, L.; Zhu, J.; Jin, T. The efficacy of vitamin D in multiple sclerosis: A meta-analysis. *Mult. Scler. Relat. Disord.* **2018**, *23*, 56–61. [CrossRef] [PubMed]

13. Camara-Lemarroy, C.R.; Metz, L.M.; Yong, V.W. Focus on the gut-brain axis: Multiple sclerosis, the intestinal barrier and the microbiome. *World J. Gastroenterol.* **2018**, *24*, 4217–4223. [CrossRef] [PubMed]

14. Probstel, A.K.; Baranzini, S.E. The Role of the Gut Microbiome in Multiple Sclerosis Risk and Progression: Towards Characterization of the "MS Microbiome". *Neurotherapeutics* **2018**, *15*, 126–134. [CrossRef]

15. Lahiri, D.K.; Maloney, B. The "LEARn" (Latent Early-life Associated Regulation) model integrates environmental risk factors and the developmental basis of Alzheimer's disease, and proposes remedial steps. *Exp. Gerontol.* **2010**, *45*, 291–296. [CrossRef]

16. Xia, Z.; Steele, S.U.; Bakshi, A.; Clarkson, S.R.; White, C.C.; Schindler, M.K.; Nair, G.; Dewey, B.E.; Price, L.R.; Ohayon, J.; et al. Assessment of Early Evidence of Multiple Sclerosis in a Prospective Study of Asymptomatic High-Risk Family Members. *JAMA Neurol.* **2017**, *74*, 293–300. [CrossRef]

17. Freedman, S.N.; Shahi, S.K.; Mangalam, A.K. The "Gut Feeling": Breaking Down the Role of Gut Microbiome in Multiple Sclerosis. *Neurotherapeutics* **2018**, *15*, 109–125. [CrossRef]

18. Picca, A.; Fanelli, F.; Calvani, R.; Mule, G.; Pesce, V.; Sisto, A.; Pantanelli, C.; Bernabei, R.; Landi, F.; Marzetti, E. Gut Dysbiosis and Muscle Aging: Searching for Novel Targets against Sarcopenia. *Mediators Inflamm.* **2018**, *2018*, 7026198. [CrossRef]

19. Ochoa-Reparaz, J.; Magori, K.; Kasper, L.H. The chicken or the egg dilemma: Intestinal dysbiosis in multiple sclerosis. *Ann. Transl. Med.* **2017**, *5*, 145. [CrossRef]

20. Blum, H.E. The human microbiome. *Adv. Med. Sci.* **2017**, *62*, 414–420. [CrossRef]

21. Mowat, A.M.; Agace, W.W. Regional specialization within the intestinal immune system. *Nat. Rev. Immunol.* **2014**, *14*, 667–685. [CrossRef] [PubMed]

22. Ghaisas, S.; Maher, J.; Kanthasamy, A. Gut microbiome in health and disease: Linking the microbiome-gut-brain axis and environmental factors in the pathogenesis of systemic and neurodegenerative diseases. *Pharmacol. Ther.* **2016**, *158*, 52–62. [CrossRef] [PubMed]

23. Fleck, A.K.; Schuppan, D.; Wiendl, H.; Klotz, L. Gut-CNS-Axis as Possibility to Modulate Inflammatory Disease Activity-Implications for Multiple Sclerosis. *Int. J. Mol. Sci.* **2017**, *18*, 1526. [CrossRef] [PubMed]

24. Vatanen, T.; Kostic, A.D.; d'Hennezel, E.; Siljander, H.; Franzosa, E.A.; Yassour, M.; Kolde, R.; Vlamakis, H.; Arthur, T.D.; Hamalainen, A.M.; et al. Variation in Microbiome LPS Immunogenicity Contributes to Autoimmunity in Humans. *Cell* **2016**, *165*, 842–853. [CrossRef]

25. Frantz, A.L.; Rogier, E.W.; Weber, C.R.; Shen, L.; Cohen, D.A.; Fenton, L.A.; Bruno, M.E.; Kaetzel, C.S. Targeted deletion of MyD88 in intestinal epithelial cells results in compromised antibacterial immunity associated with downregulation of polymeric immunoglobulin receptor, mucin-2, and antibacterial peptides. *Mucosal. Immunol.* **2012**, *5*, 501–512. [CrossRef]

26. Nieuwenhuis, E.E.; Matsumoto, T.; Lindenbergh, D.; Willemsen, R.; Kaser, A.; Simons-Oosterhuis, Y.; Brugman, S.; Yamaguchi, K.; Ishikawa, H.; Aiba, Y.; et al. Cd1d-dependent regulation of bacterial colonization in the intestine of mice. *J. Clin. Investig.* **2009**, *119*, 1241–1250. [CrossRef]

27. Suzuki, K.; Meek, B.; Doi, Y.; Muramatsu, M.; Chiba, T.; Honjo, T.; Fagarasan, S. Aberrant expansion of segmented filamentous bacteria in IgA-deficient gut. *Proc. Natl. Acad. Sci. USA* **2004**, *101*, 1981–1986. [CrossRef]

28. Hapfelmeier, S.; Lawson, M.A.; Slack, E.; Kirundi, J.K.; Stoel, M.; Heikenwalder, M.; Cahenzli, J.; Velykoredko, Y.; Balmer, M.L.; Endt, K.; et al. Reversible microbial colonization of germ-free mice reveals the dynamics of IgA immune responses. *Science* **2010**, *328*, 1705–1709. [CrossRef]

29. Dias, J.; Leeansyah, E.; Sandberg, J.K. Multiple layers of heterogeneity and subset diversity in human MAIT cell responses to distinct microorganisms and to innate cytokines. *Proc. Natl. Acad. Sci. USA* **2017**, *114*, E5434–E5443. [CrossRef]

30. Franchi, L.; Kamada, N.; Nakamura, Y.; Burberry, A.; Kuffa, P.; Suzuki, S.; Shaw, M.H.; Kim, Y.G.; Nunez, G. NLRC4-driven production of IL-1beta discriminates between pathogenic and commensal bacteria and promotes host intestinal defense. *Nat. Immunol.* **2012**, *13*, 449–456. [CrossRef]

31. Ivanov, I.I.; Atarashi, K.; Manel, N.; Brodie, E.L.; Shima, T.; Karaoz, U.; Wei, D.; Goldfarb, K.C.; Santee, C.A.; Lynch, S.V.; et al. Induction of intestinal Th17 cells by segmented filamentous bacteria. *Cell* **2009**, *139*, 485–498. [CrossRef]

32. Atarashi, K.; Tanoue, T.; Shima, T.; Imaoka, A.; Kuwahara, T.; Momose, Y.; Cheng, G.; Yamasaki, S.; Saito, T.; Ohba, Y.; et al. Induction of colonic regulatory T cells by indigenous Clostridium species. *Science* **2011**, *331*, 337–341. [CrossRef] [PubMed]

33. Shaw, M.H.; Kamada, N.; Kim, Y.G.; Nunez, G. Microbiota-induced IL-1beta, but not IL-6, is critical for the development of steady-state TH17 cells in the intestine. *J. Exp. Med.* **2012**, *209*, 251–258. [CrossRef] [PubMed]

34. Berer, K.; Boziki, M.; Krishnamoorthy, G. Selective accumulation of pro-inflammatory T cells in the intestine contributes to the resistance to autoimmune demyelinating disease. *PLoS ONE* **2014**, *9*, e87876. [CrossRef]

35. Sano, T.; Huang, W.; Hall, J.A.; Yang, Y.; Chen, A.; Gavzy, S.J.; Lee, J.Y.; Ziel, J.W.; Miraldi, E.R.; Domingos, A.I.; et al. An IL-23R/IL-22 Circuit Regulates Epithelial Serum Amyloid A to Promote Local Effector Th17 Responses. *Cell* **2015**, *163*, 381–393. [CrossRef] [PubMed]

36. Tanoue, T.; Atarashi, K.; Honda, K. Development and maintenance of intestinal regulatory T cells. *Nat. Rev. Immunol.* **2016**, *16*, 295–309. [CrossRef]

37. Kim, M.; Kim, C.H. Regulation of humoral immunity by gut microbial products. *Gut. Microbes* **2017**, *8*, 392–399. [CrossRef] [PubMed]

38. Haase, S.; Haghikia, A.; Wilck, N.; Muller, D.N.; Linker, R.A. Impacts of microbiome metabolites on immune regulation and autoimmunity. *Immunology* **2018**, *154*, 230–238. [CrossRef] [PubMed]

39. Camara-Lemarroy, C.R.; Metz, L.; Meddings, J.B.; Sharkey, K.A.; Wee Yong, V. The intestinal barrier in multiple sclerosis: Implications for pathophysiology and therapeutics. *Brain* **2018**, *141*, 1900–1916. [CrossRef]

40. Berer, K.; Mues, M.; Koutrolos, M.; Rasbi, Z.A.; Boziki, M.; Johner, C.; Wekerle, H.; Krishnamoorthy, G. Commensal microbiota and myelin autoantigen cooperate to trigger autoimmune demyelination. *Nature* **2011**, *479*, 538–541. [CrossRef]

41. Yokote, H.; Miyake, S.; Croxford, J.L.; Oki, S.; Mizusawa, H.; Yamamura, T. NKT cell-dependent amelioration of a mouse model of multiple sclerosis by altering gut flora. *Am. J. Pathol.* **2008**, *173*, 1714–1723. [CrossRef] [PubMed]

42. Atarashi, K.; Tanoue, T.; Oshima, K.; Suda, W.; Nagano, Y.; Nishikawa, H.; Fukuda, S.; Saito, T.; Narushima, S.; Hase, K.; et al. Treg induction by a rationally selected mixture of Clostridia strains from the human microbiota. *Nature* **2013**, *500*, 232–236. [CrossRef] [PubMed]

43. Berer, K.; Gerdes, L.A.; Cekanaviciute, E.; Jia, X.; Xiao, L.; Xia, Z.; Liu, C.; Klotz, L.; Stauffer, U.; Baranzini, S.E.; et al. Gut microbiota from multiple sclerosis patients enables spontaneous autoimmune encephalomyelitis in mice. *Proc. Natl. Acad. Sci. USA* **2017**, *114*, 10719–10724. [CrossRef] [PubMed]

44. Cekanaviciute, E.; Yoo, B.B.; Runia, T.F.; Debelius, J.W.; Singh, S.; Nelson, C.A.; Kanner, R.; Bencosme, Y.; Lee, Y.K.; Hauser, S.L.; et al. Gut bacteria from multiple sclerosis patients modulate human T cells and exacerbate symptoms in mouse models. *Proc. Natl. Acad. Sci. USA* **2017**, *114*, 10713–10718. [CrossRef] [PubMed]

45. Lavasani, S.; Dzhambazov, B.; Nouri, M.; Fak, F.; Buske, S.; Molin, G.; Thorlacius, H.; Alenfall, J.; Jeppsson, B.; Westrom, B. A novel probiotic mixture exerts a therapeutic effect on experimental autoimmune encephalomyelitis mediated by IL-10 producing regulatory T cells. *PLoS ONE* **2010**, *5*, e9009. [CrossRef] [PubMed]

46. Kwon, H.K.; Kim, G.C.; Kim, Y.; Hwang, W.; Jash, A.; Sahoo, A.; Kim, J.E.; Nam, J.H.; Im, S.H. Amelioration of experimental autoimmune encephalomyelitis by probiotic mixture is mediated by a shift in T helper cell immune response. *Clin. Immunol.* **2013**, *146*, 217–227. [CrossRef] [PubMed]

47. Takata, K.; Kinoshita, M.; Okuno, T.; Moriya, M.; Kohda, T.; Honorat, J.A.; Sugimoto, T.; Kumanogoh, A.; Kayama, H.; Takeda, K.; et al. The lactic acid bacterium Pediococcus acidilactici suppresses autoimmune encephalomyelitis by inducing IL-10-producing regulatory T cells. *PLoS ONE* **2011**, *6*, e27644. [CrossRef]

48. Rezende, R.M.; Oliveira, R.P.; Medeiros, S.R.; Gomes-Santos, A.C.; Alves, A.C.; Loli, F.G.; Guimaraes, M.A.; Amaral, S.S.; da Cunha, A.P.; Weiner, H.L.; et al. Hsp65-producing Lactococcus lactis prevents experimental autoimmune encephalomyelitis in mice by inducing CD4+LAP+ regulatory T cells. *J. Autoimmun.* **2013**, *40*, 45–57. [CrossRef]

49. Mangalam, A.; Shahi, S.K.; Luckey, D.; Karau, M.; Marietta, E.; Luo, N.; Choung, R.S.; Ju, J.; Sompallae, R.; Gibson-Corley, K.; et al. Human Gut-Derived Commensal Bacteria Suppress CNS Inflammatory and Demyelinating Disease. *Cell Rep.* **2017**, *20*, 1269–1277. [CrossRef]

50. Gold, R.; Linington, C.; Lassmann, H. Understanding pathogenesis and therapy of multiple sclerosis via animal models: 70 years of merits and culprits in experimental autoimmune encephalomyelitis research. *Brain* **2006**, *129*, 1953–1971. [CrossRef]

51. Pollinger, B.; Krishnamoorthy, G.; Berer, K.; Lassmann, H.; Bosl, M.R.; Dunn, R.; Domingues, H.S.; Holz, A.; Kurschus, F.C.; Wekerle, H. Spontaneous relapsing-remitting EAE in the SJL/J mouse: MOG-reactive transgenic T cells recruit endogenous MOG-specific B cells. *J. Exp. Med.* **2009**, *206*, 1303–1316. [CrossRef] [PubMed]

52. Krishnamoorthy, G.; Wekerle, H. EAE: An immunologist's magic eye. *Eur. J. Immunol.* **2009**, *39*, 2031–2035. [CrossRef] [PubMed]

53. Rumah, K.R.; Linden, J.; Fischetti, V.A.; Vartanian, T. Isolation of Clostridium perfringens type B in an individual at first clinical presentation of multiple sclerosis provides clues for environmental triggers of the disease. *PLoS ONE* **2013**, *8*, e76359. [CrossRef]

54. Miyake, S.; Kim, S.; Suda, W.; Oshima, K.; Nakamura, M.; Matsuoka, T.; Chihara, N.; Tomita, A.; Sato, W.; Kim, S.W.; et al. Dysbiosis in the Gut Microbiota of Patients with Multiple Sclerosis, with a Striking Depletion of Species Belonging to Clostridia XIVa and IV Clusters. *PLoS ONE* **2015**, *10*, e0137429. [CrossRef] [PubMed]

55. Tremlett, H.; Fadrosh, D.W.; Faruqi, A.A.; Hart, J.; Roalstad, S.; Graves, J.; Spencer, C.M.; Lynch, S.V.; Zamvil, S.S.; Waubant, E. Associations between the gut microbiota and host immune markers in pediatric multiple sclerosis and controls. *BMC Neurol.* **2016**, *16*, 182. [CrossRef]

56. Tremlett, H.; Fadrosh, D.W.; Faruqi, A.A.; Zhu, F.; Hart, J.; Roalstad, S.; Graves, J.; Lynch, S.; Waubant, E. Gut microbiota in early pediatric multiple sclerosis: A case-control study. *Eur. J. Neurol.* **2016**, *23*, 1308–1321. [CrossRef] [PubMed]

57. Jangi, S.; Gandhi, R.; Cox, L.M.; Li, N.; von Glehn, F.; Yan, R.; Patel, B.; Mazzola, M.A.; Liu, S.; Glanz, B.L.; et al. Alterations of the human gut microbiome in multiple sclerosis. *Nat. Commun.* **2016**, *7*, 12015. [CrossRef]

58. Chen, J.; Chia, N.; Kalari, K.R.; Yao, J.Z.; Novotna, M.; Paz Soldan, M.M.; Luckey, D.H.; Marietta, E.V.; Jeraldo, P.R.; Chen, X.; et al. Multiple sclerosis patients have a distinct gut microbiota compared to healthy controls. *Sci Rep.* **2016**, *6*, 28484. [CrossRef]

59. Mentis, A.A.; Dardiotis, E.; Grigoriadis, N.; Petinaki, E.; Hadjigeorgiou, G.M. Viruses and Multiple Sclerosis: From Mechanisms and Pathways to Translational Research Opportunities. *Mol. Neurobiol* **2017**, *54*, 3911–3923. [CrossRef]

60. Mentis, A.A.; Dardiotis, E.; Grigoriadis, N.; Petinaki, E.; Hadjigeorgiou, G.M. Viruses and endogenous retroviruses in multiple sclerosis: From correlation to causation. *Acta Neurol. Scand.* **2017**, *136*, 606–616. [CrossRef]

61. Kozhieva, M.K.; Melnikov, M.V.; Rogovsky, V.S.; Oleskin, A.V.; Kabilov, M.R.; Boyko, A.N. Gut human microbiota and multiple sclerosis. *Zh Nevrol. Psikhiatr. Im S S Korsakova* **2017**, *117*, 11–19. [CrossRef] [PubMed]

62. Mirza, A.; Forbes, J.D.; Zhu, F.; Bernstein, C.N.; Van Domselaar, G.; Graham, M.; Waubant, E.; Tremlett, H. The multiple sclerosis gut microbiota: A systematic review. *Mult. Scler. Relat. Disord.* **2020**, *37*, 101427. [CrossRef] [PubMed]

63. Kozhieva, M.; Naumova, N.; Alikina, T.; Boyko, A.; Vlassov, V.; Kabilov, M.R. Primary progressive multiple sclerosis in a Russian cohort: Relationship with gut bacterial diversity. *BMC Microbiol.* **2019**, *19*, 309. [CrossRef]

64. Riccio, P.; Rossano, R. Diet, Gut Microbiota, and Vitamins D + A in Multiple Sclerosis. *Neurotherapeutics* **2018**, *15*, 75–91. [CrossRef] [PubMed]

65. Borody, T.J.; Brandt, L.J.; Paramsothy, S. Therapeutic faecal microbiota transplantation: Current status and future developments. *Curr. Opin. Gastroenterol.* **2014**, *30*, 97–105. [CrossRef]

66. Makkawi, S.; Camara-Lemarroy, C.; Metz, L. Fecal microbiota transplantation associated with 10 years of stability in a patient with SPMS. *Neurol. Neuroimmunol. Neuroinflamm.* **2018**, *5*, e459. [CrossRef]

67. Cammarota, G.; Ianiro, G.; Tilg, H.; Rajilic-Stojanovic, M.; Kump, P.; Satokari, R.; Sokol, H.; Arkkila, P.; Pintus, C.; Hart, A.; et al. European consensus conference on faecal microbiota transplantation in clinical practice. *Gut* **2017**, *66*, 569–580. [CrossRef]

68. Chin, S.M.; Sauk, J.; Mahabamunuge, J.; Kaplan, J.L.; Hohmann, E.L.; Khalili, H. Fecal Microbiota Transplantation for Recurrent Clostridium difficile Infection in Patients with Inflammatory Bowel Disease: A Single-Center Experience. *Clin. Gastroenterol. Hepatol.* **2017**, *15*, 597–599. [CrossRef]

69. Paramsothy, S.; Kamm, M.A.; Kaakoush, N.O.; Walsh, A.J.; van den Bogaerde, J.; Samuel, D.; Leong, R.W.L.; Connor, S.; Ng, W.; Paramsothy, R.; et al. Multidonor intensive faecal microbiota transplantation for active ulcerative colitis: A randomised placebo-controlled trial. *Lancet* **2017**, *389*, 1218–1228. [CrossRef]

70. Jayasinghe, T.N.; Chiavaroli, V.; Holland, D.J.; Cutfield, W.S.; O'Sullivan, J.M. The New Era of Treatment for Obesity and Metabolic Disorders: Evidence and Expectations for Gut Microbiome Transplantation. *Front. Cell Infect. Microbiol.* **2016**, *6*, 15. [CrossRef]

71. Bajaj, J.S.; Kassam, Z.; Fagan, A.; Gavis, E.A.; Liu, E.; Cox, I.J.; Kheradman, R.; Heuman, D.; Wang, J.; Gurry, T.; et al. Fecal microbiota transplant from a rational stool donor improves hepatic encephalopathy: A randomized clinical trial. *Hepatology* **2017**, *66*, 1727–1738. [CrossRef]

72. Choi, H.H.; Cho, Y.S. Fecal Microbiota Transplantation: Current Applications, Effectiveness, and Future Perspectives. *Clin. Endosc.* **2016**, *49*, 257–265. [CrossRef] [PubMed]

73. Lawson Health Research Institute. Fecal Microbial Transplantation in Relapsing Multiple Sclerosis Patients. Available online: https://clinicaltrials.gov/ct2/show/NCT03183869 (accessed on 5 April 2020).

74. Rumah, K.R.; Vartanian, T.K.; Fischetti, V.A. Oral Multiple Sclerosis Drugs Inhibit the In vitro Growth of Epsilon Toxin Producing Gut Bacterium, Clostridium perfringens. *Front. Cell Infect. Microbiol.* **2017**, *7*, 11. [CrossRef] [PubMed]

75. Linden, J.R.; Ma, Y.; Zhao, B.; Harris, J.M.; Rumah, K.R.; Schaeren-Wiemers, N.; Vartanian, T. Clostridium perfringens Epsilon Toxin Causes Selective Death of Mature Oligodendrocytes and Central Nervous System Demyelination. *MBio* **2015**, *6*, e02513. [CrossRef] [PubMed]

76. Katz Sand, I.; Zhu, Y.; Ntranos, A.; Clemente, J.C.; Cekanaviciute, E.; Brandstadter, R.; Crabtree-Hartman, E.; Singh, S.; Bencosme, Y.; Debelius, J.; et al. Disease-modifying therapies alter gut microbial composition in MS. *Neurol. Neuroimmunol. Neuroinflamm.* **2019**, *6*, e517. [CrossRef] [PubMed]

77. Giles, E.M.; Stagg, A.J. Type 1 Interferon in the Human Intestine-A Co-ordinator of the Immune Response to the Microbiota. *Inflamm. Bowel Dis.* **2017**, *23*, 524–533. [CrossRef]

78. LeMessurier, K.S.; Hacker, H.; Chi, L.; Tuomanen, E.; Redecke, V. Type I interferon protects against pneumococcal invasive disease by inhibiting bacterial transmigration across the lung. *PLoS Pathog.* **2013**, *9*, e1003727. [CrossRef]

79. Nakahashi-Oda, C.; Udayanga, K.G.; Nakamura, Y.; Nakazawa, Y.; Totsuka, N.; Miki, H.; Iino, S.; Tahara-Hanaoka, S.; Honda, S.; Shibuya, K.; et al. Apoptotic epithelial cells control the abundance of Treg cells at barrier surfaces. *Nat. Immunol.* **2016**, *17*, 441–450. [CrossRef]

80. Castillo-Alvarez, F.; Perez-Matute, P.; Oteo, J.A.; Marzo-Sola, M.E. The influence of interferon beta-1b on gut microbiota composition in patients with multiple sclerosis. *Neurologia* **2018**. [CrossRef]

81. Aharoni, R.; Sonego, H.; Brenner, O.; Eilam, R.; Arnon, R. The therapeutic effect of glatiramer acetate in a murine model of inflammatory bowel disease is mediated by anti-inflammatory T-cells. *Immunol. Lett.* **2007**, *112*, 110–119. [CrossRef]

82. Yablecovitch, D.; Shabat-Simon, M.; Aharoni, R.; Eilam, R.; Brenner, O.; Arnon, R. Beneficial effect of glatiramer acetate treatment on syndecan-1 expression in dextran sodium sulfate colitis. *J. Pharmacol. Exp. Ther.* **2011**, *337*, 391–399. [CrossRef] [PubMed]

83. Shahi, S.K.; Freedman, S.N.; Murra, A.C.; Zarei, K.; Sompallae, R.; Gibson-Corley, K.N.; Karandikar, N.J.; Murray, J.A.; Mangalam, A.K. Prevotella histicola, A Human Gut Commensal, Is as Potent as COPAXONE(R) in an Animal Model of Multiple Sclerosis. *Front. Immunol.* **2019**, *10*, 462. [CrossRef] [PubMed]

84. Cantarel, B.L.; Waubant, E.; Chehoud, C.; Kuczynski, J.; DeSantis, T.Z.; Warrington, J.; Venkatesan, A.; Fraser, C.M.; Mowry, E.M. Gut microbiota in multiple sclerosis: Possible influence of immunomodulators. *J. Investig. Med.* **2015**, *63*, 729–734. [CrossRef] [PubMed]

85. Ma, N.; Wu, Y.; Xie, F.; Du, K.; Wang, Y.; Shi, L.; Ji, L.; Liu, T.; Ma, X. Dimethyl fumarate reduces the risk of mycotoxins via improving intestinal barrier and microbiota. *Oncotarget* **2017**, *8*, 44625–44638. [CrossRef] [PubMed]

86. Pitarokoili, K.; Bachir, H.; Sgodzai, M.; Gruter, T.; Haupeltshofer, S.; Duscha, A.; Pedreiturria, X.; Motte, J.; Gold, R. Induction of Regulatory Properties in the Intestinal Immune System by Dimethyl Fumarate in Lewis Rat Experimental Autoimmune Neuritis. *Front. Immunol.* **2019**, *10*, 2132. [CrossRef]

87. Ochoa-Reparaz, J.; Colpitts, S.L.; Kircher, C.; Kasper, E.J.; Telesford, K.M.; Begum-Haque, S.; Pant, A.; Kasper, L.H. Induction of gut regulatory CD39(+) T cells by teriflunomide protects against EAE. *Neurol Neuroimmunol. Neuroinflamm.* **2016**, *3*, e291. [CrossRef] [PubMed]

88. Biswas, S.; Bryant, R.V.; Travis, S. Interfering with leukocyte trafficking in Crohn's disease. *Best Pract. Res. Clin. Gastroenterol.* **2019**, *38–39*, 101617. [CrossRef]

89. Kunisawa, J.; Kurashima, Y.; Higuchi, M.; Gohda, M.; Ishikawa, I.; Ogahara, I.; Kim, N.; Shimizu, M.; Kiyono, H. Sphingosine 1-phosphate dependence in the regulation of lymphocyte trafficking to the gut epithelium. *J. Exp. Med.* **2007**, *204*, 2335–2348. [CrossRef]

90. Deguchi, Y.; Andoh, A.; Yagi, Y.; Bamba, S.; Inatomi, O.; Tsujikawa, T.; Fujiyama, Y. The S1P receptor modulator FTY720 prevents the development of experimental colitis in mice. *Oncol. Rep.* **2006**, *16*, 699–703. [CrossRef]

91. Huang, Y.; Mao, K.; Chen, X.; Sun, M.A.; Kawabe, T.; Li, W.; Usher, N.; Zhu, J.; Urban, J.F., Jr.; Paul, W.E.; et al. S1P-dependent interorgan trafficking of group 2 innate lymphoid cells supports host defense. *Science* **2018**, *359*, 114–119. [CrossRef]

92. Vidal-Martinez, G.; Vargas-Medrano, J.; Gil-Tommee, C.; Medina, D.; Garza, N.T.; Yang, B.; Segura-Ulate, I.; Dominguez, S.J.; Perez, R.G. FTY720/Fingolimod Reduces Synucleinopathy and Improves Gut Motility in A53T Mice: CONTRIBUTIONS OF PRO-BRAIN-DERIVED NEUROTROPHIC FACTOR (PRO-BDNF) AND MATURE BDNF. *J. Biol. Chem.* **2016**, *291*, 20811–20821. [CrossRef] [PubMed]

93. Bonitz, J.A.; Son, J.Y.; Chandler, B.; Tomaio, J.N.; Qin, Y.; Prescott, L.M.; Feketeova, E.; Deitch, E.A. A sphingosine-1 phosphate agonist (FTY720) limits trauma/hemorrhagic shock-induced multiple organ dysfunction syndrome. *Shock* **2014**, *42*, 448–455. [CrossRef] [PubMed]

94. Garcia, J.G.; Liu, F.; Verin, A.D.; Birukova, A.; Dechert, M.A.; Gerthoffer, W.T.; Bamberg, J.R.; English, D. Sphingosine 1-phosphate promotes endothelial cell barrier integrity by Edg-dependent cytoskeletal rearrangement. *J. Clin. Investig.* **2001**, *108*, 689–701. [CrossRef]

95. Wang, X.; Maruvada, R.; Morris, A.J.; Liu, J.O.; Wolfgang, M.J.; Baek, D.J.; Bittman, R.; Kim, K.S. Sphingosine 1-Phosphate Activation of EGFR As a Novel Target for Meningitic *Escherichia coli* Penetration of the Blood-Brain Barrier. *PLoS Pathog.* **2016**, *12*, e1005926. [CrossRef] [PubMed]

96. Cruz-Orengo, L.; Daniels, B.P.; Dorsey, D.; Basak, S.A.; Grajales-Reyes, J.G.; McCandless, E.E.; Piccio, L.; Schmidt, R.E.; Cross, A.H.; Crosby, S.D.; et al. Enhanced sphingosine-1-phosphate receptor 2 expression underlies female CNS autoimmunity susceptibility. *J. Clin. Investig.* **2014**, *124*, 2571–2584. [CrossRef] [PubMed]

97. Choi, J.W.; Gardell, S.E.; Herr, D.R.; Rivera, R.; Lee, C.W.; Noguchi, K.; Teo, S.T.; Yung, Y.C.; Lu, M.; Kennedy, G.; et al. FTY720 (fingolimod) efficacy in an animal model of multiple sclerosis requires astrocyte sphingosine 1-phosphate receptor 1 (S1P1) modulation. *Proc. Natl. Acad. Sci. USA* **2011**, *108*, 751–756. [CrossRef]

98. Colombo, E.; Di Dario, M.; Capitolo, E.; Chaabane, L.; Newcombe, J.; Martino, G.; Farina, C. Fingolimod may support neuroprotection via blockade of astrocyte nitric oxide. *Ann. Neurol.* **2014**, *76*, 325–337. [CrossRef]

99. Gohda, M.; Kunisawa, J.; Miura, F.; Kagiyama, Y.; Kurashima, Y.; Higuchi, M.; Ishikawa, I.; Ogahara, I.; Kiyono, H. Sphingosine 1-phosphate regulates the egress of IgA plasmablasts from Peyer's patches for intestinal IgA responses. *J. Immunol.* **2008**, *180*, 5335–5343. [CrossRef]

100. Kunisawa, J.; Kurashima, Y.; Gohda, M.; Higuchi, M.; Ishikawa, I.; Miura, F.; Ogahara, I.; Kiyono, H. Sphingosine 1-phosphate regulates peritoneal B-cell trafficking for subsequent intestinal IgA production. *Blood* **2007**, *109*, 3749–3756. [CrossRef]

101. Coles, A.J.; Cohen, J.A.; Fox, E.J.; Giovannoni, G.; Hartung, H.P.; Havrdova, E.; Schippling, S.; Selmaj, K.W.; Traboulsee, A.; Compston, D.A.S.; et al. Alemtuzumab CARE-MS II 5-year follow-up: Efficacy and safety findings. *Neurology* **2017**, *89*, 1117–1126. [CrossRef]

102. Havrdova, E.; Horakova, D.; Kovarova, I. Alemtuzumab in the treatment of multiple sclerosis: Key clinical trial results and considerations for use. *Ther. Adv. Neurol. Disord.* **2015**, *8*, 31–45. [CrossRef] [PubMed]

103. Holmoy, T.; Fevang, B.; Olsen, D.B.; Spigset, O.; Bo, L. Adverse events with fatal outcome associated with alemtuzumab treatment in multiple sclerosis. *BMC Res. Notes* **2019**, *12*, 497. [CrossRef] [PubMed]

104. Baker, D.; Giovannoni, G.; Schmierer, K. Marked neutropenia: Significant but rare in people with multiple sclerosis after alemtuzumab treatment. *Mult. Scler. Relat. Disord.* **2017**, *18*, 181–183. [CrossRef] [PubMed]

105. Vijiaratnam, N.; Rath, L.; Xu, S.S.; Skibina, O. Pancolitis a novel early complication of Alemtuzumab for MS treatment. *Mult. Scler. Relat. Disord.* **2016**, *7*, 83–84. [CrossRef] [PubMed]

106. Qu, L.L.; Lyu, Y.Q.; Jiang, H.T.; Shan, T.; Zhang, J.B.; Li, Q.R.; Li, J.S. Effect of alemtuzumab on intestinal intraepithelial lymphocytes and intestinal barrier function in cynomolgus model. *Chin. Med. J. (Engl.)* **2015**, *128*, 680–686. [CrossRef] [PubMed]

107. Li, Q.; Zhang, Q.; Wang, C.; Jiang, S.; Li, N.; Li, J. The response of intestinal stem cells and epithelium after alemtuzumab administration. *Cell Mol. Immunol.* **2011**, *8*, 325–332. [CrossRef]

108. Qu, L.; Li, Q.; Jiang, H.; Gu, L.; Zhang, Q.; Wang, C.; Li, J. Effect of anti-mouse CD52 monoclonal antibody on mouse intestinal intraepithelial lymphocytes. *Transplantation* **2009**, *88*, 766–772. [CrossRef]

109. Li, Q.R.; Wang, C.Y.; Tang, C.; He, Q.; Li, N.; Li, J.S. Reciprocal interaction between intestinal microbiota and mucosal lymphocyte in cynomolgus monkeys after alemtuzumab treatment. *Am. J. Transplant.* **2013**, *13*, 899–910. [CrossRef]

110. Metz, L.M.; Li, D.K.B.; Traboulsee, A.L.; Duquette, P.; Eliasziw, M.; Cerchiaro, G.; Greenfield, J.; Riddehough, A.; Yeung, M.; Kremenchutzky, M.; et al. Trial of Minocycline in a Clinically Isolated Syndrome of Multiple Sclerosis. *N. Engl. J. Med.* **2017**, *376*, 2122–2133. [CrossRef]

111. Mentis, A.A.; Pantelidi, K.; Dardiotis, E.; Hadjigeorgiou, G.M.; Petinaki, E. Precision Medicine and Global Health: The Good, the Bad, and the Ugly. *Front. Med. (Lausanne)* **2018**, *5*, 67. [CrossRef]

15

Current Advances in Pediatric Onset Multiple Sclerosis

Kristen S. Fisher [1], Fernando X. Cuascut [2], Victor M. Rivera [2] and George J. Hutton [2,*

[1]   Baylor College of Medicine, Texas Children's Hospital, Houston, TX 77030, USA; kristen.fisher@bcm.edu
[2]   Baylor College of Medicine, Maxine Mesinger Multiple Sclerosis Center, Houston, TX 77030, USA;
     fernando.cuascut@bcm.edu (F.X.C.); vrivera@bcm.edu (V.M.R.)
*   Correspondence: ghutton@bcm.edu;

Abstract: Multiple sclerosis (MS) is an autoimmune inflammatory disease affecting the central nervous system leading to demyelination. MS in the pediatric population is rare, but has been shown to lead to significant disability over the duration of the disease. As we have learned more about pediatric MS, there has been a development of improved diagnostic criteria leading to earlier diagnosis, earlier initiation of disease-modifying therapies (DMT), and an increasing number of DMT used in the treatment of pediatric MS. Over time, treatment with DMT has trended towards the initiation of higher efficacy treatment at time of diagnosis to help prevent further disease progression and accrual of disability over time, and there is evidence in current literature that supports this change in treatment patterns. In this review, we discuss the current knowledge in diagnosis, treatment, and clinical outcomes in pediatric MS.

Keywords: multiple sclerosis; pediatric multiple sclerosis; neuroimmunology; demyelinating disease; pediatric neurology; child neurology

1. Introduction

Multiple sclerosis (MS) is a chronic autoimmune disease of the central nervous system resulting in inflammation and demyelination in the brain and spinal cord. Although it is most commonly seen in adults, between 3–5% of patients have an onset of disease under the age of 18, and less than 2% of patients under 10 years of age [1–4]. Pediatric MS is rare, much less common than adult MS. The incidence of pediatric MS has been reported in ranges of 0.13 to 0.6 cases per 100,000 children per year [5]. Due to this, there have been fewer research, publications, and natural history data on pediatric MS. With the development of the International Pediatric MS Study Group (IPMSSG) in 2005, the knowledge base surrounding pediatric MS has increased. While the pathophysiology of the disease in the pediatric population is in line with that of the adult population, there are different challenges in the diagnosis, treatment, disease course, and clinical outcomes. In this review, we discuss the currently known environmental and genetic risk factors of pediatric MS, varying clinical presentations, diagnostic criteria and differential diagnoses, diagnostic evaluations, current treatment options, cognitive impairments and psychiatric comorbidity, disease course, and outcomes.

2. Epidemiology

In the pediatric MS population diagnosed before puberty, the number of males and females diagnosed is relatively equivalent [6,7]. In adolescents, the ratio of females to males with MS increases to 2 to 3:1, which may suggest that the onset of menarche plays some role in the pathogenesis of MS [6]. Additionally, the prevalence of MS increases after age 10 [8]. A diverse racial and ethnic population are diagnosed with pediatric MS, one study reporting 67% self-identifying as white and 20.6% as African

American [9]. In this cohort, 30.2% identified as Hispanic, while other cohorts have reported up to 52% of pediatric patients with MS or CIS as Hispanic [9,10]. There has been a significant link to the role of obesity in MS and it has been shown that adolescent obesity is a risk factor for pediatric MS [11]. Not only was adolescent obesity a risk to develop MS, but one study found that in pediatric MS, obesity was present in early childhood years [12]. Obesity has been shown to promote an inflammatory state, which could contribute to not only the pathogenesis of MS, but could also play a role in the risk of relapse and long-term management. A retrospective cohort study performed comparing pediatric MS patients who were obese vs. those with normal BMI showed that obese patients had statistically significant higher relapse rates on first-line treatments, and higher relapse rates on second-line treatments [13]. Low levels of vitamin D have been associated with an increased risk of pediatric MS and with increased rates of relapse [14,15]. In the adult population it has been shown that there is an increased risk of MS in those who smoke cigarettes, and coinciding with this, children who are exposed to smoking in the home have been shown to be more likely to develop pediatric MS than a control population [16,17]. Epstein-Barr virus (EBV) may play a role in pathogenesis and risk of MS and pediatric MS, although the mechanism remains unclear at this time [15,18]. Historically, a correlation between EBV and MS was proposed due to the similarities in the epidemiology of the diseases, and studies have shown a strong correlation in support of this [19]. EBV infection can occur at any age, and is generally asymptomatic in young children. The presence of MS-mimics such as Neuromyelitis Optica Spectrum Disorder (NMOSD) and anti-myelin oligodendrocyte antibody syndrome, may contribute to a higher frequency of EBV seronegative- antibody children diagnosed with MS. One of the main genetic risk factors found in pediatric MS is HLA DRB1*1501 [20,21]. HLA DRB1*1501 is additionally seen as a genetic risk factor in adult MS, and postulated to be associated with earlier age of onset in the adult population, although there has been varying evidence in support of this, and thus at this time cannot be attributed to age of onset. The HLA class II proteins play a role in cell-mediated immunity, leading to the suspicion that it could be a genetic marker or predisposition to developing MS [22]. There are 57 previously identified single nucleotide polymorphisms that have been associated with adult-onset MS that have also been identified in a large cohort of children with demyelinating diseases and found to be associated with increased risk of pediatric-onset MS [23]. One recently published cohort identified 32% of patients with at least one relative with MS [22], with a report of incidence in a first-degree relative of 2–5% [24]. In monozygotic twins, a concordance rate of 27% is reported vs. dizygotic twins with a rate of 2.3% [24]. There have been numerous correlated factors in pediatric MS, and likely more that have yet to be determined. Many of these factors also overlap, and more studies are needed in order to determine if there are additional genetic etiologies that may lead to a predisposition to development of pediatric MS in the context of certain environmental factors.

3. Clinical Presentation

In a subset of patients at the initial presentation of a demyelinating event, a diagnosis of pediatric MS can be made. Younger children will often present with multifocal symptoms, but entering adolescence it becomes more common to present with single focal symptoms more similar to that of adults [25,26]. The most commonly reported symptoms in children include sensory (15–30%), motor (30%), and brainstem dysfunction (25–41%) [27]. The clinical course in 95–98% of pediatric MS patients is relapsing remitting, compared to 85–90% in adults [27–29]. Less than 3% of pediatric MS cases are reported as primary progressive, compared to 10–15% in the adult population [28–30]. In children with a progressive course, other diagnoses should be considered. Children have been reported to have a higher relapse rate compared to adult-onset MS, especially within the first few years of diagnosis [31,32]. Studies have reported 2.3–2.8 times higher relapse rate in pediatric MS, and higher rates of relapse early in the disease if without treatment or on lower efficacy treatment [32–34]. These findings suggest that those with pediatric MS have a more significant inflammatory component than those with adult-onset MS [32]. Due to these factors, more recent treatment has trended toward initiation with higher efficacy medications at time of diagnosis to help target this increased inflammatory state, decrease relapse rate, and prevent accrual of disability.

4. Diagnosis

To make the diagnosis of MS, at least one clinical event with symptoms lasting at least 24 h must be present. Dissemination in space is the development of lesions in distinct regions of the CNS, including periventricular, cortical or juxtacortical, infratentorial brain regions, and the spinal cord [35]. Dissemination in time is demonstrated by the presence of enhancing and non-enhancing lesions at any time, or by new T2 hyperintense lesions on follow up MRI [35]. In 2007, the IPMSSG created a consensus definition for pediatric MS, which was updated in 2012 following the publication of the revised 2010 McDonald criteria for the diagnosis of MS [36]. Per the IPMSSG, pediatric MS has been defined by occurrence of any of the following [37]:

1. Two or more clinically isolated syndromes (CIS) separated by greater than 30 days involving multiple areas of the CNS;
2. One CIS associated with MRI findings consistent with dissemination in space and a follow up MRI showing at least one new lesion consistent with dissemination in time;
3. One acute disseminated encephalomyelitis (ADEM) attack followed by 1 CIS more than 3 months after symptom onset with new MRI findings consistent with dissemination in space;
4. CIS with MRI findings consistent with dissemination in time and space if the patient is at least 12 years of age.

In children with acute demyelinating attacks consistent with MS, the 2010 McDonald criteria have been studied and shown to have high sensitivity, specificity, and positive predictive value for children at least 11 years of age [38]. The criteria have only a 55% positive predictive value in children under 11, and should not be applied to those with an ADEM presentation [38]. More recently, the revised 2017 McDonald criteria were compared to the prior 2010 criteria in a pediatric cohort and demonstrated improvement in accuracy (87.2% vs 66.7%) and sensitivity (84.0% vs 46.8%), but the 2017 criteria remain unvalidated in children under 12 years of age [39]. Although there is improved accuracy and sensitivity with these revised criteria, there continues to be misdiagnosis due to overlapping features with numerous mimickers of MS including multiphasic ADEM, NMOSD, vasculitis and other neuroinflammatory diseases, metabolic disorders, and leukodystrophies.

In the pediatric population, there is a wide array of alternative diagnoses to be considered when evaluating a patient for possible pediatric MS. Most commonly reported indications of an alternative etiology include progressive course at disease onset, encephalopathy, fever, negative oligoclonal bands, and significantly elevated CSF white blood cells or protein [40]. Typical lesions are ovoid in shape, and are asymmetric in hemispheric involvement. Typically, lesions are located in periventricular and juxtacortical white matter, corpus callosum, pons, cerebellum and middle cerebellar peduncle, and spinal cord (more commonly the cervical cord). MRI features that could indicate a diagnosis other than pediatric MS include symmetric bilateral lesions, large gray matter involvement at the onset, DWI abnormalities, meningeal enhancement, presence of hemorrhage, prolonged period of contrast enhancement, and presence of edema or mass effect [40]. If the MRI and clinical presentation fall within the criteria for diagnosis, in general, lumbar puncture may not be required to aid in diagnosis; however, lumbar puncture for CSF analysis should be considered in those with atypical presentations. As there are limitations in current diagnostic criteria, evaluation for other mimics of pediatric MS, should be assessed at time of presentation with Aquaporin-4 and anti-MOG antibodies. Anti-MOG antibody can also be present in monophasic and multiphasic ADEM, which differ from MS and NMOSD in prognosis and management. Other studies to be performed at time of presentation may include (if indicated per clinical judgement) the C-reactive protein, erythrocyte sedimentation rate, anti-nuclear antibody, angiotensin-converting enzyme level, folate, vitamin B12, and thyroid-stimulating hormone. Those with a progressive course should be evaluated for mitochondrial, metabolic, and neurodegenerative disorders including leukodystrophies. Other considerations include other autoimmune conditions, including systemic lupus erythematosus, neurosarcoidosis, or Sjogren syndrome.

Clinically Isolated Syndrome (CIS) in pediatrics has been defined by the IPMSSG as a monofocal or polyfocal CNS event of presumed inflammatory/demyelinating cause in a child without encephalopathy and no prior history of CNS demyelination. The MRI should not meet the criteria for MS diagnosis, with both dissemination in time and space absent. Optic neuritis is the most common CIS presentation in pediatrics, followed by transverse myelitis and brainstem syndromes [41]. In a cohort of 770 patients with pediatric CIS who were followed for 10 years to assess the risk of conversion to MS, female gender and multifocal symptoms at onset were risk factors for the occurrence of a second attack [42]. In pediatric optic neuritis, rates of conversion to MS range from 13.8–32% [43,44]. There has been a higher risk of conversion to MS reported in those with abnormal brain MRI at the onset of optic neuritis, bilateral optic neuritis, and those with recurrent optic neuritis [43–45]. Transverse myelitis, similarly, is typically a monophasic disorder. Reported risk factors for relapse of pediatric transverse myelitis include female gender and abnormal brain MRI, which is consistent with that reported in adult studies [46].

Acute disseminated encephalomyelitis (ADEM) is most commonly a monophasic demyelinating disease preceded by viral infection or vaccination. Patients typically present with multifocal symptoms and encephalopathy, and seizures can also be present. MRI findings play a large role in the differentiation of ADEM from MS: diffuse bilateral lesions with ill-defined borders are more commonly seen in ADEM [47]. Susceptibility weighted imaging has been used in the identification of multiple sclerosis, but also has been looked at as a possible tool in helping differentiate ADEM and MS [48]. In patients with multiphasic ADEM, anti-myelin oligodendrocyte glycoprotein (MOG) antibodies can be evaluated to help differentiate from MS. Anti-MOG associated disorders can present as optic neuritis, monophasic ADEM or a neuromyelitis optica spectrum disorder (NMOSD). While some patients with anti-MOG associated disorders will respond to an initial course of steroids, some will require longer-term immunomodulation [49].

Most commonly, patients with NMOSD present with transverse myelitis and optic neuritis. MRI findings are used in differentiating pediatric MS from NMOSD. Patients with NMOSD can have brain MRI abnormalities, most commonly reported in the diencephalic region, dorsal medulla (area postrema), and peri-ependymal circumventricular areas. Typical characteristics of optic nerve lesions in NMOSD include involvement of the optic chiasm and lesions extending greater than half the length of the optic nerve [50]. In NMOSD, spinal cord lesions extend at least three vertebral segments, which is seen in 10% of patients with pediatric MS [47]. Additionally, it has been seen that contrast enhancement in spinal cord lesions in NMO display a rim-enhancement as compared to MS where more uniform enhancement is seen [51]. Due to selective involvement in the area postrema, 38% of pediatric NMO patients present with vomiting [52]. CSF can display significant pleocytosis with neutrophilic or lymphocytic predominance, and oligoclonal bands are less frequently seen than in MS [53,54].

5. Diagnostic Evaluations

MRI is an important tool in pediatric MS and aids in the diagnosis. MRI findings are used for the assessment of dissemination in time and space. Spinal cord imaging typically shows cervical cord lesions, short segment lesions (< 3 vertebral segments in length) that involve only a portion of the diameter of the cord [55]. While MRI brain and spine are the most valuable test in supporting the diagnosis of MS, the MRI spine may be less useful in the diagnosis of pediatric MS, with one study only showing 10% of patients meeting the criteria of dissemination in time and space based on the addition of MRI spine [56]. Based on the initial MRI, pediatric MS patients show a higher number of T2 lesions than adults and more frequently have cerebellar and brainstem involvement [57]. Additionally, pediatric patients have lesions that are larger and more ill-defined [58]. The presence of at least one periventricular white matter lesion and at least one T1 hypointensity on initial MRI can predict progression to MS at the time of presentation [59].

Cerebrospinal fluid (CSF) pleocytosis is present in 53–66% of patients, with cell count reported as high as 61 [60,61]. A lymphocytic predominance is more commonly seen, but in children under 11 years of age, an elevated neutrophil count may be seen [8]. The presence of oligoclonal bands in the CSF is significant for ongoing neuroinflammation and has been reported in numerous CNS inflammatory conditions, including pediatric and adult MS. The presence of oligoclonal IgG bands in the CSF has been reported in 64% to 92% of pediatric MS patients, and is seen to be less frequent in younger children [60]. Oligoclonal bands in the CSF can be used to aid in the diagnosis of pediatric MS. In children aged 12–17 years old with clinical suspicion of MS, the presence of oligoclonal bands strongly supports a diagnosis [62]. In patients with a pediatric radiologically isolated syndrome, the presence of oligoclonal bands increases the specificity of MRI criteria, and can help in predicting conversion to MS [63]. It is important to note that while oligoclonal bands can be used to make the diagnosis of pediatric MS, other conditions that are classified as mimickers of pediatric MS can also have a presence of oligoclonal bands, thus, this presence does not eliminate other diagnoses.

6. Treatment Options

The primary goal of treatment with disease modifying therapy is to achieve a state of no evidence of clinical or radiographic disease activity. No evidence of disease activity (NEDA) is characterized by the absence of clinical relapses, no progression of clinical disability, no new or enlarging T2 lesions on MRI, and no contrast-enhancing lesions on MRI [64]. There are varying approaches to disease modifying therapy, including an escalation or "step-up" vs. an induction or "step-down" approach [6]. The first approach involves starting with what is considered to be first-line therapy, and escalating treatment if the patient were to have evidence of clinical relapse or interval development of new demyelinating lesions on MRI despite patient compliance with the medication and adequate duration of treatment [6]. The second involves using the more efficacious treatments first to induce a state of no evidence of disease activity. At this time, fingolimod is the only FDA approved treatment for pediatric MS, but other treatments, including interferons, glatiramer acetate, dimethyl fumarate, teriflunomide, natalizumab, rituximab, and cyclophosphamide, have been used and reports have shown the benefits of these treatments. Currently, consensus statements suggest first-line therapies as interferons or glatiramer acetate, but more recent studies have led to a discussion of the need for revision of these guidelines in light of studies showing that a large number of patients on injectable therapies require escalation of therapy [65,66]. Additionally, there is no standard definition of treatment failure across treatment centers, and with this, no guidelines for the transition of medications. The IPMSSG has proposed definitions for breakthrough disease, including an increase or no reduction in relapse rate, development of new T2 or contrast-enhancing lesions on MRI, or two or greater clinical or MRI relapses within 12 months [67]. Some children achieve a state of NEDA on first-line medications, but some require a transition of medications due to the breakthrough of disease, while other patients may change medications due to poor tolerance or non-compliance.

Interferons in injectable formulations along with glatiramer acetate are commonly used first-line treatments in pediatric MS as has been displayed with observational studies [68]. Interferons are well tolerated, with 25–35% of children reporting flu-like symptoms [69,70]. To mitigate adverse effects, the dose can be titrated over 4 weeks until reaching full dose, and pretreatment with analgesics is recommended. Regulatory laboratory monitoring is required as interferon beta can result in elevation of liver transaminases, thyroid function abnormalities and decreased peripheral blood cell counts [69–72]. Interferons should be used with caution in children with a known history of depression as there have been reported mood side effects [6]. In 44 pediatric MS patients treated with interferon-beta-1b, no serious adverse events were reported [70]. In a retrospective study named REPLAY, adult doses of interferon beta-1a were tolerated without adverse reactions in pediatric MS [69].

Glatiramer acetate is a synthetic amino acid polymer that resembles myelin basic protein, which is delivered via subcutaneous injection. Retrospective studies have shown reduction of annualized relapse rate (ARR) similar to those of the adult trials ranging from 0.2–0.25 [73,74]. In the pediatric population, full adult dosing is used and generally well-tolerated [75]. The most commonly reported side effect are injection site reactions. Rarely, an immediate post-injection systemic reaction occurs with flushing, chest pain, palpitations, and shortness of breath, but this usually self-resolves. Regular laboratory monitoring is not required. As interferons and glatiramer acetate are generally well tolerated and shown to decrease relapse rates in retrospective studies, they were commonly used as first line treatments until the more recent development and introduction of newer treatment options.

Fingolimod, a once-daily oral medication, was approved by the FDA in 2018 as a first-line treatment in pediatric MS based on the results of the PARADIGMS trial. Fingolimod binds to sphingosine-1-phosphate receptors, sequestering lymphocytes in the lymph node and prevents activated lymphocytes from crossing into the CNS. In pediatric MS, an 82% reduction in annualized relapse rate in comparison to those treated with interferon beta-1a was demonstrated [76]. Additionally, over a two-year interval at all time points, patients treated with fingolimod had lower EDSS scores compared to those treated with interferon beta-1a [77]. While the PARADIGMS trial showed improved efficacy of treatment and improved EDSS at follow up with treatment with fingolimod compared to interferon beta-1a, it additionally has increased risks with treatment. The serious adverse events in the pediatric population included leukopenia and seizures. It is required that patients be monitored for bradycardia for 6 h with the first dose. Patients should be monitored for macular edema with annual ophthalmology exams, although there was only one report of macular edema in the PARADIGMS trial [76]. Routine laboratory monitoring of liver transaminases and lymphocyte counts are recommended. Additionally, there is a risk for progressive multifocal leukoencephalopathy (PML), which has been more commonly reported in patients on fingolimod for longer duration and with positive John Cunningham Virus (JCV) antibodies. PML is an opportunistic infection of the CNS that is potentially fatal and is caused by the reactivation of latent JCV.

Dimethyl fumarate is a twice-daily oral medication that was approved by the FDA in 2013 for the treatment of MS in adults. The specific mechanism of action is unknown, but it is shown to affect cytokines and lower lymphocyte counts. Phase 3 studies in adults have shown dimethyl fumarate significantly reduces relapse rates and the development of new T2 hyperintense lesions on MRI. Common side effects include flushing, which can be abated with pretreatment with aspirin. There have been cases of PML in patients on dimethyl fumarate, all occurring in patients with lymphocyte counts under 800, thus, routine laboratory monitoring is recommended. An open-label study, FOCUS, was performed to evaluate the effect of dimethyl fumarate on MRI activity in the pediatric population, and showed a reduction in the development of new T2 hyperintense lesions [78]. While there are data showing a reduction in the breakthrough disease on MRI, there are yet to be data on the reduction of clinical relapse in the pediatric MS population. CONNECT is an open-label randomized controlled study comparing dimethyl fumarate versus interferon beta-1a in the pediatric population that is currently ongoing [79].

Teriflunomide is a once-daily oral pill that reduces the activation and proliferation of lymphocytes by inhibiting pyrimidine synthesis. In studies in the adult MS population, teriflunomide has been shown to significantly reduce the relapse rate, disability progression, and new activity on MRI in comparison to placebo [80]. Common side effects include hair thinning, nausea, diarrhea, and elevated liver transaminases. There is a significant risk of teratogenicity, and if pregnancy is desired. a period of washout with cholestyramine should be performed. Teriflunomide is not commonly prescribed in the pediatric population. TERIKIDS, a randomized, double-blind, placebo-controlled trial, is currently ongoing, evaluating efficacy and safety of teriflunomide in pediatric MS [79].

Natalizumab is a humanized monoclonal antibody that has been shown to decrease clinical relapse by 68% and decrease the development of new T2 hyperintense lesions by 83% compared to placebo in adults, and small open-label studies in pediatric MS population have shown good efficacy and tolerability [81–84]. In a study of 55 pediatric patients, only three relapses occurred, all within 6 months of initiation of natalizumab [82]. At one year follow up, 83% were free of new T2 lesions on MRI and 74% at two years follow up [82]. No serious adverse effects were reported in this study group. Additionally, a recently published cohort of 20 treatment naïve pediatric MS patients showed that over a treatment period of 24 months with natalizumab, patients had a significant reduction in mean EDSS overall, and NEDA-3 plus status (no evidence of relapse, no disease progression, no new MRI activity, and no cognitive decline) was maintained in 80% of patients, demonstrating natalizumab as a highly effective treatment in pediatric MS [85]. JCV antibodies should be monitored at least every 6 months given the elevated risk of PML in those who are JCV antibody positive, and if seroconversion were to occur, then transitioning to alternative therapy should be considered. Additional risk factors in the setting of positive JCV status include prolonged duration of natalizumab use and prior immunosuppression.

Rituximab is a monoclonal antibody that depletes CD20+ B cells that has been shown in both pediatric and adult MS populations to reduce both clinical relapses and MRI lesions [86,87]. In a case series of 14 pediatric MS patients treated with rituximab, no patients had subsequent relapses [88]. The most common adverse effects include hypogammaglobulinemia and infusion reactions [87,89]. The risk of PML is present with rituximab; however, in pediatric MS a larger population and longer follow up is needed to better understand this risk [89].

Cyclophosphamide, an alkylating agent, has been shown to be effective in reducing the relapse rate in pediatric MS patients with aggressive disease [90]. It is given as a monthly infusion, and affects cytokine expression, in addition to T-cell and B-cell function [80]. While it is effective, there are significant risks of secondary malignancies, infection, and sterility [90]. Additional side effects include nausea, vomiting, alopecia, osteoporosis, and amenorrhea [80].

7. Cognitive Impairment, Fatigue, and Psychiatric Comorbidities

Cognitive function is affected in approximately 30% of pediatric MS patients. Children present with differing deficits than those with adult MS, as children can show greater deficits in vocabulary and language-based cognition [91]. Other commonly reported impairments in those with longer disease duration include attention, processing speed, visual-motor skills, executive functions, and memory [92]. Cohorts of pediatric MS patients who have undergone neuropsychology evaluation have found a strong association between cognitive impairment and EDSS score, number of relapses, and disease duration [93]. Studies have looked at cognitive functioning at the time of diagnosis and in follow up. One recent study compared initial neuropsychological evaluations in 19 patients who were either treatment naïve or on solely interferon beta, all of which had follow up assessments performed. Six patients were escalated to a higher efficacy treatment (three to natalizumab and three fingolimod), and the remainder did not require escalation of treatment (10 on interferon beta-1a, two on glatiramer acetate, and one on dimethyl fumarate). While cognitive impairment was seen early in the disease at initial evaluation, those patients who did not have an escalation of treatment had a higher degree of impairment at time of follow up in comparison to those who had an escalation of therapy [94]. Studies additionally have shown that those with pediatric MS are at a higher risk of cognitive disability than adult MS patients [95,96]. Cognitive impairment is more significant in the pediatric MS population, and findings show that those who have been escalated to a higher efficacy treatment to have a lower degree of cognitive impairment; thus, this argues towards an induction or "step-down" treatment approach to help protect from development or further cognitive decline, although larger studies are warranted to confirm this hypothesis.

There are additional features of pediatric MS that can impact everyday functioning. Fatigue is a common complaint in the MS population and can significantly affect daily functioning and can also be a contributing factor in cognitive functioning. In one study comparing pediatric MS patients with healthy controls, there was no significant difference between the two groups in regard to self-reported fatigue, although an additional study reported that at least half of pediatric MS patients report at least mild fatigue [97,98]. Importantly in this study, self- and parent-reported fatigue were associated with higher scores on the Children's Depression Inventory [97]. Additional studies have shown signs of depression are higher in the pediatric MS population [99,100]. In combination, depression or anxiety disorders are present in approximately half of pediatric MS patients. The most commonly reported psychiatric diagnoses are anxiety disorders, attention deficit hyperactivity disorder, and mood disorders [101]. When looking at overall quality of life, one study reported that approximately half of pediatric MS patients reported difficulties in school and emotional functioning [99]. Additional studies have shown that in addition to fatigue and depression, increased EDSS can contribute to decrease in health-related quality of life [102].

8. Clinical Outcomes

Despite elevated relapse rates, the pediatric population tends to have a complete recovery from relapse within 12 months with little accrual of disability during childhood years [36]. Generally, as children do not accumulate disability, they will not develop secondary progressive MS in childhood years, and it generally will take the pediatric MS population approximately 10 years longer than the adult MS population to convert to secondary progression [28,103]. Despite this, the time of progression from mild to severe disability is the same in adults and children [28]. Given this, those with pediatric MS will reach disability milestones at a younger age than those with adult-onset MS [30,103,104]. An increased risk of disability in pediatric MS was associated with a progressive course at onset and an increased number of relapses in the first five years, while a reduced risk was present in those that had complete remission from the initial event [103]. These findings further support the importance of early recognition and treatment in pediatric MS.

Patients with pediatric MS have a smaller brain volume than expected for their age [105], and this carries into adulthood. In comparing the adult brain volume of pediatric MS patients with age-matched adult MS patients, those with the pediatric-onset disease have reduced brain and deep grey matter volume, particularly thalamic volume [106].

9. Conclusions

Pediatric MS is a rare disorder, but the long-term clinical implications in those who are diagnosed lead to significant cognitive and physical disability in adulthood, even with current first-line treatments. The ultimate aim of the treatment of pediatric MS is to reach a state of NEDA. More recently, the goals have been aimed towards NEDA-4, which is a state of no clinical relapse, no disease progression, no new MRI activity, no cognitive decline, and no evidence of brain atrophy present [107,108]. Given the elevated annualized relapse rate, increased rate of cognitive disability, and younger age at reaching disability milestones in pediatric MS, to achieve NEDA-4, the treatment paradigm may need to shift towards that of treatment with higher efficacy medications.

Author Contributions: K.S.F. designed and wrote the manuscript. F.X.C. reviewed the manuscript. V.M.R. reviewed the manuscript. G.J.H. reviewed the manuscript. All authors have read and agreed to the published version of the manuscript.

References

1.   Boiko, A.; Vorobeychik, G.; Paty, D.; Devonshire, V.; Sadovnick, D.; UBC MS Clinic Neurologists. Early onset multiple sclerosis: A longitudinal study. *Neurology* **2002**, *59*, 1006–1010. [CrossRef] [PubMed]
2.   Bigi, S.; Banwell, B. Pediatric multiple sclerosis. *J. Child. Neurol.* **2012**, *27*, 1378–1383. [CrossRef]
3.   Tenembaum, S. Multiple sclerosis in childhood and adolescence. *J. Neurol. Sci.* **2011**, *311*, S53–S57. [CrossRef]
4.   Gordon-Lipkin, E.; Banwell, B. An update on multiple sclerosis in children: Diagnosis, therapies, and prospects for the future. *Expert Rev. Clin. Immunol.* **2017**, *13*, 975–989. [CrossRef] [PubMed]
5.   Waldman, A.; Ghezzi, A.; Bar-Or, A.; Mikaeloff, Y.; Tardieu, M.; Banwell, B. Multiple sclerosis in children: An update on clinical diagnosis, therapeutic strategies, and research. *Lancet Neurol.* **2014**, *13*, 936–948. [CrossRef]
6.   Wang, C.X.; Greenberg, B.M. Pediatric Multiple Sclerosis: From Recognition to Practical Clinical Management. *Neurol. Clin.* **2018**, *36*, 135–149. [CrossRef] [PubMed]
7.   Huppke, B.; Ellenberger, D.; Rosewich, H.; Friede, T.; Gärtner, J.; Huppke, P. Clinical presentation of pediatric multiple sclerosis before puberty. *Eur. J. Neurol.* **2014**, *21*, 441–446. [CrossRef]

8. Chitnis, T.; Krupp, L.; Yeh, A.; Rubin, J.; Kuntz, N.; Strober, J.B.; Chabas, D.; Weinstock-Guttman, B.; Ness, J.; Rodriguez, M.; et al. Pediatric Multiple Sclerosis. *Neurol. Clin.* **2011**, *29*, 481–505. [CrossRef]

9. Belman, A.L.; Krupp, L.B.; Oslen, C.S.; Rose, J.W.; Aaen, G.; Benson, L.; Chitnis, T.; Gorman, M.; Graves, J.; Harris, Y.; et al. Network of Pediatric MS Centers. Characteristics of children and adolescents with multiple sclerosis. *Pediatrics* **2016**, *138*, 1–8. [CrossRef]

10. Langer-Gould, A.; Brara, S.M.; Beaber, B.E.; Koebnick, C. Childhood obesity and risk of pediatric multiple sclerosis and clinically isolated syndrome. *Neurology* **2013**, *80*, 548–552. [CrossRef]

11. Chitnis, T.; Graves, J.; Weinstock-Guttman, B.; Belman, A.; Olsen, C.; Misra, M.; Aaen, G.; Benson, L.; Candee, M.; Gorman, M.; et al. Network of Pediatric MS Centers. Distinct effects of obesity and puberty on risk and age at onset of pediatric MS. *Ann. Clin. Transl.Neurol.* **2016**, *3*, 897–907. [CrossRef] [PubMed]

12. Brenton, J.N.; Woolbright, E.; Briscoe-Abath, C.; Qureshi, A.; Conaway, M.; Goldman, M.D. Body mass index trajectories in pediatric multiple sclerosis. *Dev. Med. Child. Neurol.* **2019**, *61*, 1289–1294. [CrossRef] [PubMed]

13. Huppke, B.; Ellenberger, D.; Hummel, H.; Stark, W.; Robl, M.; Gartner, J.; Huppke, P. Association of Obesity with Multiple Sclerosis Risk and Response to First-line Disease Modifying Drugs in Children. *JAMA Neurol.* **2019**, *76*, 1157–1165. [CrossRef] [PubMed]

14. Mowry, E.M.; Krupp, L.B.; Milazzo, M.; Chabas, D.; Strober, J.B.; Belman, A.L.; McDonald, J.C.; Oksenberg, J.R.; Bacchetti, P.; Waubant, E. Vitamin D status is associated with relapse rate in pediatric-onset multiple sclerosis. *Ann. Neurol.* **2010**, *67*, 618–624. [CrossRef] [PubMed]

15. Banwell, B.; Bar-Or, A.; Arnold, D.L.; Sadovnick, D.; Narayanan, S.; McGowan, M.; O'Mahony, J.; Magalhaes, S.; Hanwell, H.; Vieth, R.; et al. Clinical, environmental, and genetic determinants of multiple sclerosis in children with acute demyelination: A prospective national cohort study. *Lancet Neurol.* **2011**, *10*, 436–445. [CrossRef]

16. Hedström, A.K.; Olsson, T.; Alfredsson, L. Smoking is a major preventable risk factor for multiple sclerosis. *Mult. Scler.* **2016**, *22*, 1021–1026. [CrossRef]

17. Mikaeloff, Y.; Caridade, G.; Tardieu, M.; Suissa, S. Parental smoking at home and the risk of childhood-onset multiple sclerosis in children. *Brain* **2007**, *130*, 2589–2595. [CrossRef]

18. Ahmed, S.I.; Aziz, K.; Gul, A.; Samar, S.S.; Bareeqa, S.B. Risk of Multiple Sclerosis in Epstein–Barr Virus Infection. *Cureus* **2019**. [CrossRef]

19. Ascherio, A.; Munger, K.L.; Lennette, E.T.; Spiegelman, D.; Hernan, M.A.; Olek, M.J.; Hankinson, S.E.; Hunter, D.J. Epstein-Barr virus antibodies and risk of multiple sclerosis: A prospective study. *J. Am. Med. Assoc.* **2001**, *286*, 3083–3088. [CrossRef]

20. Waubant, W.; Ponsonby, A.L.; Pugliatti, M.; Hanwell, H.; Mowry, E.M.; Hintzen, R.Q. Environmental and genetic factors in pediatric inflammatory demyelinating diseases. *Neurology* **2016**, *87*, S20–S27. [CrossRef]

21. Gianfrancesco, M.A.; Stridh, P.; Shao, X.; Rhead, B.; Graves, J.S.; Chitnis, T.; Waldman, A.; Lotze, T.; Schreiner, T.; Belman, A.; et al. Genetic risk factors for pediatric-onset multiple sclerosis. *Mult. Scler. J.* **2018**, *24*, 1825–1834. [CrossRef] [PubMed]

22. Boiko, A.N.; Gusev, E.I.; Sudomoina, M.A.; Alekseenkov, A.D.; Kulakova, O.G.; Bikova, O.V.; Maslova, O.I.; Guseva, M.R.; Boiko, S.Y.; Guseva, M.E.; et al. Association and linkage of juvenile MS with HLA-DR2(15) in Russians. *Neurology* **2002**, *58*, 658–660. [CrossRef] [PubMed]

23. van Pelt, E.D.; Mescheriakova, J.Y.; Makhani, N.; Ketelslegers, I.A.; Neuteboom, R.F.; Kundu, S.; Broer, L.; Janssens, C.; Catsman-Berrevoets, C.E.; van Duijn, C.M.; et al. Risk genes associated with pediatric-Onset MS but not with monophasic acquired CNS demyelination. *Neurology* **2013**, *81*, 1996–2001. [CrossRef] [PubMed]

24. Vargas-Lowy, D.; Chitnis, T. Pathogenesis of pediatric multiple sclerosis. *J. Child. Neurol.* **2012**, *27*, 1394–1407. [CrossRef] [PubMed]

25. Mikaeloff, Y.; Suissa, S.; Vallee, L.; Lubetzki, C.; Ponsot, G.; Confavreux, C.; Tardieu, M.; KIDMUS Study Group. First episode of acute CNS inflammatory demyelination in childhood: Prognostic factors for multiple sclerosis and disability. *J. Pediatr.* **2004**, *144*, 246–252. [CrossRef] [PubMed]

26. Gadoth, N. Multiple sclerosis in children. *Brain Dev.* **2003**, *25*, 229–232. [CrossRef]

27. Banwell, B.; Ghezzi, A.; Bar-Or, A.; Mikaeloff, Y.; Tardieu, M. Multiple sclerosis in children: Clinical diagnosis, therapeutic strategies, and future directions. *Lancet Neurol.* **2007**, *6*, 887–902. [CrossRef]

28. Renoux, C.; Vukusic, S.; Mikaeloff, Y.; Edan, G.; Clanet, M.; Dubois, B.; Debouverie, M.; Brochet, B.; Lebrun-Frenay, C.; Pelletier, J.; et al. Natural history of multiple sclerosis with childhood onset. *N. Engl. J. Med.* **2007**, *356*, 2603–2613. [CrossRef]

29. Miller, D.H.; Leary, S.M. Primary-progressive multiple sclerosis. *Lancet Neurol.* **2007**, *6*, 903–912. [CrossRef]

30. Harding, K.E.; Liang, K.; Cossburn, M.D.; Ingram, G.; Hirst, C.L.; Pickersgill, T.P.; Te Water Naude, J.; Wardle, M.; Ben-Shlomo, Y.; Robertson, N.P. Long-term outcome of paediatric-onset multiple sclerosis: A population-based study. *J. Neurol. Neurosurg. Psychiatry* **2013**, *84*, 141–147. [CrossRef]

31. Waldman, A.; Ness, J.; Pohl, D.; Simone, I.L.; Anlar, B.; Pia Amato, M.; Ghezzi, A. Pediatric multiple sclerosis Clinical features and outcome. *Neurology* **2016**, *87*, S74–S81. [CrossRef] [PubMed]

32. Gorman, M.P.; Healy, B.C.; Polgar-Turcsanyi, M.; Chitnis, T. Increased relapse rate in pediatric-onset compared with adult-onset multiple sclerosis. *Arch. Neurol.* **2009**, *66*, 54–59. [CrossRef] [PubMed]

33. Yeh, E.A.; Chitnis, T.; Krupp, L.; Ness, J.; Chabas, D.; Kuntz, N.; Waubant, E. Pediatric multiple sclerosis. *Nat. Rev. Neurol.* **2009**, *5*, 621–631. [CrossRef] [PubMed]

34. Benson, L.A.; Healy, B.C.; Gorman, M.P.; Baruch, N.F.; Gholipour, T.; Musallam, A.; Chitnis, T. Elevated relapse rates in pediatric compared to adult MS persist for at least 6 years. *Mult. Scler. Relat. Disord.* **2014**, *3*, 186–193. [CrossRef] [PubMed]

35. Thompson, A.J.; Banwell, B.L.; Barkhof, F.; Carroll, W.M.; Coetzee, T.; Comi, G.; Correale, J.; Fazekas, F.; Filippi, M.; Freedman, M.S.; et al. Diagnosis of multiple sclerosis: 2017 revisions of the McDonald criteria. *Lancet Neurol.* **2018**, *17*, 162–173. [CrossRef]

36. Narula, S. New Perspectives in Pediatric Neurology-Multiple Sclerosis. *Curr. Probl. Pediatr. Adolesc. Health Care* **2016**, *46*, 62–69. [CrossRef]

37. Tardieu, M.; Banwell, B.; Wolinsky, J.S.; Pohl, D.; Krupp, L. Consensus definitions for pediatric MS and other demyelinating disorders in childhood. *Neurology* **2016**, *87*, S8–S11. [CrossRef]

38. Sadaka, Y.; Verhey, L.H.; Shroff, M.M.; Branson, H.M.; Arnold, D.L.; Narayanan, S.; Sled, J.G.; Bar-Or, A.; Sadovnick, A.D.; McGowan, M.; et al. 2010 McDonald criteria for diagnosing pediatric multiple sclerosis. *Ann. Neurol.* **2012**, *72*, 211–223. [CrossRef]

39. Hacohen, Y.; Brownlee, W.; Mankad, K.; Chong, W.K.K.; Thompson, A.; Lim, M.; Wassmer, E.; Hemingway, C.; Barkhof, F.; Ciccarelli, O. Improved performance of the 2017 McDonald criteria for diagnosis of multiple sclerosis in children in a real-life cohort. *Mult. Scler.* **2018**, 1–9. [CrossRef]

40. Padilha, I.G.; Fonseca, A.P.A.; Pettengill, A.L.M.; Fragoso, D.C.; Pacheco, F.T.; Nunes, R.H.; Maia, A.C.M., Jr.; da Rocha, A.J. Pediatric multiple sclerosis: From clinical basis to imaging spectrum and differential diagnosis. *Pediatric Radiology* **2020**. [CrossRef]

41. Trabatti, C.; Foiadelli, T.; Valentina Sparta, M.; Gagliardone, C.; Rinaldi, B.; Delmonte, M.; Lozza, A.; Savasta, S. Paediatric clinically isolated syndromes: Report of seven cases, differential diagnosis and literature review. *Childs Nerv. Syst.* **2016**, *32*, 69–77. [CrossRef] [PubMed]

42. Iaffaldano, P.; Simone, M.; Lucisano, G.; Ghezzi, A.; Coniglio, G.; Brescia Morra, V.; Salemi, G.; Patti, F.; Lugaresi, A.; Izquierdo, G.; et al. Prognostic indicators in pediatric clinically isolated syndrome. *Ann. Neurol.* **2017**, *81*, 729–739. [CrossRef] [PubMed]

43. Lee, J.Y.; Han, J.; Yang, M.; Oh, S.Y. Population-based Incidence of Pediatric and Adult Optic Neuritis and the Risk of Multiple Sclerosis. *Ophthalmology* **2019**, 1–9. [CrossRef] [PubMed]

44. Absoud, M.; Cummins, C.; Desai, N.; Gika, A.; McSweeney, N.; Munot, P.; Hemingway, C.; Lim, M.; Nischal, K.K.; Wassmer, E. Childhood optic neuritis clinical features and outcome. *Arch. Dis Child.* **2011**, *96*, 860–862. [CrossRef]

45. Lucchinetti, C.F.; Kiers, L.; O'Duffy, A.; Gomez, M.R.; Cross, S.; Leavitt, J.A.; O'Brien, P.; Rodriguez, M. Risk factors for developing multiple sclerosis after childhood optic neuritis. *Neurology* **1997**, *49*, 1413–1418. [CrossRef]

46. Absoud, M.; Greenberg, B.M.; Lim, M.; Lotze, T.; Thomas, T.; Deiva, K. Pediatric transverse myelitis. *Neurology* **2016**, *87*, S46–S52. [CrossRef]

47. Banwell, B.; Arnold, D.L.; Tillema, J.; Rocca, M.A.; Filippi, M.; Weinstock-Guttman, B.; Zivadinov, R.; Pia Sormani, M. MRI in the evaluation of pediatric multiple sclerosis. *Neurology* **2016**, *87*, S88–S96. [CrossRef]

48. Kelly, J.E.; Mar, S.; D'Angelo, G.; Zhou, G.; Rajderkar, D.; Benzinger, T.L.S. Susceptibility-weighted imaging helps to discriminate pediatric multiple sclerosis from acute disseminated encephalomyelitis. *Pediatr. Neurol.* **2015**, *52*, 36–41. [CrossRef]

49. Narayan, R.; Simpson, A.; Fritsche, K.; Salama, S.; Pardo, S.; Mealy, M.; Paul, F.; Levy, M. MOG antibody disease: A review of MOG antibody seropositive neuromyelitis optica spectrum disorder. *Mult. Scler. Relat. Disord.* **2018**, *25*, 66–72. [CrossRef]

50. Wingerchuk, D.M.; Banwell, B.; Bennett, J.L.; Cabre, P.; Carroll, W.; Chitnis, T.; de Seze, J.; Fujihara, K.; Greenberg, B.; Jacob, A.; et al. International consensus diagnostic criteria for neuromyelitis optica spectrum disorders. *Neurology* **2015**, *85*, 177–189. [CrossRef]

51. Lotze, T.E.; Northrop, J.L.; Hutton, G.J.; Ross, B.; Schiffman, J.S.; Hunter, J.V. Spectrum of pediatric neuromyelitis optica. *Pediatrics* **2008**, *122*. [CrossRef] [PubMed]

52. Galardi, M.M.; Gaudioso, C.; Ahmadi, S.; Evans, E.; Gilbert, L.; Mar, S. Differential Diagnosis of Pediatric Multiple Sclerosis. *Children* **2019**, *6*, 75. [CrossRef] [PubMed]

53. Chitnis, T.; Ness, J.; Krupp, L.; Waubant, E.; Hunt, T.; Olsen, C.S.; Rodriguez, M.; Lotze, T.; Gorman, M.; Benson, L.; et al. Clinical features of neuromyelitis optica in children US Network of Pediatric MS Centers report. *Neurology* **2015**, *86*, 245–252. [CrossRef] [PubMed]

54. Bradshaw, M.J.; Vu, N.; Hunley, T.E.; Chitnis, T. Child Neurology: Neuromyelitis optica spectrum disorders. *Neurology* **2017**, *88*, e10–e13. [CrossRef]

55. Verhey, L.H.; Branson, H.M.; Makhija, M.; Shroff, M.; Banwell, B. Magnetic resonance imaging features of the spinal cord in pediatric multiple sclerosis: A preliminary study. *Neuroradiology* **2010**, *52*, 1153–1162. [CrossRef]

56. Hummel, H.M.; Brück, W.; Dreha-Kulaczewski, S.; Gärtner, J.; Wuerfel, J. Pediatric onset multiple sclerosis: McDonald criteria 2010 and the contribution of spinal cord MRI. *Mult. Scler. J.* **2013**, *19*, 1330–1335. [CrossRef]

57. Waubant, E.; Chabas, D.; Okuda, D.; Glenn, O.; Mowry, E.; Henry, R.G.; Strober, J.B.; Soares, B.; Wintermark, M.; Pelletier, D. Difference in disease burden and activity in pediatric patients on brain magnetic resonance imaging at time of multiple sclerosis onset vs adults. *Arch. Neurol.* **2019**, *66*, 967–971. [CrossRef]

58. Langille, M.M.; Rutatangwa, A.; Francisco, C. Pediatric Multiple Sclerosis: A. Review. *Adv. Pediatr.* **2019**, *66*, 209–229. [CrossRef]

59. Verhey, L.H.; Branson, H.M.; Shroff, M.M.; Callen, D.J.A.; Sled, J.G.; Narayanan, S.; Sadovnick, A.D.; Var-Or, A.; Arnold, D.L.; Marrie, R.A.; et al. MRI parameters for prediction of multiple sclerosis diagnosis in children with acute CNS demyelination: A prospective national cohort study. *Lancet Neurol.* **2011**, *10*, 1065–1073. [CrossRef]

60. Pohl, D.; Rostasy, K.; Reiber, H.; Hanefeld, F. CSF characteristics in early-onset multiple sclerosis. *Neurology* **2004**, *63*, 1966–1967. [CrossRef]

61. Krajnc, N.; Oražem, J.; Rener-Primec, Z.; Kržan, M.J. Multiple sclerosis in pediatric patients in Slovenia. *Mult. Scler. Relat. Disord.* **2018**, *20*, 194–198. [CrossRef] [PubMed]

62. Boesen, M.S.; Born, A.P.; Hylgaard Jensen, P.E.; Sellebjerg, F.; Blinkenberg, M.; Lydolph, M.C.; Jorgensen, M.K.; Rosenberg, L.; Thomassen, J.Q.; Borresen, M.L. Diagnostic Value of Oligoclonal Bands in Children: A Nationwide Population-Based Cohort Study. *Pediatr. Neurol.* **2019**, *97*, 56–63. [CrossRef] [PubMed]

63. Makhani, N.; Lebrun, C.; Siva, A.; Narula, S.; Wassmer, E.; Brassat, D.; Brenton, J.N.; Cabre, P.; Dalliere, C.C.; de Seze, J.; et al. Oligoclonal bands increase the specificity of MRI criteria to predict multiple sclerosis in children with radiologically isolated syndrome. *Mult. Scler. J. Exp. Transl. Clin.* **2019**, *5*, 1–9. [CrossRef] [PubMed]

64. Havrdova, E.; Galetta, S.; Stefoski, D.; Comi, G. Freedom from disease activity in multiple sclerosis. *Neurology* **2010**, *74*, 3–7. [CrossRef] [PubMed]

65. Krupp, L.B.; Vieira, M.C.; Toledano, H.; Peneva, D.; Druyts, E.; Wu, P.; Boulos, F.C. A Review of Available Treatments, Clinical Evidence, and Guidelines for Diagnosis and Treatment of Pediatric Multiple Sclerosis in the United States. *J. Child. Neurol.* **2019**, *34*, 612–620. [CrossRef]

66. Baroncini, D.; Zaffaroni, M.; Moiola, L.; Lorefice, L.; Fenu, G.; Iaffaldano, P.; Simone, M.; Fanelli, F.; Patti, F.; D'Amico, E.; et al. Long-term follow-up of pediatric MS patients starting treatment with injectable first-line agents: A multicentre, Italian, retrospective, observational study. *Mult. Scler. J.* **2019**, *25*, 399–407. [CrossRef]

67. Macaron, G.; Feng, J.; Moodley, M.; Rensel, M. Newer Treatment Approaches in Pediatric-Onset Multiple Sclerosis. *Curr. Treat. Options Neurol.* **2019**, *21*. [CrossRef]

68. Krysko, K.M.; Graves, J.; Rensel, M.; Weinstock-Guttman, B.; Aaen, G.; Benson, L.; Chitnis, T.; Gormna, M.; Goyal, M.; Krupp, L.; et al. Use of newer disease-modifying therapies in pediatric multiple sclerosis in the US. *Neurology* **2018**, *91*, E1778–E1787. [CrossRef]

69. Tenembaum, S.N.; Banwell, B.; Pohl, D.; Krupp, L.B.; Boyko, A.; Meinel, M.; Lehr, L.; Rocak, S.; Verdun di Cantogno, E.; Stam Maraga, M. Subcutaneous interferon beta-1a in pediatric multiple sclerosis: A retrospective study. *J. Child. Neurol.* **2013**, *28*, 849–856. [CrossRef]

70. Banwell, B.; Reder, A.T.; Krupp, L.; Tenembaum, S.; Eraksoy, M.; Alexey, B.; Pohl, D.; Freedman, M.; Schelensky, L.; Antonijevic, I. Safety and tolerability of interferon beta-1b in pediatric multiple sclerosis. *Neurology* **2006**, *66*, 472–476. [CrossRef]

71. Francis, G.; Grumser, Y.; Alteri, E.; Micaleff, A.; O'Brien, F.; Alsop, J.; Moraga, M.; Kaplowitz, N. Hepatic reactions during treatment of multiple sclerosis with interferon-β-1a: Incidence and clinical significance. *Drug Saf.* **2003**, *26*, 815–827. [CrossRef] [PubMed]

72. Pohl, D.; Rostasy, K.; Gärtner, J.; Hanefeld, F. Treatment of early onset multiple sclerosis with subcutaneous interferon beta-1a. *Neurology* **2005**, *64*, 888–890. [CrossRef] [PubMed]

73. Ghezzi, A.; Amato, M.P.; Capobianco, M.; Gallo, P.; Marrosu, G.; Martinelli, V.; Milani, N.; Milanese, C.; Moiola, L.; Patti, F.; et al. Disease-modifying drugs in childhood-juvenile multiple sclerosis: Results of an Italian co-operative study. *Mult. Scler.* **2005**, *11*, 420–424. [CrossRef] [PubMed]

74. Ghezzi, A.; Pia Amato, M.; Annovazzi, P.; Capobianco, M.; Gallo, P.; La Mantia, L.; Marrosu, M.G.; Martinelli, V.; Milani, N.; Moiola, L.; et al. Long-term results of immunomodulatory treatment in children and adolescents with multiple sclerosis: The Italian experience. *Neurol. Sci.* **2009**, *30*, 193–199. [CrossRef]

75. Kornek, B.; Bernert, G.; Balassy, C.; Geldner, J.; Prayer, D.; Feucht, M. Glatiramer acetate treatment in patients with childhood and juvenile onset multiple sclerosis. *Neuropediatrics* **2003**, *34*, 120–126. [CrossRef] [PubMed]

76. Chitnis, T.; Arnold, D.L.; Banwell, B.; Bruck, W.; Ghezzi, A.; Giovannoni, G.; Greenberg, B.; Krupp, L.; Rostasy, K.; Tardieu, M.; et al. Trial of fingolimod versus interferon beta-1a in pediatric multiple sclerosis. *N. Engl. J. Med.* **2018**, *379*, 1017–1027. [CrossRef] [PubMed]

77. Deiva, K.; Huppke, P.; Banwell, B.; Chitnis, T.; Gartner, J.; Krupp, L.; Waubant, E.; Stites, T.; Pearce, G.L.; Merschhemke, M. Consistent control of disease activity with fingolimod versus IFN β-1a in paediatric-onset multiple sclerosis: Further insights from PARADIG MS. *J. Neurol. Neurosurg. Psychiatry* **2020**, *91*, 58–66. [CrossRef]

78. Alroughani, R.; Das, R.; Penner, N.; Pultz, J.; Taylor, C.; Eraly, S. Safety and Efficacy of Delayed-Release Dimethyl Fumarate in Pediatric Patients With Relapsing Multiple Sclerosis (FOCUS). *Pediatr. Neurol.* **2018**, *83*, 19–24. [CrossRef]

79. Waubant, E.; Banwell, B.; Wassmer, E.; Sormani, M.P.; Amato, M.P.; Hintzen, R.; Krupp, L.; Rostasy, K.; Tenembaum, S.; Chitnis, T. Clinical trials of disease-modifying agents in pediatric MS: Opportunities, challenges, and recommendations from the IPMSSG. *Neurology* **2019**, *92*, E2538–E2549. [CrossRef]

80. Brenton, J.N.; Banwell, B.L. Therapeutic Approach to the Management of Pediatric Demyelinating Disease: Multiple Sclerosis and Acute Disseminated Encephalomyelitis. *Neurotherapeutics* **2016**, *13*, 84–95. [CrossRef]

81. Polman, C.H.; Paul, M.D.; Havrdova, E.; Hutchinson, M.; Kappos, L.; Miller, D.; Phillips, T.; Lublin, F.D.; Giovannoni, G.; Wajgt, A.; et al. A randomized, placebo-controlled trial of natalizumab for relapsing multiple sclerosis. *N. Engl. J. Med.* **2006**, *354*, 899–910. [CrossRef] [PubMed]

82. Ghezzi, A.; Pozzilli, C.; Grimaldi, L.M.E.; Moiola, L.; Brescia-Morra, V.; Lugaresi, A.; Lus, G.; Rinaldi, F.; Rocca, M.A.; Trojano, M.; et al. Natalizumab in pediatric multiple sclerosis: Results of a cohort of 55 cases. *Mult. Scler. J.* **2013**, *19*, 1106–1112. [CrossRef] [PubMed]

83. Ghezzi, A.; Pozzilli, C.; Grimaldi, L.M.E.; Brescia Morra, V.; Bortolon, F.; Capra, R.; Filippi, M.; Moiola, L.; Rocca, M.A.; Rottoli, M.; et al. Safety and efficacy of natalizumab in children with multiple sclerosis. *Neurology* **2010**, *75*, 912–917. [CrossRef] [PubMed]

84. Ghezzi, A.; Moiola, L.; Pozzilli, C.; Brescia-Morra, V.; Gallo, P.; Grimaldi, L.M.E.; Filippi, M.; Comi, G.G. Natalizumab in the pediatric MS population: Results of the Italian registry. *BMC Neurol.* **2015**, *15*, 1–6. [CrossRef] [PubMed]

85. Margoni, M.; Rinaldi, F.; Riccardi, A.; Franciotta, S.; Perini, P.; Gallo, P. No evidence of disease activity including cognition (NEDA-3 plus) in naïve pediatric multiple sclerosis patients treated with natalizumab. *J. Neurol.* **2020**, *267*, 100–105. [CrossRef] [PubMed]

86. Hauser, S.L.; Waubant, E.; Arnold, D.L.; Vollmer, T.; Antel, J.; Fox, R.J.; Bar-Or, A.; Panzar, M.; Sarkar, N.; Agarwal, S.; et al. B-cell depletion with rituximab in relapsing-remitting multiple sclerosis. *N Engl. J. Med.* **2008**, *358*, 676–688. [CrossRef]

87. Beres, S.J.; Graves, S.; Waubant, E. Rituximab use in pediatric central demyelinating disease. *Pediatr. Neurol.* **2014**, *51*, 114–118. [CrossRef]

88. Salzer, J.; Lycke, J.; Wickström, R.; Naver, H.; Piehl, F.; Svenningsson, A. Rituximab in paediatric onset multiple sclerosis: A case series. *J. Neurol.* **2016**, *263*, 322–326. [CrossRef]

89. Dale, R.D.; Brilot, F.; Duffy, L.V.; Twilt, M.; Waldman, A.T.; Narula, S.; Muscal, E.; Deiva, K.; Andersen, E.; Eyre, M.R.; et al. Utility and safety of rituximab in pediatric autoimmune and inflammatory CNS disease. *Neurology* **2014**, *83*, 142–150. [CrossRef]

90. Makhani, N.; Gorman, M.P.; Branson, H.M.; Stazzone, L.; Banwell, B.L.; Chitnis, T. Cyclophosphamide therapy in pediatric multiple sclerosis. *Neurology* **2009**, *72*, 2076–2082. [CrossRef]

91. Parrish, J.B.; Farooq, O.; Weinstock-Guttman, B. Cognitive deficits in pediatric-onset multiple sclerosis: What does the future hold? *Neurodegener. Dis. Manag* **2014**, *4*, 137–146. [CrossRef] [PubMed]

92. Ekmekci, O. Pediatric Multiple Sclerosis and Cognition: A Review of Clinical, Neuropsychologic, and Neuroradiologic Features. *Behav. Neurol.* **2017**. [CrossRef] [PubMed]

93. MacAllister, W.; Belman, A.; Milazzo, M.; Weisbrot, D.; Christodoulou, C.; Scherl, W.; Preston, T.; Cianciulli, C.; Krupp, L. Cognitive functioning in children and adolescents with multiple sclerosis. *Neurology* **2005**, *64*, 1422–1425. [CrossRef] [PubMed]

94. Johnen, A.; Elpers, C.; Riepl, E.; Landmeyer, N.C.; Kramer, J.; Polzer, P.; Lohmann, H.; Omran, H.; Wiendl, H.; Gobel, K.; et al. Early effective treatment may protect from cognitive decline in paediatric multiple sclerosis. *Eur. J. Paediatr. Neurol.* **2019**, *23*, 783–791. [CrossRef] [PubMed]

95. Ruano, L.; Branco, M.; Portaccio, E.; Goretti, B.; Niccolai, C.; Patti, F.; Chisari, C.; Gallo, P.; Grossi, P.; Ghezzi, A.; et al. Patients with paediatric-onset multiple sclerosis are at higher risk of cognitive impairment in adulthood: An Italian collaborative study. *Mult. Scler. J.* **2018**, *24*, 1234–1242. [CrossRef] [PubMed]

96. McKay, K.A.; Manouchehrinia, A.; Berrigan, L.; Fisk, J.D.; Olsson, T.; Hillert, J. Long-term Cognitive Outcomes in Patients with Pediatric-Onset vs Adult-Onset Multiple Sclerosis. *JAMA Neurol.* **2019**, *76*, 1028–1034. [CrossRef]

97. Goretti, B.; Portaccio, E.; Ghezzi, A.; Lori, S.; Moiola, L.; Falautano, M.; Viterbo, R.; Patti, F.; Vecchio, R.; Pozzilli, C.; et al. Fatigue and its relationships with cognitive functioning and depression in paediatric multiple sclerosis. *Mult. Scler. J.* **2012**, *18*, 329–334. [CrossRef]

98. MacAllister, W.S.; Christodoulou, C.; Troxell, R.; Milazzo, M.; Block, P.; Preston, T.E.; Bender, H.A.; Belman, A.; Krupp, L.B. Fatigue and quality of life in pediatric multiple sclerosis. *Mult Scler* **2009**, *15*, 1502–1508. [CrossRef]

99. Florea, A.; Maurey, H.; Le Sauter, M.; Bellesme, C.; Sevin, C.; Deiva, K. Fatigue, depression, and quality of life in children with multiple sclerosis: A comparative study with other demyelinating diseases. *Dev. Med. Child. Neurol.* **2020**, *62*, 241–244. [CrossRef]

100. Weisbrot, D.M.; Ettinger, A.B.; Gadow, K.D.; Belman, A.L.; MacAllister, W.S.; Milazzo, M.; Reed, M.L.; Serrano, D.; Krupp, L.B. Psychiatric comorbidity in pediatric patients with demyelinating disorders. *J. Child. Neurol.* **2010**, *25*, 192–202. [CrossRef]

101. Weisbrot, D.; Charvet, L.; Serafin, D.; Milazzo, M.; Preston, T.; Cleary, R.; Moadel, T.; Seibert, M.; Belman, A.; Krupp, L. Psychiatric diagnoses and cognitive impairment in pediatric multiple sclerosis. *Mult. Scler. J.* **2014**, *20*, 588–593. [CrossRef] [PubMed]

102. Storm van's Gravesande, K.; Blaschek, A.; Calabrese, P.; Rostasy, K.; Huppke, P.; Kessler, J.; Kalbe, E.; Mall, V. Fatigue and depression predict health-related quality of life in patients with pediatric-onset multiple sclerosis. *Mult. Scler. Relat. Disord.* **2019**, *36*, 101368. [CrossRef] [PubMed]

103. McKay, K.A.; Hillert, J.; Manouchehrinia, A. Long-term disability progression of pediatric-onset multiple sclerosis. *Neurology* **2019**, *92*, E2764–E2773. [CrossRef] [PubMed]

104. Ghezzi, A.; Amato, M.P. Pediatric multiple sclerosis: Conventional first-line treatment and general management. *Neurology* **2016**, *87*, 2068. [CrossRef]

105. Kerbrat, A.; Aubert-Broche, B.; Fonov, V.; Narayanan, S.; Sled, J.G.; Arnold, D.A.; Banwell, B.; Collins, D.L. Reduced head and brain size for age and disproportionately smaller thalami in child-onset MS. *Neurology* **2012**, *78*, 194–201. [CrossRef]

106. Fenu, G.; Lorefice, L.; Loi, L.; Sechi, V.; Contu, F.; Coghe, G.; Frau, J.; Spinicci, G.; Barracciu, M.A.; Marrosu, M.G.; et al. Adult brain volume in multiple sclerosis: The impact of paediatric onset. *Mult. Scler. Relat. Disord.* **2018**, *21*, 103–107. [CrossRef]

107. Pandit, L. No evidence of disease activity (NEDA) in multiple sclerosis-Shifting the goal posts. *Ann. Indian Acad. Neurol.* **2019**, *22*, 261–263. [CrossRef]

108. Kappos, L.; De Stefano, N.; Freedman, M.; Cree, B.; Radue, E.; Sprenger, T.; Sormani, M.; Smith, T.; Haring, D.; Piani Meier, D.; et al. Inclusion of brain volume loss in a revised measure of 'no evidence of disease activity' (NEDA-4) in relapsing-remitting multiple sclerosis. *Mult. Scler.* **2016**, *22*, 1297–1305. [CrossRef]

Permissions

The contributors of this book come from diverse backgrounds, making this book a truly international effort. This book will bring forth new frontiers with its revolutionizing research information and detailed analysis of the nascent developments around the world.

We would like to thank all the contributing authors for lending their expertise to make the book truly unique. They have played a crucial role in the development of this book. Without their invaluable contributions this book wouldn't have been possible. They have made vital efforts to compile up to date information on the varied aspects of this subject to make this book a valuable addition to the collection of many professionals and students.

This book was conceptualized with the vision of imparting up-to-date information and advanced data in this field. To ensure the same, a matchless editorial board was set up. Every individual on the board went through rigorous rounds of assessment to prove their worth. After which they invested a large part of their time researching and compiling the most relevant data for our readers.

The editorial board has been involved in producing this book since its inception. They have spent rigorous hours researching and exploring the diverse topics which have resulted in the successful publishing of this book. They have passed on their knowledge of decades through this book. To expedite this challenging task, the publisher supported the team at every step. A small team of assistant editors was also appointed to further simplify the editing procedure and attain best results for the readers.

Apart from the editorial board, the designing team has also invested a significant amount of their time in understanding the subject and creating the most relevant covers. They scrutinized every image to scout for the most suitable representation of the subject and create an appropriate cover for the book.

The publishing team has been an ardent support to the editorial, designing and production team. Their endless efforts to recruit the best for this project, has resulted in the accomplishment of this book. They are a veteran in the field of academics and their pool of knowledge is as vast as their experience in printing. Their expertise and guidance has proved useful at every step. Their uncompromising quality standards have made this book an exceptional effort. Their encouragement from time to time has been an inspiration for everyone.

The publisher and the editorial board hope that this book will prove to be a valuable piece of knowledge for researchers, students, practitioners and scholars across the globe.

List of Contributors

Lucia Ziccardi, Lucilla Barbano and Vincenzo Parisi
IRCCS—Fondazione Bietti, Via Livenza 1, 00198 Rome, Italy

Laura Boffa and Maria Albanese
Unit of Neurology, Fondazione Policlinico Tor Vergata, Via Oxford 81, 00133 Rome, Italy

Carolina Gabri Nicoletti and Doriana Landi
Multiple Sclerosis Clinical and Research Unit, Department of Systems Medicine, Tor Vergata University, Via Montpellier 1, 00133 Rome, Italy

Andrzej Grzybowski
Department of Ophthalmology, University of Warmia and Mazury, Michała Oczapowskiego 2, 10455 Olsztyn, Poland
Institute for Research in Ophthalmology, Foundation for Ophthalmology Development, Collegium Maius Fredry 10, 61701 Poznań, Poland

Benedetto Falsini
Ophthalmology Department, IRCCS—Fondazione Policlinico Universitario A. Gemelli, Catholic University, Largo F. Vito 1, 00168 Rome, Italy

Girolama Alessandra Marfia and Diego Centonze
Multiple Sclerosis Clinical and Research Unit, Department of Systems Medicine, Tor Vergata University, Via Montpellier 1, 00133 Rome, Italy
Unit of Neurology and Neurorehabilitation, IRCCS—Neuromed, Via Atinense 18, 86077 Pozzilli (IS), Italy

Nicola Capasso, Roberta Lanzillo, Antonio Carotenuto, Maria Petracca, Rosa Iodice, Aniello Iovino, Francesco Aruta, Vincenzo Brescia Morra and Marcello Moccia
Multiple Sclerosis Clinical Care and Research Centre, Department of Neuroscience, Reproductive Sciences and Odontostomatology, University of Naples "Federico II", 80138 Naples, Italy

Raffaele Palladino
Department of Public Health, University of Naples "Federico II", 80138 Naples, Italy
Department of Primary Care and Public Health, Imperial College London, London W68RP, UK

Emma Montella
Department of Hygiene, Preventive and Industrial Medicine, University Hospital "Federico II", 80138 Naples, Italy

Francesca Pennino, Viviana Pastore and Maria Triassi
Department of Public Health, University of Naples "Federico II", 80138 Naples, Italy

Antonio Riccardo Buonomo and Emanuela Zappulo
Section of Infectious Diseases, Department of Clinical Medicine and Surgery, University of Naples "Federico II", 80138 Naples, Italy

Ivan Gentile
Section of Infectious Diseases, Department of Clinical Medicine and Surgery, University of Naples "Federico II", 80138 Naples, Italy
Health Education and Sustainable Development, University of Naples "Federico II", 80138 Naples, Italy

Mariano Marrodan, María I. Gaitán and Jorge Correale
Neurology Department, Fleni, C1428AQK Buenos Aires, Argentina

María Célica Ysrraelit
Department of Neurology, FLENI, Buenos Aires 1428, Argentina

Antonio Capacchione
Medical Affairs Department, Merck, 00176 Rome, Italy

Fortunata Carbone
Neuroimmunology Unit, IRCCS Fondazione Santa Lucia, 00142 Rome, Italy
Laboratory of Immunology, Institute of Experimental Endocrinology and Oncology, National Research Council (IEOS-CNR), 80131 Naples, Italy

Teresa Micillo
Department of Biology, Federico II University, 80131 Naples, Italy

Giuseppe Matarese
Laboratory of Immunology, Institute of Experimental Endocrinology and Oncology, National Research Council (IEOS-CNR), 80131 Naples, Italy
Treg Cell Lab, Department of Molecular Medicine and Medical Biotechnologies, Federico II University, 80131 Naples, Italy

Joanna Tarasiuk, Alina Kułakowska and Jan Kochanowicz
Department of Neurology, Medical University of Bialystok, M. Skłodowskiej—Curie 24A St., 15-276 Bialystok, Poland

Marco A. Lana-Peixoto and Natália Talim
CIEM MS Research Center, Federal University of Minas Gerais Medical School, Belo Horizonte, MG 30130-090, Brazil

Monika Gudowska-Sawczuk
Department of Biochemical Diagnostics, Medical University of Bialystok, Waszyngtona 15A St., 15-269 Bialystok, Poland

Barbara Mroczko
Department of Biochemical Diagnostics, Medical University of Bialystok, Waszyngtona 15A St., 15-269 Bialystok, Poland
Department of Neurodegeneration Diagnostics, Medical University of Bialystok, Waszyngtona 15A St., 15-269 Bialystok, Poland

Vicki Mercado
Immunology and Microbiology Graduate Program, Baylor College of Medicine, Houston, TX 77030, USA
Medical Scientist Training Program, Baylor College of Medicine, Houston, TX 77030, USA
Center of Excellence in Health Equity, Training and Research Program, Baylor College of Medicine, Houston, TX 77030, USA

Deepa Dongarwar
Center of Excellence in Health Equity, Training and Research Program, Baylor College of Medicine, Houston, TX 77030, USA

Kristen Fisher
Texas Children Hospital, Blue Bird Circle Clinic for Multiple Sclerosis, Houston, TX 77030, USA

Hamisu M. Salihu
Department of Family & Community Medicine, Baylor College of Medicine, Houston, TX 77030, USA

George J. Hutton
Baylor College of Medicine, Maxine Mesinger Multiple Sclerosis Center, Houston, TX 77030, USA

Fernando X. Cuascut
Center of Excellence in Health Equity, Training and Research Program, Baylor College of Medicine, Houston, TX 77030, USA
Baylor College of Medicine, Maxine Mesinger Multiple Sclerosis Center, Houston, TX 77030, USA

Athanasios Metaxakis and Dionysia Petratou
Institute of Molecular Biology and Biotechnology, Foundation for Research and Technology Hellas, Nikolaou Plastira 100, 70013 Heraklion, Greece

Nektarios Tavernarakis
Institute of Molecular Biology and Biotechnology, Foundation for Research and Technology Hellas, Nikolaou Plastira 100, 70013 Heraklion, Greece
Department of Basic Sciences, Faculty of Medicine, University of Crete, 71110 Heraklion, Greece

Victor M. Rivera
Department of Neurology, Baylor College of Medicine, Houston, TX 77030, USA
Baylor College of Medicine, Maxine Mesinger Multiple Sclerosis Center, Houston, TX 77030, USA

Efstathios Deskoulidis, Sousana Petrouli and Emmanuel Topoglidis
Materials Science Department, University of Patras, 26504 Patras, Greece

Vasso Apostolopoulos
Institute for Health and Sport, Victoria University, Melbourne, VIC 3030, Australia

John Matsoukas
Institute for Health and Sport, Victoria University, Melbourne, VIC 3030, Australia
Newdrug, Patras Science Park, 26500 Patras, Greece
Department of Physiology and Pharmacology, Cumming School of Medicine, University of Calgary, Alberta, AB T2N 4N1, Canada

André Huss, Makbule Senel, Jan Kassubek, Albert C. Ludolph and Markus Otto
Department of Neurology, University Hospital of Ulm, Oberer Eselsberg 45, 89081 Ulm, Germany

Ahmed Abdelhak
Department of Neurology, University Hospital of Ulm, Oberer Eselsberg 45, 89081 Ulm, Germany
Department of Neurology and Stroke, University Hospital of Tübingen, Hoppe-Seyler-Alle 3, 72076 Tübingen, Germany
Hertie institute of clinical of clinical brain research, University of Tübingen, Hoppe-Seyler-Alle 3, 72076 Tübingen, Germany

Benjamin Mayer
Institute of Epidemiology and Medical Biometry, Ulm University, Schwabstraße 13, 89075 Ulm, Germany

Anna Ferretta, Silvia Russo, Maddalena Ruggieri, Piergiorgio Lasorella, Damiano Paolicelli, Maria Trojano and Anna Signorile
Department of Basic Medical Sciences, Neurosciences and Sense Organs, University of Bari "Aldo Moro", 70124 Bari, Italy

Hayrettin Tumani
Department of Neurology, University Hospital of Ulm, Oberer Eselsberg 45, 89081 Ulm, Germany
Speciality Clinic of Neurology Dietenbronn, Dietenbronn 7, 88477 Schwendi, Germany

Marina Kleopatra Boziki, Evangelia Kesidou, Paschalis Theotokis, Eleni Karafoulidou and Nikolaos Grigoriadis
2nd Neurological University Department, Aristotle University of Thessaloniki, AHEPA General Hospital, 54634 Thessaloniki, Greece

Alexios-Fotios A. Mentis
Public Health Laboratories, Hellenic Pasteur Institute, Athens 11521, Greece
Laboratory of Microbiology, University Hospital of Larissa, School of Medicine, University of Thessaly, 41110 Larissa, Greece

Domenico De Rasmo
CNR-Institute of Biomembranes, Bioenergetics and Molecular Biotechnologies, 70126 Bari, Italy

Mikhail Melnikov, Anastasia Sviridova and Alexey Boyko
Department of Neurology, Neurosurgery and Medical Genetics, Pirogov Russian National Research Medical University, Moscow 117997, Russia
Department of Neuroimmunology, Federal Center of Cerebrovascular Pathology and Stroke, Moscow 117342, Russia

Vladimir Rogovski
Department of Molecular Pharmacology and Radiobiology, Pirogov Russian National Research Medical University, Moscow 117997, Russia

Kristen S. Fisher
Baylor College of Medicine, Texas Children's Hospital, Houston, TX 77030, USA

Index

Printed in the USA
CPSIA information can be obtained
at www.ICGtesting.com
JSHW051404091023
49903JS00006B/277